T0179579

Working with Refugee Families

Trauma and Exile in Family Relationships

Working with Refugee Families

Trauma and Exile in Family Relationships

Edited by

Lucia De Haene
University of Leuven, Belgium

Cécile Rousseau
McGill University, Canada

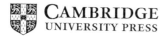

CAMBRIDGE
UNIVERSITY PRESS

CAMBRIDGE
UNIVERSITY PRESS

University Printing House, Cambridge CB2 8BS, United Kingdom

One Liberty Plaza, 20th Floor, New York, NY 10006, USA

477 Williamstown Road, Port Melbourne, VIC 3207, Australia

314–321, 3rd Floor, Plot 3, Splendor Forum, Jasola District Centre, New Delhi – 110025, India

79 Anson Road, #06–04/06, Singapore 079906

Cambridge University Press is part of the University of Cambridge.

It furthers the University's mission by disseminating knowledge in the pursuit of
education, learning, and research at the highest international levels of excellence.

www.cambridge.org
Information on this title: www.cambridge.org/9781108429030
DOI: 10.1017/9781108602105

© Cambridge University Press 2020

First published 2020

Printed in the United Kingdom by TJ International Ltd, Padstow Cornwall

A catalogue record for this publication is available from the British Library.

Library of Congress Cataloging-in-Publication Data
Names: Haene, Lucia de, editor. | Rousseau, Cécile, editor.
Title: Working with refugee families : coping with trauma and displacement in family relationships / edited
by Lucia De Haene, Assistant Professor, Director of Refugee Trauma Care, University of Leuven, Belgium,
Cécile Rousseau, Professor of Psychiatry, McGill University, Canada.
Description: Cambridge, United Kingdom ; New York, NY : Cambridge University Press, 2020. | Includes
bibliographical references and index.
Identifiers: LCCN 2019047078 (print) | LCCN 2019047079 (ebook) | ISBN 9781108429030 (hardback) |
ISBN 9781108602105 (ebook)
Subjects: LCSH: Refugees – Mental health. | Psychic trauma – Treatment. | Refugee families – Psychological
aspects. | Emigration and immigration – Psychological aspects.
Classification: LCC RC451.4.R43 W67 2020 (print) | LCC RC451.4.R43 (ebook) | DDC 616.85/210086914–dc23
LC record available at https://lccn.loc.gov/2019047078
LC ebook record available at https://lccn.loc.gov/2019047079

ISBN 978-1-108-42903-0 Hardback

....

On the cover of this volume: Co-constructing representations of suffering and hope in refugee families

In editing this volume, *Working with Refugee Families: Trauma and Exile in Family Relationships*, we have been privileged to receive inspirational images and to collaborate with several artists on the creation of the cover image.

As a gift by Professor Peter Adriaenssens, a picture of two men carrying young children through a street destroyed by war violence in the Salihin neighborhood of eastern Aleppo by Syrian photographer Ameer Alhabi (Ameer Alhabi/AFP) was integrated into a drawing by Belgian artist and sculptor Willy Peeters. In the drawing, the photographical form of Alhabi's picture is brought together with a coal-based drawing of an original clay sculpture by Paul De Haene.

Our collaboration on the cover design developed into an intensive dialogue between us, with the artist Willy Peeters, and with our research and clinical teams at the University of Leuven and McGill University. In our initial reflections on compiling the cover design based on original work in photography and sculpture, we imagined a cover design that would represent both the suffering evoked by predicaments of collective violence and the power of family relationships in restoring security in the face of injustice and destruction. In developing and co-editing the volume, the role of clinical and psychosocial practice in supporting refugee family relationships as a space of post-trauma reconstruction underpinned our engagement in our shared editorial work, emphasizing family relationships as a space of containment, affective regulation, restorative meaning-making, and reconstructing future perspectives.

In this process, an initial design generated questions on the extent to which the image was echoing suffering too extensively, with divergent impressions between us. We consulted our teams in Leuven and Montreal, inviting a range of reflective responses on the design. These addressed how the initial image evoked resonances of parental protection in the face of threat, the role of male community members as representatives of safety and cohesion, the absent presence of transnational and transgenerational family relationships and lived experiences of loss and guilt in relation to those left behind, the intrusive void provoked by traumatization, and the alienation that may be part of uprooting. Further, we reflected on how the image's integration of the different visual modalities of photography, drawing, and sculpture may mirror the fragmentation that is evoked by traumatic memories, balancing vivid, literal images with distant echoes of the disruption of meaning systems and trustful human relationships. As part of these resonances, fears that the picture could be retraumatizing for refugees were shared, along with concerns that the cover image may unwillingly participate in a depiction of refugees as mere helpless victims. These reflections spurred dialogue between us and provided the basis for further collaboration with the artist Willy Peeters, in which we tried to articulate those meanings we deemed important to convey in the volume's cover. Throughout this dialogue, Willy Peeters' careful engagement with our thoughts and sensitivities was enriched by his artistic knowledge and his emphasis on shaping a cover design that honoured the original artistic works by Ameer Alhabi and Paul De Haene.

Our dialogue illustrated the complexities of assuming responsibility for shaping a clinical encounter that does not reactivate traumatic suffering but that ensures a safe distance in which survivors can invest traumatic experience with layers of meaning that allow them to feel reinscribed in meaningful perspectives. It resonated clinical dilemmas where, as clinicians, we often witness difficulties in mobilizing the promise of continuity and restoration in the face of adversity and encounter how holding both suffering and hope as profound expressions of humanity is a delicate exercise.

Encountering these dilemmas in the depiction of refugees also extends into a reflection on representing refugees in the broader social space. The intensity of our dialogue invites to address the intricate ways in which our position as clinicians and academics is imbued with both personal and social dimensions that we, at least in part, represent in our academic and health care institutions. Here, our conversation about the editorial choices on the cover design illustrates the intricate balance between reiterating or counteracting stereotypical depictions of refugees (as, for example, in our joint appreciation of the absence of female figures on the cover, where the representation of male figures may not only evoke cultural notions of male protection and provision but could equally counteract stereotypical images of refugee men in current western host societies). From this perspective of our social position as clinicians and academics, our dialogue underlines the complexity of advocating for refugees within broader social spaces that are increasingly marked by polarized representations of refugee individuals and families. Our conversation on the cover resonates how 'working with refugee families' is marked by exploring ways of endorsing a social voice on the encounter with refugee families – as an ongoing search for how we can participate in shaping a community of listeners and witnesses engaging in dialogue.

We profoundly thank the three artists who collaborated on this work and who provided new vocabularies and voices in reflecting on our clinical and social practice with refugee families.

Contents

Part III – Intersectoral Psychosocial Interventions in Working with Refugee Families

Conclusion

Contributors

Peter Adriaenssens is Clinical Professor in Child and Adolescent Psychiatry at the Faculty of Medicine, KU Leuven, and is responsible for the department of residential child psychiatry and the Confidential Center for Child Abuse and Neglect, University Hospital Leuven, Leuven, Belgium.

Kjerstin Almqvist is Professor in Psychology at the Department for Psychology, Karlstad University, Karlstad, Sweden. Kjerstin is also Research Leader at the Centre for Clinical Research, Värmland, Sweden, a licensed psychologist and a licensed child psychotherapist.

Lisa Andermann, MPhil, MDCM, FRCPC is a psychiatrist at Mount Sinai Hospital and Associate Professor in the Equity, Gender and Populations Division, Department of Psychiatry, University of Toronto, Canada. She works with an Ethnocultural Assertive Community Treatment team, refugee mental health clinics at the Centre for Addiction and Mental Health (CAMH) and the Canadian Centre for Victims of Torture (CCVT).

Winny Ang, MD, is a child and adolescent psychiatrist at the Faculty of Medicine and Health Sciences, University of Antwerp, Antwerp, Belgium and works in child and adolescent psychiatry in private practice.

Julia Bala, PhD, is a clinical psychologist, psychotherapist, independent consultant and former staff member of Foundation Centrum '45, partner in the Arq National Psychotrauma Expert Group in the Netherlands. Julia's main fields of interest include intergenerational consequences of trauma and strengthening the resilience of refugee children and families.

Aïcha Cissé is a clinical psychology doctoral student at Fordham University, New York, USA, where she conducts research on culture, migration, and community. Aïcha is also completing a clinical externship at the Mount Sinai Hospital Child and Family Institute in New York, USA.

Lucia De Haene is Associate Professor at the Faculty of Psychology and Educational Sciences at the University of Leuven, Belgium. Lucia conducts research on refugee family relationships and on clinical practice with refugees. She coordinates the Refugee Trauma Care Team at the Faculty Clinical Centre PraxisP. She is a licensed family therapist involved in family therapy training and coordinator of the postgraduate program in psychotraumatherapy at the University of Leuven.

Ilse Derluyn is Professor at Ghent University, Belgium, researching topics concerning the wellbeing of young refugees, war-affected children and victims of trafficking. Ilse holds an ERC-SG and coordinates a H2020 project alongside co-directing the Centre for Children in Vulnerable Situations and managing the Centre for the Social Study of Migration and Refugees.

Nele Deruddere is a family therapist in the Refugee Trauma Care Team at the Faculty Clinical Centre PraxisP, Faculty of Psychology and Educational Sciences,

University of Leuven, Belgium. Nele is equally involved in process- and outcome evaluations of refugee care modalities.

Elisabetta Dozio, PhD, is a clinical psychologist and mental health advisor at Action Contre la Faim, a MHPSS (Mental Health and Psychosocial Support) consultant and trainer, and a researcher at the University Paris Descartes, Paris, France.

Mayssa' El Husseini is an Adjunct Professor at the University of Picardie Jules Verne, Amiens, France, researcher at the CHSSC EA 4289, a clinical psychologist at Maison de Solenn, Cochin Hospital, Paris, France, and a consultant for Doctors without Borders.

Mina Fazel is an Associate Professor in the Department of Psychiatry at the University of Oxford and a consultant child and adolescent psychiatrist in the Department of Children's Psychological Medicine at Oxford University Hospitals NHS Foundation Trust. Her research concerns service provision, school-based mental health services, and improving access to evidence-based trauma therapies.

Marion Feldman is a clinical psychologist and Professor of Psychoanalytic Psychopathology at Paris Nanterre University, Nanterre, France. Marion is also a researcher at CLInique PSYchanalyse Développement (CLIPSYD), studying approaches in psychoanalytic psychopathology.

Kenneth Fung is a psychiatrist and Clinical Director of Asian Initiative in Mental Health, University Health Network; Associate Professor at the Department of Psychiatry, University of Toronto, Toronto, Canada; a consultant at Hong Fook Mental Health Association; and President of the Society for the Study of Psychiatry and Culture.

Jaswant Guzder is Professor at the Department of Psychiatry, Division of Child Psychiatry and Division of Social and Transcultural Psychiatry, McGill University, Montreal, Canada. Jaswant is also a cofounder and senior clinician at the Jewish General Hospital Cultural Consultation Service and former head of child psychiatry.

Matthew Hodes is Honorary Clinical Senior Lecturer in Child and Adolescent Psychiatry at the Centre for Psychiatry, Imperial College London and a consultant in child and adolescent psychiatry at the Westminster Child and Adolescent Mental Health Service, Central and North West London NHS Foundation Trust, UK.

Marie Høgh Thøgersen, PhD, is a researcher and clinical psychologist at the Danish Institute Against Torture (DIGNITY), Copenhagen, Denmark. Marie specializes in psychotraumatology and is currently heading the Danish Trauma and Refugee Database (DTD). Her clinical and academic work focuses on the long-term consequences of refugee trauma.

Nasima Hussain is a consultant family and systemic psychotherapist in the Westminster Child and Adolescent Mental Health Service (CAMHS), Head of Systemic Psychotherapy Discipline in the Central and North West London NHS Foundation Trust (CNWL), and Course Director of Systemic Psychotherapy in the Central and North London NHS Foundation Trust, UK.

Rukiya Jemmott is a systemic psychotherapist and social worker. Rukiya is a course lead and tutor at the Tavistock and Portman NHS Foundation Trust, London, UK, where she works therapeutically with families identified as refugees and in adult mental health services. She has a particular interest in the use of genograms in systemic psychotherapy.

Eva Keatley, PhD, obtained her doctoral degree from the University of Windsor in clinical psychology with a specialization in neuropsychology. She is currently completing a postdoctoral fellowship at Johns Hopkins University School of Medicine in rehabilitation neuropsychology.

Ruth Kevers, PhD, is a researcher at the Faculty of Psychology and Educational Sciences, University of Leuven (KU Leuven) Belgium. As a family therapy trainee at KU Leuven, Ruth works in the Refugee Trauma Care Team at the Faculty's Clinical Centre PraxisP.

Inga-Britt Krause is the lead of the Systemic Psychotherapy Doctoral Programme in the Tavistock and Portman NHS Foundation Trust, London, UK, where she also practises as a consultant systemic psychotherapist. From initially training in social anthropology, Inga has worked with issues of race, culture, and equality in mental health services in the UK for 30 years.

Vanessa Lemire has an MA in special education and is a researcher and research coordinator at the University of Montreal, Canada.

Caterina Mamprin is a PhD student, research assistant and lecturer at the University of Montreal, Canada. Caterina's main research interests focus on social support and teachers' wellbeing in collective activities.

Malika Mansouri, PhD, is Assistant Professor in Clinical Psychology at Paris Descartes University, France, and a researcher at the Laboratory of Clinical Psychology, Psychopathology, and Psychoanalysis (PCPP). Malika also works

as a clinical psychologist in a Safe Childhood Association.

Mony Mok is a mental health worker at Hong Fook Mental Health Association, Toronto, Canada, providing case management services for the Cambodian community in Toronto, Canada, for over 20 years.

Edith Montgomery, PhD, DMSc, is a specialist in child psychology and psychotherapy and has previously worked at the Danish Institute Against Torture for almost 30 years. Now she is partly retired and affiliated with the Research Centre for Migration, Ethnicity and Health at the University of Copenhagen, Denmark.

Trudy Mooren, PhD, is a clinical psychologist at Foundation Centrum '45, partner in the Arq National Psychotrauma Expert Group, and Senior Researcher at the Department of Clinical Psychology, Faculty of Social Sciences, Utrecht University. Trudy is also president of the Dutch Society of Traumatic Stress Studies and a board member of the European Society of Traumatic Stress Studies.

Marie Rose Moro is Professor of Child and Adolescent Psychiatry at Paris Descartes University and Head of Department of the House of Adolescents of Cochin, House of Solenn (AP-HP), Paris, France.

Aoife O'Higgins, PhD, is a research associate at Magdalen College and the Department of Experimental Psychology, University of Oxford, UK. Her research investigates mechanisms that explain the psychosocial outcomes of young people in care, including refugee children.

Garine Papazian-Zohrabian is a member of the Order of Psychologists of Quebec, an associate professor at the University of Montreal, Canada, and a researcher at the research centre SHERPA. Garine's clinical and academic work focuses on loss and trauma among immigrant and refugee students and school mental health.

Venerable Vireak Phorn is a Buddhist monk and a social service worker of Khmer Buddhist Temple of Ontario, Canada. He also provides language support for Hong Fook Mental Health Association and co-leads ACT-Buddhism therapy groups.

Priyadarshani Raju is a psychiatrist working with various marginalized populations in Toronto, Canada. At the SickKids Centre for Community Mental Health, she provides consultation to newcomer and refugee families. She is an Assistant Professor at the University of Toronto.

Andrew Rasmussen is Associate Professor of Psychology at Fordham University, New York, USA. His research focuses on the distress experienced by forced migrants and immigrants, how cultural features interact with service delivery, and the well-being of the communities in which they resettle.

Sissel Reichelt[†] was Professor Emeritus in clinical psychology, Department of Psychology, University of Oslo, Norway, and had a clinical practice with adults and families. She worked particularly with refugee families for some years in a project developed together with Nora Sveaass. Reichelt has worked with, and done research on, various groups of client families.

Karin Riber, PhD, Psychologist specialist in psychotherapy, has worked as a clinical psychologist in the Mental Health Services of the Capital region of Denmark for a decade, including work with complex refugee trauma and TF-CBT at the Competence Centre for Transcultural Psychiatry. Karin is trained in the Adult Attachment Interview and a certified coder of Reflective Functioning on the AAI, and specializes in mentalization-based therapy and compassion-focused therapy. She is currently working as a psychologist at The Danish National Center for Grief.

Peter Rober is Professor at the Institute for Family and Sexuality Studies, Medical School University of Leuven (KU Leuven), Belgium. Peter is responsible for Context, the Centre of Marital and Family Therapy at the University Psychiatric Centre KU Leuven, Belgium.

Cécile Rousseau is Professor of Psychiatry at McGill University, Montreal, Canada, and Scientific Director of the Research Institute on Health and Cultural Diversity SHERPA. She coordinates an academic mental health care centre (CLSC ParcExtension) and leads and supervises a clinical team working with immigrant and refugee families in close collaboration with primary care settings.

Radhika Santhanam-Martin is a clinical psychologist who works in the field of trauma. Radhika works in Melbourne, Australia, supporting systems and providing services across three sectors: refugees and asylum seekers; Indigenous families; and diverse communities.

Ditte Shapiro, PhD, is Assistant Professor in Psychology at the Centre for Social Work and Administration, University College Absalon, Roskilde, Denmark. Ditte is an authorized psychologist with clinical experience in the Red Cross Asylum Department, Copenhagen, Denmark.

Debra Stein is a child and adolescent psychiatrist at the Sickkids Centre for Community Mental Health in Toronto, Canada, where she provides consultation to newcomer and refugee families. Debra is also an assistant professor in the

Department of Psychiatry, University of Toronto, Toronto, Canada.

Nora Sveaass is Professor in clinical psychology at the University of Oslo, Norway. She has worked clinically with refugees at the Psychosocial Centre for Refugees at the University of Oslo. She is head of the board of the NGO Health and Human Rights Info and vice-chair of the UN Subcommittee for the Prevention of Torture. In 2009 she was awarded an Amnesty International Award; she received the University of Oslo's Human Rights Prize in 2018 and was appointed in 2019 to Knight 1st Class of the Royal Norwegian Order of St. Olav by the King of Norway for her work on human rights.

Nina Thorup Dalgaard, PhD, is a psychologist currently working as a researcher at VIVE, the Danish Centre for Social Science Research, Copenhagen, Denmark. Nina previously worked as a clinical psychologist for the Danish Red Cross and as a researcher and psychologist at Dignity – Danish Institute Against Torture.

Alyssa Turpin-Samson is a PhD student, research assistant, and lecturer at the University of Montreal, Montreal, Canada. Alyssa's research focuses on traumas and their influence on the school experience of refugee (MA) and First Nation students.

Foreword

Caminante, no hay camino,
Se hace camino al andar.[1]

(Antonio Machado)

Lucia De Haene and Cécile Rousseau have succeeded in convening for this volume a remarkable kaleidoscope of programs developed on behalf of refugees at different moments in their harrowing peregrinations in search of a better future. This collection of chapters provides us with an updated cross-cultural panorama of systematic efforts at helping refugees at different points of transition across one of the most jarring existential experiences – that of seeking refuge away from our hearth.

The programs described and evaluated in this book are notable humanitarian efforts at welcoming human beings trapped between loss and hope, between despair and resilience, and aim at undertaking the complex task of helping refugees to reconstruct their shaken identity and their undermined agency, allowing them to be able to recapture their future.

The map of the journey transited by the refugee is extraordinarily varied and complex. We are born wherever we are born, not by choice but by chance: it happens to occur where our mother, parents, extended family, clan, or tribe were when we came into this world. As time passes, we develop attachments to people, habits, creeds, and places, and we internalize them and make them ours as we expand our reach from the sensorial (our mother's touch, skin texture, scent, voice) and the instinctive (the connection with those around us that soothe or trigger our distress) to the relational and the social. We may develop a family of our own, expanding our social attachment to include several generations. It becomes our homeland, a part of our core identity – until that covenant is broken.

That journey – transited by millions of us human beings each year – starts when the taken-for-granted covenant between us and our homeland is breached by social violence, political indifference, or, frequently, natural disasters that shake our roots, materializing our need to leave. This realization may appear into our life abruptly, as an imminent danger sometimes imposed, as when we are expelled by force; sometimes as a slow realization when our meager means of subsistence wane.

It continues into the actual departure on a scarcely designed, unmapped, and frequently unpredictable journey. The exit may be planned and mindful, or abrupt and chaotic. We may choose to leave voluntarily, for a variety of benign reasons, the town or country where we were born – nomadic habits of our tribe, improvement (or, occasionally, decline) in our job, a mixed blessing attached to marriage in many cultures, or the need of access to education. However, that move can be forced upon us – as for millions of people each year in a multiplicity of scenarios. A war between factions in our region is endangering us, our family, our livelihood. A dictatorial regime threatens to get rid of whoever belongs to our ideology, activity, profession, or creed, and people have already 'disappeared': we have to escape to survive. A persistent drought has destroyed our agrarian livelihood and unleashed a famine that will kill us all. Gangs are terrorizing our towns with impunity

---

1 Traveler, there is no road,
  You make your own path as you walk.

under the indifferent or complicit eyes of a weak central government. Our children are in danger. There isn't any future – education, jobs, security – in our place: we have to leave for survival and, if possible, in search of a better life.

The departure and transit may be filled with actual dangers which we may not be prepared to recognize and know how to defend ourselves from. In all our peregrination, we may be alone and longing for the succor of loved ones left behind, or caught in the ambivalent trap of the comfort and responsibility of sharing our journey with our nuclear bunch of loved ones. That whole sequence may take a short time but sometimes years to unfold. It may place us in neighboring, familiar territory or a distant, foreboding world with different languages and social rules.

Our journey may be graspable or hallucinatory; once forced to leave, our transit to a destination varies enormously, depending on context. We may try to sneak into a neighboring country without a fixed goal, perhaps counting only on an address of a distant relative. We may participate in harrowing stampedes toward a foreign embassy in search of asylum; cross jungles, deserts, swamps; walk for days to then sneak under barbed wire to uncertain destinations. We may participate in interminable caravans of refugees to then be detained at the border. We may have embarked in dangerously overcrowded boats – from Vietnam years ago; nowadays perhaps from the Maghreb, from Turkey, Myanmar, Haiti. We end up transiting through sometimes harrowing intermediate stations – refugee camps, structured or unstructured encampments – that may become a limbo without a definite time or mode of exit, spending months or years being 'processed' and, meanwhile, just managing to survive. Alas, a few may arrive by car or by plane, entering through the doors of the privileged, encountering friendly officers rather than overworked bureaucratic functionaries that look at us with glazed eyes and ask us for documents that we cannot provide.

And we may arrive in the country of our choice, or the one that admitted us, or the one that was assigned to us, or wherever we could. We may share the language, or at least we may understand one another, or we may stare at each other with blank expressions when one of us or one of them tries to explain something. Their clothing and social habits may be similar to ours, or our (or their) looks and behaviors may decry our alienation; we know how to organize our future in the new environment, or we are like children, lost in a seemingly chaotic world without clear signals of what is what and where to go.

Whatever our departure, our journey, and our arrival, a forced migration propels us into a turmoiled imbalance between hope and despair and a significant disruption of our identity, as our self is rooted in the predictable continuity of our context. And the process of forced emigration is a liminal situation that unavoidably challenges to the extreme the resources required to retain, and in many cases only reconstitute, the refugees' humanity, their identity, agency, and the resources to become in turn a source of strength for his or her own and us all.

As I commented in the first paragraph of these notes, many of the programs detailed in this rich collection are located at different pivotal stations within the journey of the refugees (rather than being bunched at the end of it, so to speak), and targeted at the vicissitudes specific to that station. The more their merit, and the merit of the selection by professors De Haene and Rousseau: these endeavors are not only restorative upon entry but provide the refugees with the resources necessary for them to go on with their individual or collective journeys toward what they are seeking: a future for them and their families, a new shared place where they may build a community.

Bravo, Lucia and Cécile! Bravo, all the authors!

Carlos E. Sluzki, MD
Clinical Professor of Psychiatry
George Washington University
Professor Emeritus of Global and Community Health
George Mason University

Acknowledgments

To all refugee families we work with in our therapeutic practice, we wish to express our sincere gratitude for all we have learned in our encounters, in listening to your voices and sharing in your stories. Working with you has been and is a precious gift that lies at the heart of this book, a book that would not have been possible without all of you. You have taught us the important role of the family in living through collective violence and displacement, where family relationships hold the promise of restoring future and dignity and convey meaning to our world. We hope this volume may represent the intricate richness of your voices, witness to the multiple diasporic, transnational, and transgenerational family relationships you live in, and invite clinicians to co-constuct further knowledge together with you.

We would like to express our sincere thankfulness to all the scholars and clinicians who have generously contributed to this volume. It was a true honor to collaborate with you, to enter into dialogue, and to share in a joint orientation towards mobilizing family relationships in supporting refugees' reconstruction in our host societies.

We wish to thank our colleagues in clinical and research practice, who share in our engagement to develop care for refugee families and join who forces in preserving clinical and social spaces for transcultural practice and dialogue. Their experiences are reflected in diverse ways in this volume and form a core element of the ongoing reflecting on and rethinking of our practices. We sincerely thank the research team at the CLSC Parc-Extension (Montreal) where the proposal for this book was developed and whose members supported the book process in diverse ways: Marie-Ève, Janique, Lucie, Marie Hélène, and Anousheh, you are among the colleagues who inspired some of the insights developed in this book. For my team at the University of Leuven, I (LDH) wish to sincerely thank my team members at the Refugee Trauma Care service at the Faculty Clinical Centre PraxisP. Nele, Sofie, Ruth, Lies, Caroline, and Jakob, thank you for all we share in developing our therapeutic practice, in constructing a shared voice, and in enabling those precious spaces of difference between our voices. I deeply cherish our joint work, close to refugee families' suffering, often piloting modes of practice, and always imbued with a profound orientation towards shaping modalities of care that enable to hold personal, collective, social, cultural, and moral dimensions that so deeply imbue refugee families' predicaments. My profound thankfulness is extended to the Board of the Faculty Clinical Centre PraxisP and the Faculty of Psychology and Educational Sciences, for supporting the development of our clinical practice with refugees. In times of managed care, the Faculty's support is more than a precious gift – it is a social expression of solidarity. Peter Rober, thank you for your kind guidance in supporting our team, for the clinical wisdom you share, and for the profound gift of your trust. Peter Adriaenssens, 'my voice will go with you' is an Ericksonian phrase you at times refer to. I am deeply grateful for all those many times when I can hear and feel your voice resonating in my work and beyond.

Our sincere thankfulness is extended to the support provided by Cambridge University Press. The coordination and progress of this volume were consistently and most kindly supported with expertise and enthusiasm by Catherine Barnes, who guided us in the process of preparing the book proposal, and Jessica Papworth and Saskia Weaver-Pronk, who provided decisive support throughout the full editorial process. To our administrative assistants in Leuven and Montreal, thank you so much for your continued help throughout all facets of our work. Maria Leon (in Leuven) and Lyne Des Rosiers (in Montreal), thank you for your patient bibliographical work.

To both our families, thank you for all you mean in what is a very dear part of our lives, being and becoming the mother of our families, every time again. Thank you for everything you taught us about what it means to be a family, and for deepening our understanding of the promise that lies in the holding within family relationships throughout development and life trajectories. You will never cease to voice what we still ignore.

As this volume originated in a special time for our family, I (LDH) would like to add an expression of my deep love and gratitude to my family: Dominic, Sybille, and Isaac. Dominic, when we moved with our family to Montreal to prepare this book, with you in full support of my visiting professorship at McGill, we did not know that the time of working on this book would also become the time of the loss of your moederke, my schoonmama, and our children's bontje. Working on this book has been marked by our grief and by reshaping our understanding of the generations that have given us life. At the same time, and always, working on this book was deeply marked by what she wrote me just before submitting the proposal for this book, her pride in you and me, and by what she gave us to *never let go* – her blessing. I deeply love you, and I cherish our journey as a couple and a family in all its steps and changes that sound '*like a whisper*' and deepen our '*never let go*'. Sybille and Isaac, this book is what made your father and me move our family to Montreal three years ago, where we discovered a new world through your eyes, where you learned to sing your *premières chansons en français* (many more to come!), where we were close enough together to face icy winds at -30°, where we wondered at stormy waves and whale tails in Newfoundland, and where you swung your way through Montreal subway on your pink and blue steps. Three years later, your discovering, learning, singing, facing, wondering, and swinging has become no less. It has amplified: amplified with meaning, in the meaningful threads you weave through your experience of our world, in all the questions you raise, in all the stories you share, and in our many shared story times, when you listen, draw, play, tell, sing (in the case of Kleine Muis), or dance (in the case of Grote Beer) stories. At all those story times (far beyond bedtime), you *never let go* to ask what the story is about, or (more frequently) share your thoughts on the stories' meaning. By the time you are big enough to read an academic volume, I don't know whether you'll ever ask me about the meaning of the stories in this book – by then it will be time for us to ask you about the meaning of the stories and worlds you bring to us. But if one day you would ask me what this book is all about, I will tell you that it's about how my work always connects me to the gift I received from you since the day you were born together seven years ago – the most profound love for you and for all the stories you will bring.

Lucia De Haene and Cécile Rousseau
Brussels and Montreal

Working with refugee families
Inscribing Suffering and Restoration in Personal and Communal Worlds

Lucia De Haene and Cécile Rousseau

Supporting Refugees in Coping with Life Histories of Violence and Exile: Locating the Therapeutic Relationship at the Intersection of Personal and Social Suffering and Healing

In the past few years, major transformations have occurred in relationships between Western societies and refugees seeking a home within their borders. A marked increase in the influx of refugees and asylum seekers into these host societies has coincided with polarization in receiving societies' collective representations of refugees, associated with socioeconomic and political dynamics shattering European and North American majorities' privileges in a globalizing world [1]. Policy responses to the growing demands of refugee reception have fueled polarized debates of both solidarity and exclusion within political discourses and local communities. This ongoing debate surrounding the increasing influx of refugees is shaped by split representations of refugees and asylum claimants, with on the one hand the more traditional figure of the refugee as a vulnerable individual in search of protection and solidarity, inherited from the Geneva Convention and prevalent after the Second World War until the 1980s, and on the other hand discourses depicting refugee individuals and communities as potentially dangerous, in which the perception of the refugee becomes permeated with images of threat and violence [2, 3]. The growing negative collective representations of refugees can be seen as an expression of a broader upsurge of xenophobia in post-9/11 Western societies [4–9]. Here, stereotyping and discriminatory views of refugees equally extend their imprint to the representation of refugee families, as for example in negative portrayals of familial gender role patterns or parental authority and support for children's school trajectories [10, 11].

In today's Western host societies, social responses of empathy and solidarity versus fear and hostility mark refugees' trajectories in resettlement where they seek protection in the aftermath of collective violence. This polarization of communal responses to refugees' resettlement calls for a reflection on how social conditions in exile may shape clinical work with refugees. In clinical literature, sensitivity to broader social predicaments encroaching upon the process and meaning of the clinical encounter with refugees forms a central therapeutic impetus [12–14]. Therapeutic processes are shaped by refugees' plights of violence and loss in their home societies as well as by social and cultural dynamics in resettlement. Therefore, supporting refugees in recovering from traumatic suffering and in mobilizing social and cultural adaptation in exile requires to take into account how clinical processes are imbued with these dynamics in refugees' social and cultural spaces within both

1

home and host societies. In delineating how broader social predicaments enter the intimate space of the clinical encounter, several interacting layers of a profound and intricate imprint of social dynamics imbuing the clinical process can be identified.

First, clinical trajectories are profoundly marked by the meaning and sequelae of social conditions of persecution, war, human rights abuses, and man-made atrocities in refugees' home countries and flight trajectories. Working with refugees inherently revolves around processes of post-trauma reconstruction, in which refugees seek to restore a sense of safety, meaning, and connectedness in the aftermath of collective violence, persecution, or pervasive fear and abuse during flight [15]. In this process of post-trauma reconstruction involving stabilization, integration, and reconnection as core modalities of reparation, the iterative negotiation of the therapeutic relationship as a safe space of holding and mentalization aims at supporting refugees in shifting from the distrust of traumatic expectations, avoidance, and powerlessness towards an agentic re-engagement with meaningful life trajectories, developmental tasks, and future perspectives in exile.

Second, social conditions in exile affect clinical trajectories in their role as sources of distress and predictors of mental health problems in refugees. Post-migration stressors of isolation, discrimination, exclusion, ostracism, asylum insecurity, and detention have consistently been documented as major predictors of psychosocial vulnerability and psychopathological conditions of depression, anxiety, post-traumatic suffering, and psychosis [16]. Negative resettlement conditions may operate as a prolongation and reactivation of pre-migration experiences of injustice, impeding the re-establishment of safety that forms a necessary condition of healing in the aftermath of trauma and, therefore, of individuals' abilities to project life courses into meaningful future perspectives in exile [17, 18].

Third, the imprint of resettlement conditions of exclusion and marginalization extends into processes of power disparity and implicit exclusionary practices that may mark clinical relationships as well as refugees' positions within health care institutions. Studies in different Western host societies have documented refugee communities' limited mental health care access and participation [19, 20]. This is caused by the interplay of different barriers at the levels of refugee communities, clinicians, and mental health institutions. Refugees' access to health care is reduced by dynamics in refugee communities, including lack of information on the landscape of psychosocial provisions and experiences of stigma revolving around mental illness. Further, studies document clinicians' reluctance to work with refugee clients as well as practices marked by subtle forms of stereotyping and exclusion both within clinical processes and institutionalized regulations [21]. In the latter, the therapeutic space itself comes to operate as a microcosm that resonates with refugees' broader social predicaments in exile, invoking the clinician's encounter with the challenge of acknowledging how tensions or hesitations within therapeutic conversations with refugees may reflect their lived social experiences of marginalization and exclusion. In addressing institutional racism, where prejudice or exclusion permeates daily organizational and regulatory practices, clinicians are confronted with negotiating fragile trade-offs between denouncing these practices and safeguarding institutional positions that preserve refugee clients' access to care [14].

Fourth, clinical work with refugees most often entails an engagement with refugees' cultural change and continuity in navigating resettlement and re-shaping future perspectives. Clinical work may explore the meanings of cultural identifications as threads of continuity in coping with the fragmentation invoked by traumatic life histories, or support refugee clients in mourning the loss of cultural meaning systems for those

communities where collective violence disrupted communal ties or where cultural meaning systems and repertoires were a source of trauma [13]. Further, engaging with culture
in the clinical space may revolve around the meaning of cultural loss and change in
ensuring future-oriented resettlement trajectories, the shaping of transnational family
interaction, or the exploration of transgenerational family dynamics [22]. Throughout
these processes, the therapeutic exploration may validate the multilayered role of cultural
practices and meaning-making in coping with trauma and exile, support refugee clients
in engaging with the intricate tensions involved in shaping hybrid identities across
different social spaces, or address the role of narratives of cultural continuity and change
in dynamics of cultural camouflage [23]. The therapeutic dialogue may also develop
a reflection on how the therapeutic relationship itself becomes a vehicle of hybridization,
where clinicians represent cultural change throughout their explicit and implicit adherence to knowledge and belief systems regarding, for example, notions of mental health
suffering or gender role behaviours. Throughout these therapeutic processes, broader
social dynamics of polarization in refugees' resettlement contexts encroach upon the
therapeutic relationship. Social predicaments of exclusion may mark refugees' lived
experience of shaping cultural belonging and creolization within personal and social
spaces and therefore resonate with their stories of distress within the clinical space.
Equally, polarization in the broader social climate may influence service delivery and
clinicians' understanding of clients' shifting forms of belonging in gender role identifications, parenting practices, religious or racial identity markers, or reactive identity mobilization [24]. In those instances, the clinical position may either create a space of carefully
expressing and exploring refugee clients' legitimate distrust in the person of the clinician
as representative of the host society or become another space where subtle micro-
interactions between clinician and clients reiterate prejudice, the experience of marginalization, and retaliation.

Finally, resettlement conditions may profoundly shape the clinical encounter when
clinicians become explicit partners in institutionalized practices influencing refugees' social
position in exile. This occurs in those frequent situations where clinicians are invited to use
their clinical expertise in challenging or condoning migratory procedures, as in requests for
the provision of medico-legal reports in support of refugee clients' asylum claims or family
reunification procedures. It is also at stake when clinicians have a role within intersectoral
care networks where they interact with partners in housing, employment, or social participation. Finally, they may be involved in advocacy to mitigate the detrimental sequelae of
detention, family separation, or the role of psychiatric knowledge in legal procedures
determining rights to residence. In all those instances, clinicians are invited to step outside
of the consultation room and to act within societal spaces in shaping resettlement conditions. For clinicians, these practices are often marked by ambiguities and fragile balances
between preserving the protective shield of the therapeutic space and endorsing social
positions of solidarity in the face of injustice.

In all these intersecting dimensions, social conditions are intricately part of the therapeutic process. The imprint of social predicaments on therapeutic trajectories is not only
fundamentally present in supporting refugees in coping with the suffering invoked by
collective violence and resettlement stressors. This imprint extends into the implicit markers of broader social dynamics encroaching upon the therapeutic process, invoking
a therapeutic relationship that at times may echo broader social processes of solidarity or
exclusion and that in a certain sense becomes part of those resettlement conditions in which

refugees seek to find security, restore dignity, and develop testimonies of their life histories of structural violence in both home and host societies.

This interest in social predicaments encroaching upon therapeutic practice invites reflection on how refugees' care needs and help-seeking strategies cannot only be understood as mere strategies of symptom reduction at the level of personal functioning but may equally be understood as profound expressions of mobilizing support in coping with social predicaments: they form accounts of searching for meaningful, restorative ways of shaping belonging and community in the face of collective violence, loss, and exile [25]. They form part of seeking social spaces of remembrance and forgetfulness in engaging with the moral imperatives of surviving human rights abuses, and they aim to mobilize the reshaping of social fabric and social position as strategies of recovery and reconnection with meaningful future perspectives. This perspective invites clinicians to shape modalities of therapeutic intervention that locate refugees' suffering within social predicaments, create relational and social vocabularies to contain distress, and mobilize strategies for engaging communal, transgenerational, transnational, and cultural spaces of witnessing and social support. Furthermore, the imprint of broader social conditions in refugees' home and host societies upon clinical relationships invites a therapeutic position that engages with complex social and moral questions, compelling the clinician to enter the realm of action in social spaces beyond the private consultation room. Navigating these complexities implies an ongoing reflection on how engaging with social action may cross familiar borders of therapeutic neutrality and its related representations of a therapeutic position marked by benevolence and a safe distance from societal dynamics [14].

Working on the Threshold between Personal and Social Dimensions of Refugees' Suffering and Restoration: Systemic Perspectives on Refugee Care

The orientation towards engaging with the intersection between personal and social dimensions of suffering and reconstruction in therapeutic practice with refugees converges with the central impetus of systemic perspectives on refugee care in resettlement [26–29]. In the developing field of refugee rehabilitation, characterized by ongoing explorations of adequate modalities of refugee care and nascent stages of process- and outcome analysis [30], a growing body of systemic approaches addresses the pivotal role of moving beyond purely medicalizing and individualizing treatment models that consist of intervention protocols embedded in a medical model of diagnosis and related treatment and which most often focus on the reduction of post-traumatic stress disorder (PTSD) and co-morbid symptoms in refugees' individual mental health. In the systemic shift beyond such medicalizing approaches, clinical scholarship has addressed the at times limited ability of diagnostic constructs of PTSD and co-morbid conditions to provide an adequate vocabulary to account for refugees' suffering and distress in the aftermath of collective violence and exile [31, 32]. Here, it is argued that the language of PTSD may have a limited capacity to capture refugees' suffering, as it fails to address their multilayered lived experiences of distress in exile and may insufficiently engage with cultural idioms of distress and cultural parameters of suffering and healing [33]. Simultaneously, scholars have emphasized that a focus on PTSD and related individual treatments may miss or minimize the fundamentally social and political nature of refugees' suffering. Individualizing a social and political predicament may aggravate the individual's disconnection from the broader social fabric that evokes and continuously shapes suffering and coping [34–38]. These arguments are complemented by a growing emphasis on holistic approaches to psychosocial care for refugee populations [39, 40], in which a focus on healing post-trauma distress is complemented by interventions supporting refugees in coping with multiple resettlement stressors (e.g., social isolation, housing or employment difficulties), thereby explicitly engaging with the social and political dimensions of their new lives in exile.

In sum, these lines of scholarship develop a systemic approach to refugee care, locating the individual's suffering and healing within the complex interconnections of personal, social, cultural, and political realities embedded in meaning-making and integration processes [13, 15, 41]. Here, the therapeutic relationship becomes both a reflection and an active agent of refugees' intra-psychic, familial, and social reconstruction trajectory.

Putting a Systemic Perspective into Focus: The Role of Refugee Families in Coping with Trauma, Culture, and Social Conditions

Within systemic approaches to psychosocial refugee care, working with refugee families has received relatively scant attention in clinical literature. Yet, an in-depth exploration of family-oriented approaches seems particularly relevant, as different dimensions of family life are profoundly shaped by this intersection between intimate, social, cultural, and political meaning-making. Indeed, family relationships operate as a central vehicle of engaging and coping with trauma, culture, and social conditions in a life history of collective violence and exile [42, 43]. Within family relationships, family members are involved in meaning-making, communication, and coping processes that revolve around dealing with a traumatic family history interwoven with complex negotiations of cultural identification and social position in a context of exile and cultural change. A growing body of scholarship increasingly documents these three, interwoven dimensions of coping with trauma, culture, and social conditions within family relationships in exile.

First, in coping with trauma within refugee family relationships, specific trauma-related family processes have been documented. Scholarly literature has indicated how family relationships may be pervasively affected by the cumulative distress provoked by pre-migration trauma, flight, and post-migration stressors (e.g., decreased parental availability and responsiveness or the development of intra-family violence), but equally how family relationships can operate as a vital source of protection and re-establishment of security in exile [44–49]. Here, intra-family communication pertaining to trauma and exile is increasingly documented as a central dynamic within parent-child and spousal relationships. This process of trauma communication is underpinned by parental orientations to maintain a sense of security in exile, avoid family members' reactivation of distress, or adhere to cultural strategies of remembrance [50, 51]. Different (and potentially shifting) patterns of silencing, disclosure, or modulated disclosure within family relationships indicate divergent strategies of coping with the transgenerational transmission of traumatic life histories [52–56]. In this respect, studies have documented how shared or partially transmitted family histories of forced migration are often characterized by the interplay between personal and collective layers of meaning, interweaving intimate, social, moral, and political dimensions in family migration narratives in exile [57–60].

Second, in processes of cultural coping and meaning-making within refugee family relationships, studies have documented how cultural models of symptom expression, symptom interpretation, explanatory models, and strategies of coping are embedded (but also potentially contested) within family relationships [23]. Equally, refugee family members in exile become involved in a complex negotiation of cultural change and cultural continuity within family dynamics and in engaging with (changing) cultural meanings in coping with traumatic life histories [61–64]. This negotiation equally involves transgenerational and transnational family ties by which refugees relate to extended family networks and communal belonging in exile [65]. Furthermore, through this negotiation of cultural change and continuity, family members also actively cope with life experiences of discrimination and racism in exile [66].

Third, in processes of negotiating social condition in exile, scientific literature shows how, as a unit, the refugee family is involved in multiple interactions with actors in the diverse collective spaces of school, employment, and the cultural community, indicating that the family unit operates at the threshold where intimate lived experiences intersect with broader dynamics within the social fabric, cultural and host society communities [67–70]. The refugee family operates as a vehicle of (access to) resources and resilience in social relationships and participation, while, simultaneously, entering social spaces marked by processes of exclusion or ostracism may evoke a reiteration of injustice and disempowerment.

This emerging body of literature documents how the refugee family operates as a central systemic niche in trauma-related, cultural, and social coping and meaning-making. The refugee family system forms a dynamic ecology in which an intricate interplay of personal and broader collective meanings shapes and mobilizes personal and social resources in dealing with life histories of violence and exile.

From the perspective of a systemic approach to refugee care and its core emphasis on supporting refugees' reconstruction from within the complex intersections between perso-nal and communal realities, the growing scholarship on the role of refugee family relation-ships invites us to explore the refugee family system as a core locus of intervention. This volume aims at furthering the growing interest in refugee family systems as a core nexus of personal, social, and cultural coping strategies in the face of collective violence and forced displacement. The edited collection builds on an integrative account of the role of refugee family relationships in shaping the sequelae of trauma and exile to develop an in-depth exploration of therapeutic, collaborative, and community-based approaches to working with refugee families. Throughout this exploration of refugee family systems in both research and clinical practice, this volume aims to strengthen a systemic approach to the provision of mental health care for refugees and further our understanding of working with refugee families as a vehicle of engaging with the intricate nexus of personal and social processes of restoration in the face of trauma and exile.

This Volume: Working with Refugee Families in Supporting Reconstruction in Exile

This volume develops an understanding of the role of refugee family relationships in promot-ing post-trauma reconstruction and explores modalities of therapeutic and community-based clinical work with refugee families. Throughout this exploration, the refugee family system is highlighted as a central niche in shaping trauma-related reconstruction, cultural belonging, and social position in exile, and explored as a core locus of intervention in transcultural psychosocial and clinical care. To this end, the volume brings together contributions that address the role of refugee family relationships in shaping reconstruction in exile from research and clinical perspectives, structured around three main sections.

Part I presents an account of empirical research on key aspects of refugee family functioning and its role in reconstruction in the aftermath of organized violence. This section documents the refugee family unit as a dynamic system of interacting personal and collective meaning systems that shapes post-trauma reconstruction through relational and cultural dynamics of coping and resilience. In particular, contributions in this section address the impact of traumatization at the micro-level of parent-child and spousal relationships and extend this micro-focus to exploring intra-family cultural and collective meaning-making and practices in coping with trauma and exile as well as the role of transnational family relationships.

Analyzing the sequelae of trauma at the micro-level of parent-child and spousal relationships (see Chapter 1 by Hodes & Hussain; Chapter 2 by Thorup Dalgaard, Høgh Thøgersen, & Riber), contributions review the intra-family processes of attachment, separation, bereavement, and intra-family violence, addressing the impact of traumatization on refugee family relationships and their role in shaping the transgenerational transmission of trauma.

This focus on the micro-level of the parent-child and spousal dyad is extended with contributions that explore the refugee family system as an ecological niche of cultural practices and meaning-making, where cultural and collective meaning systems are mobilized and negotiated in shaping adaptation in the face of post-trauma suffering, bereavement, and exile-related distress. Here, contributions present original empirical accounts on dynamics of families coping with pre- and post-migration stressors and the role of cultural continuity and change in shaping family resilience (see Chapter 3 by Cissé, De Haene, Keatley, & Rasmussen) as well as the particular role of collective, political and cultural identifications in supporting post-trauma reconstruction within family functioning (see Chapter 4 by Kevers & Rober). These empirical analyses provide an insight into the multilayered role of cultural belonging in coping with trauma as well as with social predicaments in exile, inviting to reflect on how this mobilizing of cultural meaning systems may interact with the growing social dynamics of stereotyping and exclusion in Western host societies.

Finally, this section focuses on the role of transnational family relationships in exile, exploring the pivotal role of transnational family processes in shaping diasporic trajectories for both refugee families (see Chapter 5 by Shapiro & Montgomery) and unaccompanied minors (see Chapter 6 by Derluyn & Ang). These accounts of the pervasive impact of family separation and the ongoing relational complexities of transnational and transgenerational loyalties in exile underscore an understanding of the refugee family system as profoundly inscribed within extended family networks, related cultural notions of a relational self in communal belonging, and the complex interaction between trauma-related grief and ongoing separation.

In Part II and Part III, the volume builds on these empirical accounts to shift towards clinical practice with refugee family systems. Part II focuses on therapeutic approaches that engage with refugee families; Part III addresses modalities of intersectoral interventions as embedded within schools, communities, and collaborative care networks, operating within refugee families' broader collective spaces of resource and participation. Parts II and III are structured around three core transversal clinical themes of post-trauma rehabilitation, coping with bereavement and loss, and therapeutic positioning, substantiating these themes with clinical accounts that reflect a diversity of voices and approaches in different settings.

The first transversal clinical theme addresses post-trauma rehabilitation modalities of stabilization, integration, and reconnection as they structure cyclic and interacting therapeutic processes around the restoration of safety, meaning, and social connectedness [52, 71, 72]. Through a differential emphasis on each of these core therapeutic processes, clinical contributions in this section share and develop an approach in which stabilization, integration, and reconnection is located and supported within family relationships.

Stabilization, or the process of regaining safety and control, is explored in reflections on the complexities of building alliance with refugee family systems, psychoeducation, enhancing parental sensitive responsivity and mentalization, and supporting adequate coping through the mobilization of social and cultural resources (see Chapter 7 by Mooren & Bala; Chapter 8 by El Husseini and Dozio, Mansouri, Feldman, & Moro). Further, a specific contribution focuses on reducing family conflict and violence as part of relational stabilization (see Chapter 12 by Almqvist).

Integration, or the reshaping of traumatic memories through the reconstruction of the trauma narrative as inscribed within a meaningful and coherent life history is addressed through an account of supporting relational processes of trauma narration in therapeutic practice with refugee families (see Chapter 9 by De Haene, Adriaenssens, Deruddere, & Rober). This process of relational trauma narration is further explored in its interconnections with refugee family members' trajectories of cultural belonging in exile: clinical accounts document the therapeutic space as a vehicle of cultural hybridization in relation to transgenerational trauma in refugee families (see Chapter 10 by Guzder) and address the mobilization of cultural and spiritual metaphors and symbols in revisiting trauma histories (see Chapter 8 and Chapter 11 by Fung, Mok, & Phorn).

Reconnection, or the mobilization of social participation and connectedness, is addressed in contributions documenting modalities of clinical work that explicitly engage refugees' social and cultural worlds and use intervention strategies that mirror the presence of extended family networks (see Chapter 7; Chapter 16 by Santhanam-Martin). Further, the thread of reconnection is equally present in this volume's exploration of school-based psychosocial care and collaborative care networks (see Chapter 17 by Fazel & O'Higgins; Chapter 18 by Papazian-Zohrabian, Mamprin, Turpin-Samson, & Lemire), which reflects an emphasis on mobilizing therapeutic trajectories as vehicles of social participation and integration in resettlement.

Second, the transversal clinical theme of coping with bereavement and loss in exile complements these core threads of stabilization, integration, and reconnection in post-trauma rehabilitation. Several contributions emphasize the central role of coping with bereavement and (ambiguous) loss in therapeutic trajectories with refugee family systems, addressing how working around trauma in the clinical space is often closely tied to supporting family members in coping with grief and bereavement. This involves multiple layers of loss, including cultural bereavement (see Chapter 8; Chapter 10), traumatic loss, ambiguous loss, transnational loss and grief (see Chapter 7; Chapter 9), and coping with forced separation and the reshaping of loss through family reunification (see Chapter 13 by Sveaass & Reichelt).

Finally, a third transversal clinical theme focuses on the clinical relationship itself, and develops an understanding of the therapeutic position in working with refugee families as an intricate space of both resonating and reconstructing refugees' post-trauma suffering. Contributions account for particular processes and meanings of reflexivity in working with refugees' traumatic life histories (see Chapter 15 by Jemmot & Krause), including a reflective stance on the complex role of providing medico-legal reports and the negotiation of this provision in ways that support refugee families' actorship rather than reiterating their powerlessness (see Chapter 14 by Stein, Raju, & Andermann). Further, contributions explore the role of refugee families' institutional trajectories in reshaping their communal belonging, with a specific focus on dynamics of traumatic re-enactment in refugee families' encounters with care systems (see Chapter 19 by Rousseau) or clinical processes that invoke colonizing power disparities through the neglect of cultural knowledge systems and vocabularies of self and community (see Chapter 10; Chapter 16). Finally, contributions adress how to avoid a diagnostic bias that fails to account for the complexity of transcultural assessment (see Chapter 17) and the role of the therapeutic encounter as a space of communal listening and witnessing (see Chapter 9). These reflections provide a window into the intricate role of the therapeutic relationship as a space for post-trauma reconstruction, balancing between the relational reiteration of violence or the reconstruction of safety and trust in the face of injustice.

Across contributions, these transversal clinical themes are explored in different forms of therapeutic and community-based practice, including family therapeutic work, infant-parent psychotherapy, multifamily therapy, school- and community-based care, and intersectoral care networks located in divergent national and cultural settings in Western host societies. Parts II and III aim to provide scholars and clinicians with a multilayered account of intervention modalities in supporting refugee families, combined with an in-depth understanding of transversal clinical themes that are key across different modalities.

Core Systemic Threads Throughout the Volume

With this empirical and clinical exploration of refugee family relationships and their role in coping with trauma, culture, and social conditions, this edited volume shows how working with refugee family systems as a core locus of intervention provides ample possibilities to engage with the intricate intersections between personal, social, cultural, and political realities in refugees' suffering and post-trauma reconstruction. In presenting this edited collection on working with refugee families as a particular operationalization of a systemic approach to refugee care, we identify several threads that may guide the reader. Below, an overview of these guiding systemic threads starts from a relational understanding of the sequelae of traumatic life histories and moves on to address a particular systemic notion of trauma as expression of social predicaments. This understanding of trauma invokes the systemic emphasis on understanding the clinical space as marked by an engagement with supporting refugees to cope with broader social predicaments and finally extends into an understanding of intervention modalities as well as the therapeutic position itself as imbued by intricate intersections between personal, relational, and social dimensions of healing.

This volume engages with a particular notion of post-trauma reconstruction, focusing on the relational impact of traumatization and the relational impetus of coping in its aftermath. Rather than an understanding of post-trauma reconstruction revolving around recovery from post-traumatic distress as individual suffering and vulnerability, this volume focuses on the relational sequelae of traumatization and displacement within family functioning and on how to mobilize relationships as vehicles of reconstruction. Across contributions, this interest is reflected in a shift from an individualizing approach to refugees' suffering towards a relational vocabulary in conceptualizing distress and recovery. This relational understanding of post-trauma suffering and coping is developed through addressing how refugees mobilize family relationships, in their interactions with their the broader social fabric, in reconstructing meaning and connectedness.

This focus on developing relational vocabularies in understanding post-trauma suffering and coping in refugee family systems locates suffering and healing at the nexus of personal and social dimensions. From this perspective, the notion of trauma does not merely refer to an individual, symptom-focused category of distress, but equally to expressions of social predicaments of atrocities, persecution, and collective violence [52]. Corresponding to this social perspective on trauma, post-trauma reconstruction is primarily situated as coping with communal social predicaments and the seeking of restoration in the face of social conditions of injustice and uprooting. This orientation towards understanding the sequelae of refugee families' social conditions explicitly includes ongoing resettlement stressors of isolation, marginalization, and increased discrimination, hereby shifting a reductive focus on pre-flight or flight-related traumatic stressors towards the inclusion of multiple forms of social, clean violence in exile [73].

This systemic perspective on locating post-trauma reconstruction at the nexus of personal and social dimensions of suffering and healing calls for an understanding of the therapeutic relationship as a space of validating refugees' suffering and help-seeking strategies as ways of coping with social conditions in home and host societies. It recognizes that relieving suffering through therapeutic practice will inherently entail the restoration of meaningful ways of belonging through the mobilization of resilience and resources in both personal and collective spaces. This orientation is amply developed throughout this volume with its iterative emphasis on the complex intersection between personal, social, cultural, and collective layers of reshaping meaning and supporting adaptation. Across the volume, this dynamic interaction of personal, familial, social, and cultural meaning-making is articulated at the level of refugee family systems and further developed in clinical explorations of intervention modalities and the therapeutic positioning itself. At the level of intervention modalities, the systemic interest in the intersection of personal, familial, social, cultural, and political coping and meaning-making explains the volume's cross-cutting emphasis on the multiplicity of voices that resonate within refugee families' stories of suffering and restoration within the therapeutic encounter: clinical accounts in this volume explore the intersection of personal and relational narratives; cultural notions of well-being, self, and community in relation to cultural practices of coping and healing; forms of communal belonging to and identification with ethnic, racial, or religious groups; and collective histories and legacies. Equally, the volume documents how transnational and transgenerational voices profoundly imbue therapeutic dialogue as well. Indeed, transnational family relationships continue to shape refugees' well-being and social integration in exile, and their stories of displacement may be part of transgenerational histories of collective violence or political oppression. From a systemic perspective, this multiplicity of voices is at stake at both intrapersonal and interpersonal levels within the therapeutic encounter [74]. As several contributions address, clinical work with refugee families involves the exploration of these multiple personal, relational, cultural, social, transnational, and transgenerational voices within individual family members' lived experiences of collective trauma and diaspora, and it engages in the creation of a dialogical space in which family members can explore, co-construct, and re-shape these multiple voices and their roles in relational stories of reconstruction. At the level of therapeutic positioning, the volume explores in several ways the interest of articulating the clinical encounter itself at the intersection between personal, familial, and social meaning. The therapeutic position is marked by transactions between the clinician's personal engagement with refugee families' distress and the resonating of broader social and cultural differences within the therapeutic encounter. This leads to an interest in exploring those relational complexities of revisiting or restoring trauma within the therapeutic relationship. Further, in engaging with the imprint of broader social predicaments in home and host societies, the therapeutic position is mobilized to cross the institutionalized boundaries of the clinical space and to become an actor within the broader sets of social relationships shaping refugee families' resettlement, engaging within intersectoral collaborations or advocacy.

These core systemic threads throughout the volume invite an understanding of how a systemic approach to working on the threshold of personal and social dimensions of suffering and healing evokes a therapeutic position that operates as a mirror image of this personal-social nexus. Through developing a therapeutic approach that explores and amplifies refugee families' intimate transgenerational and cultural engagement with social and political predicaments of violence and exile, the therapeutic space may provide a space for holding and mentalizing containment of the sequelae of atrocity, loss, and displacement [52]. In validating and witnessing refugee families' predicaments of a pervasive disruption of both personal and communal worlds, in mobilizing bridges between personal and communal worlds as spaces of restoration, the therapeutic space may support family members to reconnect to a sense of shared humanity, holding the promise of rebuilding those worlds.

References

1. M. J. da Silva Rebelo, M. Fernández and J. Achotegui, Mistrust, anger, and hostility in refugees, asylum seekers, and immigrants: A systematic review. *Canadian Psychology/ Psychologie Canadienne*, 59(3)(2018), 239.

2. J. Anderson, J. Hollaus, A. Lindsay and C. Williamson, (2014).The culture of disbelief: An ethnographic approach to understanding an under-theorised concept in the UK asylum system. Refugee Studies Centre Working Paper.

3. L. J. Kirmayer, Refugees and forced migration: Hardening of the arteries in the global reign of insecurity. *Transcultural Psychiatry*, 44(3) (2007), 307–10.

4. M. Bayoumi, *How Does It Feel to Be a Problem? Being Young and Arab in America* (New York: Penguin, 2009).

5. C. Rousseau, G. Hassan, N. Moreau and B. Thombs, Perceived discrimination and its association with psychological distress in newly arrived immigrants before and after September 11, 2001. *American Journal of Public Health*, 101(5) (2011), 909–15.

6. C. Rousseau, U. Jamil, B. Kamaldeep and M. Boudjarane, Consequences of 9/11 and the war on terror on children's and young adults' mental health: A systematic review of the past 10 years. *Clinical Child Psychology and Psychiatry*, 20(2) (2015), 173–93.

7. C. Rousseau, Addressing mental health needs of refugees. *The Canadian Journal of Psychiatry*, 63(5) (2018), 287–9.

8. R. Kronick and C. Rousseau, Rights, compassion and invisible children: A critical discourse analysis of the parliamentary debates on the mandatory detention of migrant children in Canada. *Journal of Refugee Studies*, 28(4) (2015), 544–69.

9. K. Müller and C. Schwarz, (2018), Fanning the Flames of Hate: Social Media and Hate Crime (CAGE Working Paper Series).

10. G. Hassan and C. Rousseau, North African and South American parents' and adolescents' perceptions of physical discipline and physical abuse: When dysnormativity begets exclusion. *Child Welfare*, 88(6) (2009), 5–22.

11. C. Rousseau and U. Jamil, Muslim families understanding and reacting to 'The War on Terror'. *American Journal of Orthopsychiatry*, 80(4) (2010), 601–9.

12. J. Bala, *Beyond the Personal Pain: Forced Migration and Mental Health* (Boston: Springer, 2005), pp. 169–82.

13. L. De Haene and P. Rober, Looking for a home: An exploration of Jacques Derrida's notion of hospitality in family therapy practice with refugees. In I. McCarthy and G. Simon, eds., *Systemic Therapy as Transformative Practice* (Farnhill: Everything Is Connected Press, 2016).

14. C. Rousseau, L. Nadeau and T. Measham, Les mains sales: Racisme et responsabilité morale en clinique. *L'autre, cliniques, cultures et sociétés*, 9(3) (2008), 349–59.

15. C. Rousseau and T. Measham, Posttraumatic suffering as a source of transformation: A clinical perspective. In L. J. Kirmayer, R. Lemelson and M. Barad, eds., *Understanding Trauma: Integrating Biological, Clinical and Cultural Perspectives* (Boston, MA: Cambridge University Press, 2007), pp. 275–93.

16. M. Beiser and F. Hou, Mental health effects of premigration trauma and postmigration discrimination on refugee youth in Canada. *The Journal of Nervous and Mental Disease*, 204(6) (2016), 464–70.

17. K. Carswell, P. Blackburn and C. Barker, The relationship between trauma, post-migration problems and the psychological well-being of refugees and asylum seekers. *International Journal of Social Psychiatry*, 57(2) (2011), 107–19.

18. E. Montgomery, Trauma, exile and mental health in young refugees. *Acta Psychiatrica Scandinavica*, 124 (2011), 1–46.

19. B. H. Ellis, A. K. Lincoln, M. E. Charney, R. Ford-Paz, M. Benson and L. Strunin, Mental health service utilization of Somali adolescents: Religion, community, and school as gateways to healing. *Transcultural Psychiatry*, 47(5) (2010), 789–811.

20. S. M. Weine, Developing preventive mental health interventions for refugee families in resettlement. *Family Process*, 50(3) (2011), 410–30.

21. C. Rousseau, Y. Oulhote, M. Ruiz-Casares, J. Cleveland and C. Greenaway, Encouraging, understanding or increasing prejudices: A cross-sectional survey of institutional influence on health personnel attitudes about refugee claimants' access to health care. *PLoS One*, 12(2) (2017). DOI: https://doi.org/10.1371/journal .pone.0170910

22. J. Bala and S. Kramer, Intercultural dimensions in the treatment of traumatized refugee families. *Traumatology*, 16(4) (2010), 153–9.

23. J. Guzder, Family systems in cultural consultation. In L. J. Kirmayer, J. Guzder and C. Rousseau, eds., *Cultural Consultation: Encountering the Other in Mental Health Care* (New York: Springer, 2014), pp. 139–61.

24. P. Rober and L. De Haene, Intercultural therapy and the limitations of a cultural competency framework: About cultural differences, universalities and the unresolvable tensions between them. *Journal of Family Therapy*, 36 (2014), 3–20.

25. L. J. Kirmayer, C. Rousseau and J. Guzder, Introduction: The place of culture in mental health services. In L. J. Kirmayer, J. Guzder and C. Rousseau, eds., *Cultural Consultation: Encountering the Other in Mental Health Care* (New York: Springer, 2014), pp. 1–20.

26. L. Nadeau, A. Jaimes, J. Jonhson-Lafleur and C. Rousseau, Perspectives of migrant youth, parents and clinicians on community-based mental health services: Negotiating safe pathways. *Journal of Child and Family Studies*, 26 (2017), 1936–48.

27. M. Benson, S. Abdi, A. Miller and H. Ellis, Trauma systems therapy for refugee children and families. In N. Morina and

A. Nickerson, eds., *Mental Health of Refugee and Conflict-Affected Populations: Theory, Research and Clinical Practice* (Cham: Springer, 2019), pp. 243–59.

28. F. Walsh, Applying a family resilience framework in training, practice, and research: Mastering the art of the possible. *Family Process*, 55(4) (2016), 616–32.

29. T. Wenzel and B. Drožđek, *An Uncertain Safety: Integrative Health Care for the 21st Century Refugees* (Cham: Springer, 2018).

30. O. Slobodin and J. T. de Jong, Mental health interventions for traumatized asylum seekers and refugees: What do we know about their efficacy? *International Journal of Social Psychiatry*, 61(1) (2015), 17–26.

31. L. J. Kirmayer, R. Lemelson and M. Barad, *Understanding Trauma: Integrating Biological, Clinical, and Cultural Perspectives* (New York: Cambridge University Press, 2007).

32. D. Summerfield, My whole body is sick . . . my life is not good: A Rwandan asylum Seeker attends a psychiatric clinic in London. In D. Ingleby, ed., *International and Cultural Psychology Series. Forced Migration and Mental Health: Rethinking the Care of Refugees and Displaced Persons* (New York: Springer, 2005), pp. 97–114.

33. L. J. Kirmayer and R. Bennegadi, Les politiques de l'altérité dans la rencontre clinique. *L'Autre*, 12(1) (2011), 16–29.

34. M. Brough, R. Schweitzer, J. Shakespeare-Finch, L. Vromans and J. King, Unpacking the micro–macro nexus: Narratives of suffering and hope among refugees from Burma recently settled in Australia. *Journal of Refugee Studies*, 26(2) (2012), 207–25.

35. A. Kleinman, V. Das and M. M. Lock, *Social Suffering* (Berkeley, CA: University of California Press, 1997).

36. C. Rousseau, Se décentrer pour cerner l'univers du possible: Penser l'intervention en psychiatrie transculturelle. *Prisme*, 8(3) (1998), 20–37.

37. C. Rousseau, L'horreur et l'humanité. *Frontières*, 15(2) (2003), 60–2.

38. S. Weine, *Testimony after Catastrophe: Narrating the Traumas of Political Violence* (Evanston, IL: Northwestern University Press, 2006).

39. K. E. Miller and A. Rasmussen, War exposure, daily stressors, and mental health in conflict and post-conflict settings: Bridging the divide between trauma-focused and psychosocial frameworks. *Social Science & Medicine*, 70 (1) (2010), 7–16.

40. M. Hynie, The social determinants of refugee mental health in the post-migration context: A critical review. *The Canadian Journal of Psychiatry*, (2017), 0706743717746666.

41. J. Cleveland, C. Rousseau and J. Guzder, Cultural consultation for refugees. In L. Kirmayer, C. Rousseau and J. Guzder, eds., *Cultural Consultation: Encountering the Other in Mental Health Care* (New York: Springer, 2014), pp. 245–68.

42. L. De Haene, H. Grietens and K. Verschueren, From symptom to context. *Hellenic Journal of Psychology*, 4 (2007), 233–56.

43. S. Weine, N. Muzurovic, Y. Kulauzovic, S. Besic, A. Lezic, A. Mujagic et al., Family consequences of refugee trauma. *Family Process*, 43(2) (2004), 147–60.

44. K. Almqvist and A. G. Broberg, Young children traumatized by organized violence together with their mothers: The critical effects of damaged internal representations. *Attachment & Human Development*, 5(4) (2003), 367–80.

45. L. De Haene, N. T. Dalgaard, E. Montgomery, H. Grietens and K. Verschueren, Attachment narratives in refugee children: Interrater reliability and qualitative analysis in pilot findings from a two-site study. *Journal of Traumatic Stress*, 26(3) (2013), 413–17.

46. A. Nickerson, R. A. Bryant, R. Brooks, Z. Steel, D. Silove and J. Chen, The familial influence of loss and trauma on refugee mental health: A multilevel path analysis. *Journal of Traumatic Stress*, 24(1) (2011), 25–33.

47. K. James, Domestic violence within refugee families: Intersecting patriarchal culture and the refugee experience. *Australian*

and *New Zealand Journal of Family Therapy*, 31(3) (2010), 275–84.

48. K. Riber, Attachment organization in Arabic-speaking refugees with post traumatic stress disorder. *Attachment & Human Development*, 18(2) (2016), 154–75.

49. C. C. Sangalang, J. Jager and T. W. Harachi, Effects of maternal traumatic distress on family functioning and child mental health: An examination of southeast Asian refugee families in the US. *Social Science & Medicine*, 184 (2017), 178–86.

50. E. Montgomery, Tortured families: A coordinated management of meaning analysis. *Family Process*, 43(3) (2004), 349–71.

51. R. Kevers, P. Rober, C. Rousseau and L. De Haene, Silencing or silent transmission? An exploratory study on trauma communication in Kurdish refugee families. *Transcultural Psychiatry*, in press.

52. L. De Haene, C. Rousseau, R. Kevers, N. Deruddere and P. Rober, Stories of trauma in family therapy with refugees: Supporting safe relational spaces of narration and silence. *Clinical Child Psychology and Psychiatry*, 23(2) (2018), 258–78.

53. N. T. Dalgaard, S. Y. Diab, E. Montgomery, S. R. Qouta and R.-L. Punamäki, Is silence about trauma harmful for children? Transgenerational communication in Palestinian families. *Transcultural Psychiatry*, 56(2) (2019), 398–427.

54. N. T. Dalgaard and E. Montgomery, Disclosure and silencing: A systematic review of the literature on patterns of trauma communication in refugee families. *Transcultural Psychiatry*, 52(5) (2015), 579–93.

55. T. Measham and C. Rousseau, Family disclosure of war trauma to children. *Traumatology*, 16(2) (2010), 14–25.

56. C. Rousseau and A. Drapeau, The impact of culture on the transmission of trauma: Refugees' stories and silence embodied in their children's lives. In Y. Danieli, ed., *International Handbook of Multigenerational Legacies of Trauma*

(New York: Plenum Press, 1998), pp. 465–86.

57. K. Bek-Pedersen and E. Montgomery, Narratives of the past and present: Young refugees' construction of a family identity in exile. *Journal of Refugee Studies*, 19(1) (2006), 94–112.

58. L. De Haene, P. Rober, P. Adriaenssens and K. Verschueren, Voices of dialogue and directivity in family therapy with refugees: Evolving ideas about dialogical refugee care. *Family Process*, 51(3) (2012), 391–404.

59. R. Kevers, P. Rober, I. Derluyn and L. De Haene, Remembering collective violence: Broadening the notion of traumatic memory in post-conflict rehabilitation. *Culture, Medicine, and Psychiatry*, 40(4) (2016), 620–40.

60. J. Walter and J. Bala, Where meanings, sorrow, and hope have a resident permit: treatment of families and children. In J. P. Wilson and B. Drozdek, eds., *Broken Spirits: The Treatment of Traumatized Asylum-Seekers, Refugees, War and Torture Victims* (New York: Brunner-Routledge, 2004), pp. 487–519.

61. R. Kevers, P. Rober, C. Rousseau and L. De Haene, (2019). Silencing or silent transmission? An exploratory study on trauma communication in Kurdish refugee families. (Manuscript under review.)

62. R. Ramsden and D. Ridge, 'It was the most beautiful country I have ever seen': The role of Somali narratives in adapting to a new country. *Journal of Refugee Studies*, 26(2) (2012), 226–46.

63. S. Roubeni, L. De Haene, E. Keatley, N. Shah and A. Rasmussen, 'If we can't do it, our children will do it one day': A qualitative study of West African immigrant parents' losses and educational aspirations for their children. *American Educational Research Journal*, 52(2) (2015), 275–305.

64. C. Rousseau, M. Rufagari, D. Bagilishya and T. Measham, Remaking family life: Strategies for re-establishing continuity among Congolese refugees during the family reunification process. *Social Science & Medicine*, 59(5) (2004), 1095–108.

65. C. E. Sluzki, *The Presence of the Absent: Therapy with Families and their Ghosts* (New York: Routledge, 2015).

66. C. Rousseau, U. Jamil, T. Ferradji and A. Mekki-Berrada, North African Muslim immigrant families in Canada: Giving meaning and coping with the war on terror. *Journal of Immigrant & Refugee Studies*, 11 (2013), 136–56.

67. B. H. Ellis, S. M. Abdi, J. Horgan, A. B. Miller, G. N. Saxe and E. Blood, Trauma and openness to legal and illegal activism among Somali refugees. *Terrorism and Political Violence*, 27(5) (2014), 1–27. DOI:https://doi.org/10.1080/09546553.2013.867849

68. C. Rousseau, L. Nadeau, A. Laurin-Lamothe and S. Deshaies, Measuring the quality of interprofessional collaboration in child mental health collaborative care. *International Journal of Integrated Care*, 12 (2012). www.ncbi.nlm.nih.gov/pmc/articles/PMC3426395/

69. R. A. Tyrer and M. Fazel, School and community-based interventions for refugee and asylum seeking children: A systematic review. *PlOS One*, 9(2) (2014), e89359.

70. S. Weine, Y. Kulauzovic, A. Klebic, S. Besic, A. Mujagic, J. Muzurovic et al., Evaluating a multiple-family group access intervention for refugees with PTSD. *Journal of Marital and Family Therapy*, 34(2) (2008), 149–64.

71. B. Drozdek and D. Silove, Psychotherapy and psychosocial support in host countries: State-of-the-art and emerging paradigms. In T. W. B. Drozdek, ed., *An Uncertain Safety: Integrative Health Care for the 21st Century Refugees* (Cham: Springer, 2019), pp. 257–82.

72. J. L. Herman, *Trauma and Recovery* (New York: Basic, Harper, 1992).

73. M. de Certeau, *Cahiers pour un temps* (Paris: Centre Georges Pompidou, 1987).

74. P. Rober, *In Therapy Together: Family Therapy as a Dialogue* (London: Palgrave Macmillan, 2017).

The Role of Family Functioning in Refugee Child and Adult Mental Health

Matthew Hodes and Nasima Hussain

Introduction

The mental health of refugees is determined by individual, family, community and wider social influences [1–4]. In this chapter, we focus on the role of family variables in refugees' mental health. Many people flee their country and seek reunification with family members by encouraging those left behind to travel to join them. The stresses they experience in migrating and re-settling may be attenuated by family relationships that may provide an important buffering role, while decreased intra-familial support may exacerbate individual suffering. There are also families in which the disruption to family and community life and experiences of adversity and abuse, sometimes linked to mental health problems, contribute to intra-familial tensions that can escalate into intra-familial violence.

The aim of this chapter is to provide an account of the ways in which the family can play a role in mediating the impact of refugee experiences, as well as increasing resilience in coping with loss and change. We also address the potential for the family to develop strained relationships that lead to the deterioration of function and even dissolution. The association between the quality of family life and mental health is a central theme. We consider the relationship between this range of family experiences and the most prevalent psychological difficulties and disorders associated with refugees' experiences, including grief and bereavement, post-traumatic stress disorder (PTSD) and depression.

We have drawn on a range of empirical studies from many fields including developmental psychopathology, cultural psychiatry, family psychology and social science. However, the relatively small body of work on this topic imposes limitations on the chapter. Research into refugee family relationships and family life has typically been carried out using single informants [5–9], although some has involved multiple members of the same family [10], with some notable exceptions [11, 12]. Few interactional studies have been carried out, apart from the recent studies of infant-parent attachment [13]. Most quantitative studies have measured family factors and variables that are relatively easy to operationalise. Few studies have integrated social anthropological and family perspectives and linked them to mental health, although some qualitative investigations have drawn on these fields [11, 14, 15].

It is useful to consider the functions of the family before discussing how these may change as a result of war experiences, displacement and resettlement. For decades, the role of the family has been understood in functionalist terms with regard to the tasks that the family carries out [16, 17]. These include meeting the material and physical needs of family members by providing a home, food or clothing. This functionalist view also includes the provision of child care for rearing the young, and caring for family members when they are sick and unable to work and contribute to the family income. For many refugee families who experience financial hardship, disruption of employment, family separations, losses and legal uncertainty, performing these basic tasks may be a great challenge and sometimes even impossible. In addition, the family also serves to stabilise the emotional state of the parental couple and provide emotional support to the offspring. Achieving this emotional stability and support requires daily conversations, confiding and care, and joint activities that are an integral part of family life. Many shared family activities can be regarded as routines, such as mealtimes, the daily departure for school or work and returning later in the day, and less frequent activities such as visiting extended family and holidays [18, 19]. Family members may also participate in and share rituals that link them to religious practice and beliefs shared by the wider community [19, 20]. Families that come to resettlement countries will experience cultural and language differences and also differences in family organisation and values [21, 22].

Of course, when closely observed, all families are different and reveal their particular family history and experiences, shaped by, and reflecting, their beliefs and practices. These components create the family meaning system that further contributes to the anchoring of family members, as well as shaping, particularly for children and adolescents, their cognitive and social development [23]. The parental couple also brings family-of-origin beliefs and narratives that contribute to the new family meanings or cultures. For families and individuals fleeing organised violence or the threat of violence and persecution, the routines, shared activities and shared meanings that maintain the family are under great threat and may for some be abruptly terminated [24]. Such changes may also take place in the context of the loss of family members because of abduction, detention, killing or involvement in combat, which further strains the family as a functioning unit.

While people have fled violence or persecution for centuries, the twentieth century saw an increased involvement of non-combatants in war and violence [25]. The Second World War was followed by the creation of the United Nations (UN) [26], which was instrumental in defining the term 'refugee' in its 1951 Convention as a person who:

> owing to well-founded fear of being persecuted for reasons of race, religion, nationality, membership of a particular social group or political opinion, is outside the country of his [sic] nationality and is unable or, owing to such fear, is unwilling to avail himself [sic] of the protection of that country; or who, not having a nationality and being outside that country of his [sic] former habitual residence as a result of such events, is unable or, owing to such fear, is unwilling to return to it.

There are some related terms that need to be defined. An asylum seeker is a person who has left their country of origin and formally applied for asylum in another country but whose application has not yet been concluded. A refused asylum seeker is a person whose asylum application has been unsuccessful and who has no other claim for protection while awaiting a decision. Some refused asylum seekers voluntarily return home, others are forcibly returned, and for some it is not safe or practical for them to return until conditions in their country change. Refugee status is awarded to an asylum seeker by a receiving country as described in the Refugee Convention. Unaccompanied children seeking asylum (UASCs) are children (under the age of 18 years) who have applied for asylum in their own right, who are outside their country of origin and who are separated from both parents or their previous/legal customary primary caregiver [27].

The number of people globally of concern to the UN Refugee Agency (UNHCR) has increased since 2010, and by 2018 had reached 68.5 million forcibly displaced people, of whom 25.4 million are refugees and 3.1 million asylum seekers [28]. Over half of the refugees are aged under 18 years. The three top countries from which refugees came were Syria, Afghanistan and South Sudan, and the top receiving countries were Turkey, Pakistan, Lebanon and Iran. While most of the children are cared for in families, there are many unaccompanied refugee children. In 2016, there were 63,300 asylum applications in EU countries from unaccompanied minors. The flow of refugees to Europe is continuing, but at a reduced rate [29]. During the months of January to June 2017, 12,239 refugee children arrived in Italy, of whom 93% (11,406) were unaccompanied or separated. In the same period, 44,300 children with parent(s) sought asylum in Germany, including 5,700 applications from UASCs. These statistics reveal the large number of children amongst the refugees as well as the high proportion of families.

The Refugee Family Experience

The experiences of people who migrate because of fear of persecution or exposure to war, and the ensuing adversities, have been detailed in numerous reports from the last century [25, 26]. Sadly, there is ongoing war in many regions of the world, which results in continuing suffering for refugees [30–33]. Some of the most important influences on refugees' adjustment have been summarised in Table 1.1.

Table 1.1 lists the experiences and adversities that might increase risk for individual refugees' psychiatric disorders and psychological distress, as well as protective factors. The table provides an accessible heuristic representation but simultaneously imposes a static quality on experiences that often arise out of dynamic intra-familial and wider social processes. The discussion here addresses some of these processes from a family perspective.

Pre-flight

Different forms of persecution and exposure to violence may have varied family impacts. In some conflicts, all family members will witness or experience violence, including killings or combat, such as those experiencing bombardment in the Syrian war [33]. Sexual violence may be an intentional aspect of a war against a community [34]. In situations of violent revolutionary social change, as occurred during the Pol Pot Khmer Rouge regime in Cambodia (1975–9), family members were deliberately separated with a view to weakening family bonds. Under Pol Pot, spouses were separated from each other, children were separated from parents and some were taught to spy on their elders to obtain extra favours or were forced to commit atrocities themselves [35, 36]. A high proportion of the refugees fleeing Eritrea are men. In this repressive regime, every Eritrean must serve an indeterminate period of 'national service', with many ending up serving for well over a decade. Eritreans are subject to arbitrary arrest and imprisonment [37].

The decision to migrate is one that will often involve family discussions with a view to assessing the best plan for the flight. There is often sharing of resources and choices made around who migrates and who does not. Conversation may be expanded to include a wider social group and community regarding the risks of travel, the prevalent need for secrecy, and how to manage danger and trust. These decisions are often very stressful and ridden with guilt, which can surface in the post-migration phase as survivor guilt [38, 39]. The

1.1 Risk and protective factors in the mental health of refugees

Time in relation to flight	Risk factors for poorer mental health	Protective factors for better mental health
Before flight	1. Persecution 2. Experience of or witnessing violence or combat 3. Loss of family or community members 4. Disruption of family/community life 5. Child cared for by parent with poor mental health	1. Belief in community cause 2. Planned departure and flight from community 3. Family survival and cohesion
In flight	1. Long arduous journeys 2. Privation (food, accommodation, schooling) 3. Ongoing exposure to violence and abuse (including sexual exploitation) 4. Detention en route to resettlement countries	1. Journeys supported by UNHCR and other organisations, often associated with more rapid entry to safe areas and flight 2. Family union/child continues in care of parents/relatives 3. Ongoing contact with supportive family members and friends, e.g., by telephone or social networking
On arrival in resettlement countries	1. Continual movement in host country, unsettled accommodation 2. Economic hardship 3. Legal uncertainties that can result in threats of deportation or actual deportation 4. Long delays in settling asylum application 5. Detention 6. Age disputes in which UASCs are categorised as adults and only given access to adult services 7. Social isolation 8. Long periods when forbidden to work/unemployed 9. Lack of fluency in language and poor opportunities to acquire new language 10. Persecution and racism 11. Intra-familial tensions, conflict and poor parenting	1. Negotiated entry to resettlement country 2. Rapid resolution of asylum claims 3. Settlement in neighbourhood with high same ethnic/language density 4. Family union/child continues in care of parents/relatives 5. Ongoing contact with family members, e.g., by telephone or social networking 6. Children successfully negotiate their 'bicultural' and bilingual identity 7. Timely and supported access to services, e.g., health and community welfare organisations 8. Sense of belonging to resettlement country

decision may relate to the availability of financial resources, the degree of danger to family members and the perceived appropriateness of certain family members, sometimes young healthy males, travelling first.

The extent to which families flee and remain together during journeys is very varied. Not all refugees manage to migrate as an intact nuclear family.

Flight

Some refugees make their own arrangements for their journeys while others negotiate their route with traffickers, but in both cases they often encounter great danger. The adversities include privation from lack of food and water, assaults, the need to sell personal belongings and take on employment to raise funds to pay for the ongoing journey, and often exposure to adverse weather conditions, including rough sea crossings. Arduous journeys were undertaken during the vast movements of people in the turbulent years of war and fascism in Europe and throughout many parts of the world since the Second World War [25, 26]. Well-documented movements occurred during the British de-colonisation of South Asia with the creation of India and Pakistan, and then afterwards associated with the wars in southeast Asia (formerly the French colonies of Indochina: Vietnam, Cambodia, Laos) [26]. Some of the most dramatic and shocking examples were the 'boat people' who left Vietnam during the 1970s and 1980s, setting off in small boats across the South China Sea seeking haven in safer countries [26]. This is reminiscent of the thousands of refugees since 2015 who have tried to cross the Mediterranean to reach European destinations, often in small and sometimes inflatable boats and at great peril [40].

Many refugees travel alone and hope that their families will join them after they have established themselves in the resettlement country. A high proportion of refugees in transit are exposed to violence, including sexual assault [30, 41]. In other cases, close family members have been killed or detained. During journeys, the ability to communicate with family, friends and people-smugglers is very important [42, 43]. Many refugees regard the mobile telephone as a lifeline for seeking help and obtaining information about their onward journey. They can call for help when catastrophe strikes in the Mediterranean and they fear their boat will sink, with the risk of drowning [42].

Those who are under 18 years old (UASCs) form a particularly important group. Their plight is highlighted in view of the high number of losses and separations from parents, carers and family that they may have experienced in their country of origin, and many are orphans as a result of war and organised violence [30, 44, 45]. Attention to their needs was stimulated by the plight of southeast Asia's unaccompanied minors, who fled Cambodia during the 1970s [26]. Since 2015, there has been a dramatic increase in UASCs coming to Europe [29].

Prior to and during journeys, family life and familiar routines may be highly disrupted. Involvement in work and school may cease. Parents or caregivers may be missing or killed. Older children may become carers for younger children. Great effort may be needed to obtain adequate food and water and temporary accommodation. Understandably, this can have massive effects on mood and the ability to cope with strained family relationships, and it challenges parents' ability to care for their children and provide adequate nurture, warmth and stimulating interaction [46].

Resettlement

The arrival of refugees in safe countries may have been negotiated by an international agreement for their resettlement. This will significantly smooth their reception, as facilities for accommodation, legal and language support and rapid granting of refugee status will enable the bread-winners to seek work and permanent housing. However, since around 2000, such programmes have been less available and there is an increasing harshness towards refugees [47]. This has been provoked by the bombing of the twin towers on 9/11 [48], the consequences of austerity for the welfare state, and the European refugee crisis, beginning with large inflows of refugees in 2014–15 [49–51]. Many countries are reluctant to accept asylum seekers and develop harsh regimes to deter them [52]. One notorious example is Australia, which has offshore detention centres [53]. Many refugees, including families, live in temporary camps or temporary accommodation without employment or adequate schooling and facilities for rearing children. In many countries, there are policies to deport asylum seekers. In 2017, across the European Union nearly half (46%) of first-application asylum decisions resulted in positive outcomes, but the proportion of such outcomes is variable across the continent [29]. Financial hardship, social isolation that may arise because of dispersal policies, and lack of fluency in the language of the host community add to the stresses that impact on family life.

These cumulative experiences during pre-flight, flight and resettlement phases impact on mental health, and the vast majority of studies document an association between asylum-seeking or refugee status and higher levels of psychiatric symptoms and prevalence of disorder. An early meta-analysis of studies carried out in Western countries found a prevalence amongst refugees of post-traumatic stress disorder (PTSD) of 9% (99% Confidence Intervals (CI) 8–10%) and 5% (4–6%) for major depression amongst adults and a prevalence of 11% (7–17%) for PTSD amongst children [54]. A larger global study of 81,866 refugees and other conflict-affected persons reported an unadjusted weighted prevalence rate for PTSD of 30.6% (95% CI, 26.3%–35.2%) and for depression of 30.8% (95% CI, 26.3%–35.6%) [55]. When looked at longitudinally five years after settlement, the prevalence rate of psychiatric disorder appears elevated compared with non-migrant peers [56]. These studies produce generalisable data, but the meta-analytic methodology averages out rates, and specific processes that may give a more nuanced understanding to study findings may be lost.

Refugee Family Processes

Case example – Disruption in attachment and its impact

Rona is a 10-year-old Iraqi Kurdish girl. She was referred by her school with concerns regarding her quiet withdrawn behaviour and constant complaints of headaches and stomachaches. Rona often expressed her physical symptoms in a very dramatic way by crying out loud, wailing and becoming hysterical. Teachers described her behaviour as very similar to the way her mother expressed her distress, as witnessed by school staff. Despite Rona's appearance as very bright, she was failing academically due to lack of concentration.

Rona lives with her mother and two sisters, one two years older than her and one two years younger. Her parents separated a few years after migrating to England. Her father had a mental breakdown and became violent towards her mother. This was explained in part by his inability to support the family. He lives near the family and children to support the family. Her mother has suffered from depressive disorder for many years. She was prescribed anti-depressants, but did not take them for fear of becoming out of control and not being able to look after the children and because of her beliefs regarding medication interfering with her brain functioning. She experienced somatic complaints not attributed to disease.

Rona's mother described experiencing very traumatic events associated with their escape from Iraq. She described fleeing to the mountains whilst pregnant with their third child, a pregnancy that she did not want to continue. She describes trying to abort the baby by hitting her stomach, punching herself and going without food. She had hoped that the stress would bring on a natural termination of the pregnancy. During the journey, additional traumatic events included privation of food for days with very little shelter and witnessing deaths and the mass destruction of villages. Her mother narrated the story in a very fragmented way and became overwhelmed in the telling process, and during that process her mental state became fragile. She was visibly shaking, crying and repeating that she could not bear her life; she was only living for the children. She could not acknowledge what the then two- and four-year-old children had witnessed and experienced and its possible psychological impact. She explained that as they were small they would not remember anything. For Rona's mother, nothing could be worse than what they had experienced during their escape from the war. Now that they were in a safe country, the children should not be having any problems. For her to accept that the children could have difficulties would mean a failure of her parenting, and she refused to accept that Rona was having difficulties. Her mother's (as well as her father's) distress contributed to the lack of emotional availability of the parental figure(s) in Rona's life. In the absence of the extended family, the impact on children's mental health becomes more fragile. Rona became the identified child who exhibited parental distress and lack of emotional availability. It is often the children's distress that brings the parents into contact with professional services.

In order to understand the ways in which past and ongoing adversities, as well as protective factors, may interact with family processes, the subsequent sections explore specific family experiences and their links with specific forms of psychopathology.

Separation and Loss

Refugees experience the loss of many aspects of their lives. First, there is often the loss of close family members, either through death, injury or separation. Death and separation from relatives causes intense sadness, pain and a sense of loss [57]. Where there has been death, the surviving family's responsibility is to dispose of the body in the appropriate culturally sanctioned way [58]. For many bereaved people, performing appropriate death rituals facilitates grieving and social mobilisation that may help to achieve some level of acceptance and closure.

Cultures and religions have very diverse ways of understanding death and its consequences. The cultural shaping of bereavement and the detrimental effect of inadequate funerary rituals have been graphically described [59–61]. One example of cultural difference is the genocide of Pol Pot in the 1970s and its impact on death, which affected many refugees. Hinton and colleagues explain that 'Cambodians worry that the Pol Pot dead are not reborn and that they wander the earth in a purgatory-like state, and moreover they believe that those who have not attained rebirth may only do so through the merit-making of their relatives or through suffering while wandering the earth, with suffering having the power to eliminate demerit' [60]. This has implications for interventions, as psychological recovery and healing requires the performance of appropriate rituals to enable rebirth and lay the soul to rest [59, 62].

Funerary rites may be impossible for many refugees to carry out while in transit. Family bereavement also cannot be fully experienced and the death rituals cannot be performed by those whose relatives have 'disappeared'. This produces a state of 'frozen bereavement' [63], or ambiguous loss [63, 64], which may be associated with persistent complex bereavement disorder. Documented accounts from Central and South America, when there was military dictatorship and thousands of people were killed, poignantly illustrate this. As one mother said: 'There are many families in Argentina destroyed by this, just like us. We have gone through 37 years of not knowing. To have a relative disappeared is a wound that does not close until the person appears again' [65]. Full grieving for the 'disappeared' is not possible because of the hope that the person will re-appear. During this time, life is 'suspended', as new relationships cannot be formed and re-marriage is not possible without the formal certification of the death of the spouse. Relatives of family members who have been killed may experience guilt about their survival while other family members perished [38, 66].

For those who survive conflict and journeys, a strong sense of loss may arise because of the cessation of contact with loved ones. Many refugees have travelled across the world to find safety in a country with prospects of a settled family life and opportunities for children. During the twentieth century, contact with those in the country of origin would have been by letter and then later in the century by telephone. The rise of the internet and widespread use of mobile telephones has substantially changed this. Telephone ownership and use is high amongst refugees [43].

When looked at from a cultural perspective, refugees often travel to countries with very different cultures, languages and religions to their own. This can add to the sense of loss, or 'cultural bereavement' [67]. In coping with cultural bereavement, the sense of loss may be mitigated by the new meaning and sense of purpose that arises in the new country [24]. Feeling connected to the new country is associated with better mental health [68]. A key challenge for families is to adapt to the new community and re-create family relationships and meanings in their lives with renewed hope. Most achieve this with some level of success, which explains why, for many refugees, depression and associated hopelessness reduces over time [69–71].

However, there are others for whom pre-migration adversity, losses and resettlement stressors are overwhelming. This can result in continuing depression, hopelessness, self-harm and suicide. Suicidal behaviour and suicide is more prevalent amongst refugees than in host community populations [72, 73], with a higher risk for those refugees with low family and social connectedness [74].

Case example – Survivor guilt and its impact on mental health

A Syrian female survivor came to the UK with her children and husband. She repeatedly attempted to take her life by trying to jump off bridges, hang herself, and various other forms of suicide attempts. During an interview with the adult mental health team, she said that it was not worth living while all her extended family members were being killed in Syria. Her mental health and attempts to take her own life arose because she was a survivor and unable to endure the guilt of living. In this case, the social structures and belief systems (such as religious and cultural) that often help individuals to manage adversity could not support her mental anguish, highlighting her underlying susceptibility to mental health difficulties, and her experiences as a refugee brought these to the forefront. The survivor may be tormented by what actions could have saved other family members, even if such actions were impossible to carry out.

Attachment

The attachment dynamic is fundamental in understanding family relationships and child development. Refugee experiences, as described above, include threatening events that will activate the attachment dynamic between child and caregiver or parent [57]. For this reason, refugee children who are separated from their parents may show increased anxiety [75], and this is apparent in pre-school children [76]. Attachment is less likely to be secure when parents are depressed [77]. Refugee children may also show insecure attachment, including disorganised attachment, when their parents have PTSD [13], shown to be related to frightening, threatening and dissociative parenting behaviour. Refugee parents may be preoccupied with and communicate their own distressing cognitions (related to grief, depressive cognitions or PTSD), which can interfere with their ability to attend to their infants' emotional needs [78]. The refugee parents may find it hard to separate from their children, for example, for nursery or school, having experienced the world as a dangerous place, and this can be communicated to the children. An attachment perspective investigating the long-term effects of the Holocaust showed that parents found it hard to separate from their children, yet at the same time they wanted them to be successful and take up all available opportunities [79].

The attachment dynamic also operates for older children, adolescents and spouses. The parent or spouse serves as a 'secure base' or attachment figure. This is consistent with substantial research showing that adult and adolescent refugees who are settled with family members are less distressed [2, 68, 80]. Secure attachment in adults is associated with lower levels of PTSD symptoms following trauma [81]. The refugee experiences described above can increase an adult's wish to seek proximity to their attachment figure, a role taken on by spouses or intimate partners. While separation anxiety disorder is usually regarded as occurring in children, it has been reported in adult refugees who came to the USA after experiencing war in Bosnia [82].

Violence Exposure, PTSD and Family Life

It has been established that the strongest predictor for the onset of PTSD in refugees is the proximity to violence, the extent of personal threat and the duration of exposure [2–4]. However, there are many other influences on this link, and the family may play an important role in protecting against PTSD and influencing the severity of PTSD symptoms. These influences need to be considered in relation to the life cycle and maturational processes.

Infants who experience exposure to violence may develop PTSD, which is observed using age-specific techniques. A study of infants from Iran showed post-traumatic functioning through play assessment: infants who experienced prolonged separations from their fathers because they were imprisoned and whose mothers had poor mental health had high levels of distress [83]. In many conflict settings, both children and parents experience exposure to traumatic events. Parental PTSD and anxiety may increase child PTSD and anxiety [84, 85]. The mechanism is likely to be through communication of emotion and reduced ability to contain and reassure the child [86]. The quality of parent-child interaction, including between fathers and children, is negatively affected by PTSD [87]. On the other hand, some studies suggest that PTSD may be associated with relatively good social function, so that parents are able to continue in their role as carers for their children [88].

Nevertheless, PTSD may be relatively stable, with some people, including infants, experiencing PTSD symptoms over many years [69, 71, 83].

Threatening events may increase PTSD intensity in family members. Most of the studies on this subject have been carried out with individuals, but nevertheless it is clear that some events will be understood and experienced as threatening by all family members. These include threats of deportation and possible return to the country that the family came from [89]. Detention is associated with the deterioration of mental health, including PTSD [90–94]. Additional examples of increased threats are the re-experiencing that occurs when people with past war trauma are exposed to reminders of this by hearing about or seeing further violence, for example, on television or in news reports.

A consistent finding on protective factors for mitigating PTSD is the presence of attachment or supportive figures that reduce PTSD, anxiety and depression [4, 68]. Children who experience war or violent events whilst in the presence of their parents or attachment figures may be protected against the risk of developing PTSD [95]. Interestingly, this also applies to UASCs who are fostered with families and who are placed in higher-support living arrangements rather than in low-support arrangements [96–98]. In the more supportive settings, the level of PTSD symptoms was lower.

The long-term effects of PTSD include the effects on offspring. In a study of survivors of the Khmer Rouge regime in Cambodia (1975–9) and their adolescent daughters, parents with PTSD had daughters who scored high on anxiety [99]. Maternal role reversal was shown to mediate the relationship between the mother's and the daughter's symptoms. Another study of survivors of the Ukrainian atrocities of genocide and starvation in the 1930s investigated second- and third-generation offspring [100]. The emotions transmitted included fear, mistrust, sadness, shame, anger, anxiety and decreased self-worth. There was also stockpiling of food and high value placed on food. Many of these features have been found in the offspring of Holocaust survivors, including overprotection, anxiety and disordered eating [101].

For a long time, the main explanation for intergenerational transmission of PTSD and anxiety was located in communication and modelling, but in recent years attention has turned to epigenetic mechanisms as a source of trauma transmission, with accumulating evidence from studies with Holocaust survivors [102–104]. One influential study showed that parental PTSD had an effect on DNA methylation of the exon 1F promoter of the glucocorticoid receptor (GR-1F) gene, and this has an effect on the neuroendocrine system [103].

Culture Change, Exile and Reconstitution of Family Life

There are numerous influences on mental health in the resettlement phase that change over time and that have an impact on family life (see Table 1.1). One of the most important is that refugees who arrive in resettlement countries and claim asylum are usually unable to apply for work and obtain work permits, and in the absence of private savings they are forced to depend on state benefits. This can impose financial hardship on the family, which itself is a cause of considerable stress [105]. In addition to the financial consequences, being out of work can have negative effects on self-esteem and increase social isolation, a sense of purposelessness and tensions between spouses. Pre-migration stressors, such as war trauma,

Case example – Loss of social status and financial security

Faizal, aged 12 years, lived with his parents and 2 older brothers. Both parents were from the Middle East, where they were both professors in mathematics in a well-established university. Faizal was referred for aggressive behaviour in school, lacking in concentration and not doing very well academically. His older brother obtained a place to study medicine in the UK but was struggling with depression, although his middle brother was managing academically. The family was very distressed, as both parents were finding it difficult to get a job in the UK. His father was trying to do some teaching in college but found it degrading, as the UK system of teaching was very different to that of the Middle East. He was preoccupied with what was happening in his country of origin and the number of academics being imprisoned and killed. This generated conflict for the father, who was relieved at his and his family's refugee status but also anguished by his own loss of professional status in the UK, as well as feeling helpless with regard to his former colleagues in his country of origin. This preoccupation had a significant impact on family dynamics, as Faizal's father became emotionally unavailable and his mother became depressed. There was an emphasis on the boys achieving well academically, which contributed to further pressure in the home.

are also associated with lower take-up of employment [106]. Some refugees with professional backgrounds, such as doctors, scientists or engineers, may find great difficulty in obtaining employment using their qualifications, and this process of de-skilling leads them to experience a sense of loss of role and disempowerment. Many men find it hard to contribute to child care. There may also be significant changes in family gender roles. Women may be the heads of households and be responsible for household income, as they are often separated from their spouses who are involved in combat, detained or killed. These changes can contribute to family tensions and affect the adjustment of children, as illustrated in this case vignette.

This case emphasises the loss of social class and privilege and the effects of having to rely on state benefits. Survivor guilt also added to their distress, as they got frequent feedback from their country about colleagues who were killed in bombings or imprisoned. This vignette is consistent with the findings of a Quebec study of adolescent refugees, who were predominantly not war-exposed [107]. A higher prevalence of disorder was found amongst the refugee group than amongst the non-refugee comparison group, and interestingly this occurred amongst the male adolescents and much of it was accounted for by conduct disorder. Difficulties were associated with paternal unemployment of more than six months and single-parent, mother-headed families. The authors suggest that there was less confidence amongst fathers and less authoritative parenting by mothers in single-parent households. These processes which strained family relationships reduced warmth and increased the criticism and conflict that may be associated with parental preoccupation, depression or PTSD and the disruptions of routines, social isolation, financial hardship and overcrowding, which are all risk factors for the development of conduct disorder [108–111].

Many refugees seek asylum in countries that are culturally different from the one they came from. This gives rise to an awareness of cultural and ethnic difference. By ethnicity is meant a combination of race, religion, cultural history, family organisation and values, attitudes to work and employment and more local cultural influences, including dietary practice [112]. Awareness of culture and ethnicity is often heightened by migration and the encounters of refugees with the host society. Refugees need to negotiate and decide the extent to which they adopt the culture and values of the host society and the extent to which they retain or distance themselves from the culture of origin [21, 113, 114]. The process of acculturation and acquisition of the new language and culture of the host society is usually different across generations. Children and adolescents who are in school or college learn very quickly. Parents, who may be isolated and not working, may struggle to learn the language and feel less adept at judging culturally appropriate behaviour and establishing age-appropriate norms for their children. Residing in an area with a clustering of immigrant communities may enable refugees to feel familiar and safe, although it could reduce the adaptation process to the host country. The differential rates of language acquisition and acculturation may set up tensions that can lead to interge-nerational conflict. However, adolescent children are aware of culturally shaped parental expectations and may try to maintain loyalty to their culture of origin as well as adopting the culture and ways of the host community [7]. They become bicultural and bilingual and may adapt their behaviour to the setting they are in [22, 115]. For this reason, there is no simple link between rates of offspring acculturation and parental acculturation and adjustment [116].

In resettlement, the process of family reunification may invoke relational complexities in coping with cultural change and adaptation. Re-uniting engenders many feelings. While there may be a yearning to restore the family to its earlier state, the situation may generate anxiety about how the other family members have changed and what reunification will mean [11]. During long separations, spouses may have had very different experiences. Some, often men who have been combatants, may have been detained, sometimes tortured, and migrate after their wives and children have arrived in resettlement countries. In this situation, wives may have started to acquire autonomy as heads of households and language fluency in the new country [11, 117]. The arrival of fathers may strain marital and family relationships. The newly formed family will need to negotiate new routines and the extent to which it will follow traditional customs or those of the host society. A further source of tension between spouses can be the difficulty of attaining intimacy, especially after women have been sexually abused. For women, assault often brings great shame and guilt, which they may feel cannot be shared with their spouse for fear of rejection and divorce [117]. Sometimes this distress is communicated through their bodies as medically unexplained symptoms [118] (see first vignette).

The strains in refugee families may result in violence, a topic that has been poorly researched. Available studies suggest that it could have a prevalence of 30–50% [5]. Risk factors for this include individual war trauma associated with psychiatric disorder including depression and PTSD, family structural variables including single-parent families, strained parent-child interaction, financial adversity, and cultural influences including patriarchal beliefs [5]. It appears that a risk accumulation model provides the best explanation.

While much of this section and earlier sections concern refugees' psychiatric and social difficulties, it is important to bear in mind that as time elapses most families will become settled, and many will experience satisfaction with their new life and will be able to see benefits. Many individuals experience 'post-traumatic growth' in which past adversities enable them to develop strengths that help them to become more resilient. 'Post-traumatic growth' is more likely to occur in the presence of a high level of family and social support and a positive outlook about the new country and planning [119–121].

Conclusion

This chapter has outlined the varied ways in which the family is affected by war, threat of violence, migration and resettlement. The family may be a buffer against these adversities. However, in some circumstances, relationships become so strained that conflict and violence can arise, and in this circumstance there will be a further detrimental effect on mental health. Over time, most refugee families in resettlement countries become less distressed, but PTSD and associated protective and fearful behaviours in parents may be communicated to offspring. Most families show surprising resilience and some show post-traumatic growth.

References

1. E. M. Cummings, C. E. Merrilees, L. K. Taylor and C. F. Mondi, Developmental and social-ecological perspectives on children, political violence, and armed conflict. *Development and Psychopathology*, 29(1) (2017), 1–10.

2. M. Fazel, R. V. Reed, C. Panter-Brick and A. Stein, Mental health of displaced and refugee children resettled in high-income countries: Risk and protective factors. *The Lancet*, 379(9812) (2012), 266–82.

3. R. V. Reed, M. Fazel, L. Jones, C. Panter-Brick and A. Stein, Mental health of displaced and refugee children resettled in low-income and middle-income countries: Risk and protective factors. *The Lancet*, 379 (9812) (2012), 250–65.

4. S. Priebe, D. Giacco and R. El-Nagib, *WHO Health Evidence Network Synthesis Report 47. Public Health Aspects of Mental Health Among Migrants and Refugees: A Review of the Evidence on Mental Health Care for Refugees, Asylum Seekers and Irregular Migrants in the WHO European Region* (Copenhagen: WHO Regional Office for Europe, 2016).

5. I. Timshel, E. Montgomery and N. T. Dalgaard, A systematic review of risk and protective factors associated with family related violence in refugee families. *Child Abuse & Neglect*, 70 (2017), 315–30.

6. M. Beiser, F. Hou, I. Hyman and M. Tousignant, Poverty, family process, and the mental health of immigrant children in Canada. *American Journal of Public Health*, 92(2) (2002), 220–7.

7. R. L. Frounfelker, M. T. Assefa, E. Smith, A. Hussein and T. S. Betancourt, 'We would never forget who we are': Resettlement, cultural negotiation, and family relationships among Somali Bantu refugees. *European Child & Adolescent Psychiatry*, 26(11) (2017), 1387–400.

8. N. T. Dalgaard and E. Montogomery, The transgenerational transmission of refugee trauma: Family functioning and children's psychosocial adjustment. *International Journal of Migration, Health and Social Care*, 13(3) (2016), 289–301.

9. L. De Haene, H. Grietens and K. Verschueren, Adult attachment in the context of refugee traumatisation: The impact of organized violence and forced separation on parental states of mind regarding attachment. *Attachment & Human Development*, 12(3) (2010), 249–64.

10. E. Montgomery, Tortured families: A coordinated management of meaning analysis. *Family Process*, 43(3) (2004), 349–71.

11. C. C. Rousseau, M. C. Rufagari, D. Bagilishya and T. Measham, Remaking family life: Strategies for re-establishing continuity among Congolese refugees during the family reunification process. *Social Science & Medicine (1982)*, 59(5) (2004), 1095–108.

12. R. Kevers, P. Rober and L. De Haene, Unraveling the mobilization of memory in research with refugees. *Qualitative Health Research*, 28(4) (2018), 659–72.

13. E. van Ee, R. J. Kleber, M. J. Jongmans, T. T. Mooren and D. Out, Parental PTSD: Adverse parenting and child attachment in a refugee sample. *Attachment & Human Development*, 18(3) (2016), 273–91.

14. S. Weine, S. Feetham, Y. Kulauzovic, K. Knafl, S. Besic, A. Klebic et al., A family beliefs framework for socially and culturally specific preventive interventions with refugee youths and families. *The American Journal of Orthopsychiatry*, 76(1) (2006), 1–9.

15. S. M. Weine, D. Raina, M. Zhubi, M Delesi, D. Huseni, S. Feetham et al., The TAFES multi-family group intervention for Kosovar refugees: A feasibility study. *The Journal of Nervous and Mental Disease*, 191 (2) (2003), 100–7.

16. T. Parsons, The social structure of the family. In R. N. Anshen, ed., *The Family: Its Functions and Destiny* (New York: Harper & Row, 1959).

17. T. Parsons, The normal American family. In S. M. Farber, ed., *Man and Civilization: The Family's Search for Survival* (New York: McGraw-Hill, 1965).

18. B. H. Fiese, T. J. Tomcho, M. Douglas, K. Josephs, S. Poltrock and T. Baker, A review of 50 years of research on naturally occurring family routines and rituals: Cause for celebration? *Journal of Family Psychology (JFP) Journal of the Division of Family Psychology of the American Psychological Association (Division 43)*, 16(4) (2002), 381–90.

19. A. M. Graybiel, Habits, rituals, and the evaluative brain. *Annual Review of Neuroscience*, 31 (2008), 359–87.

20. C. J. Falicov, *Latino Families in Therapy* (New York: Guildford Press, 1998).

21. J. W. Berry, Acculturation strategies and adaptation. In J. E. Lansford, K. Deater-Deckard and M. C. Bornstein, eds., *Immigrant Families in Contemporary Society* (New York: Guilford Press, 2007), pp. 69–82.

22. S. J. Schwartz, J. B. Unger, B. L. Zamboanga and J. Szapocznik, Rethinking the concept of acculturation: Implications for theory and research. *The American Psychologist*, 65(4) (2010), 237–51.

23. L. Hoffman, Constructing realities: An art of lenses. *Family Process*, 29(1) (1990), 1–12.

24. F. Walsh, Traumatic loss and major disasters: Strengthening family and community resilience. *Family Process*, 46 (2007), 207–27.

25. T. Kushner and K. Knox, *Refugees in an Age of Genocide* (London: Frank Cass, 1999).

26. UNHCR, *The State of the World's Refugees* (Oxford: Oxford University Press, 2000).

27. UNHCR, *Guidelines on Policies and Procedures in Dealing with Unaccompanied Children Seeking Asylum* (Geneva: UNHCR, 1997).

28. UNHCR, (2018). Figures at a glance. Geneva UNHCR. www.unhcr.org/uk/figures-at-a-glance.html

29. Eurostat, (2018). Asylum statistics. Eurostat. http://ec.europa.eu/eurostat/statistics-explained/index.php/Asylum_statistics

30. J. DeJong, F. Sbeity, J. Schlecht, M. Harfouche, R. Yamout, F. M. Fouad et al., Young lives disrupted: Gender and well-being among adolescent Syrian refugees in Lebanon. *Conflict and Health*, 11(Suppl. 1) (2017), 23.

31. T. S. Betancourt, E. A. Newnham, D. Birman, R. Lee, B. H. Ellis and C. M. Layne, Comparing trauma exposure, mental health needs, and service utilization across clinical samples of refugee, immigrant, and US-origin children. *Journal of Traumatic Stress*, 30(3) (2017), 209–18.

32. V. Cetorelli, I. Sasson, N. Shabila and G. Burnham, Mortality and kidnapping estimates for the Yazidi population in the area of Mount Sinjar, Iraq, in August 2014: A retrospective household survey. *PLoS Medicine*, 14(5) (2017), e1002297.

33. A. H. Mokdad, Intentional injuries in the Eastern Mediterranean Region, 1990–2015: Findings from the Global Burden of Disease 2015 study. *International Journal of Public Health* 63(1) (2017), 39–46.

34. I. Skjelsbaek, Sexual violence and war: Mapping out a complex relationship. *European Journal of International Relations*, 7(2) (2001), 211–37.

35. G. Clarke, W. H. Sack and B. Goff, Three forms of stress in Cambodian adolescent refugees. *Journal of Abnormal Child Psychology*, 21(1) (1993), 65–77.

36. J. D. Kinzie and W. Sack, Severely traumatized Cambodian children: Research findings and clinical implications. In F. L. Ahearn and J. L. Athey, eds., *Refugee Children: Theory, Research, Services* (Baltimore, MA: Johns Hopkins University Press, 1991), pp. 92–105.

37. Human Rights Watch, (2018). *World Report 2018: Eritrea, 18 January 2018*, (accessed 26 October 2018). www .refworld.org/docid/5a61ee79c.html

38. R. F. Mollica, *Healing Invisible Wounds* (Nashville, TN: Vanderbilt University Press, 2006).

39. J. Goveas and S. Coomarasamy, Why am I still here? The impact of survivor guilt on the mental health and settlement process of refugee youth. In S. Pashang, N. Khanlou and J. Clarke, eds., *Today's Youth and Mental Health: Hope, Power, and Resilience* (Cham: Springer International Publishing, 2018), pp. 101–17.

40. UNHCR, *Desperate Journeys* (Geneva: UNHCR, 2017).

41. J. Ben Farhat, K. Blanchet, P. Juul Bjertrup, A. Veizis, C. Perrin, R. M. Coulborn et al., Syrian refugees in Greece: Experience with violence, mental health status, and access to information during the journey and while in Greece. *BMC Medicine*, 16(1) (2018), 40.

42. Migrants with mobiles. *The Economist* (2017). www.economist.com/interna tional/2017/02/11/phones-are-now-indispensable-for-refugees

43. UNHCR, *Connecting Refugees* (Geneva: UNHCR, 2016).

44. A. Crepet, F. Rita, A. Reid, W. Van den Boogaard, P. Deiana, G. Quaranta et al., Mental health and trauma in asylum seekers landing in Sicily in 2015: A descriptive study of neglected invisible wounds. *Conflict and Health*, 11 (2017), 1.

45. J. K. Felsman, F. T. Leong, M. C. Johnson and I. C. Felsman, Estimates of psychological distress among Vietnamese refugees: Adolescents, unaccompanied minors and young adults. *Social Science & Medicine (1982)*, 31(11) (1990), 1251–6.

46. UNHCR, *Global Report 2016* (Geneva: UNHCR, 2017).

47. L. J. Kirmayer, Refugees and forced migration: Hardening of the arteries in the global reign of insecurity. *Transcultural Psychiatry*, 44(3) (2007), 307–10.

48. F. Crepeau, D. Nakache and I. Atak, International migration: Security concerns and human rights standards. *Transcultural Psychiatry*, 44(3) (2007), 311–37.

49. D. C. Anagnostopoulos, G. Giannakopoulos and N. G. Christodoulou, The synergy of the refugee crisis and the financial crisis in Greece: Impact on mental health. *The International Journal of Social Psychiatry*, (2017), 20764017700444.

50. M. Hodes, M. M. Vasquez, D. Anagnostopoulos, K. Triantafyllou, D. Abdelhady, K. Weiss et al., Refugees in Europe: National overviews from key countries with a special focus on child and adolescent mental health. *European Child & Adolescent Psychiatry*, 27(4) (2018), 389–99.

51. L. Lucassen, The refugee crisis in historical perspective. In ZentIM-Congress, Key Elements of Model Communities for Refugees and Immigrants: An Interdisciplinary Perspective (Essen: 21–23 June 2017). http://www.inzentim.de /wp-content/uploads/ftp/07-2017/Abstrac t_InZentIM-Tagung_Lucassen.pdf

52. D. Silove, Z. Steel and C. Watters, Policies of deterrence and the mental health of asylum seekers. *The Journal of the American Medical Association*, 284(5) (2000), 604–11.

53. Australia RCo, Recent changes in Australian refugee policy (Surry Hills, NSW: Refugee Council of Australia, 2010). www.refugeecouncil.org.au/publica tions/recent-changes-australian-refugee-policy/

54. M. Fazel, J. Wheeler and J. Danesh, Prevalence of serious mental disorder in 7000 refugees resettled in western countries: A systematic review. *The Lancet*, 365(9467) (2005), 1309–14.

55. Z. Steel, T. Chey, D. Silove, C. Marnane, R. A. Bryant and M. van Ommeren, Association of torture and other

potentially traumatic events with mental health outcomes among populations exposed to mass conflict and displacement: A systematic review and meta-analysis. *The Journal of the American Medical Association*, 302(5) (2009), 537–49.

56. M. Bogic, A. Njoku and S. Priebe, Long-term mental health of war-refugees: A systematic literature review. *BMC International Health and Human Rights*, 15 (2015), 29.

57. C. Murray Parkes, J. Stevenson-Hinde and P. Marris, *Attachment Across the Life Cycle* (London: Tavistock/Routledge, 1991).

58. M. Eisenbruch, Cross-cultural aspects of bereavement. I: A conceptual framework for comparative analysis. *Culture, Medicine and Psychiatry*, 8(3) (1984), 283–309.

59. D. E. Hinton, N. P. Field, A. Nickerson, R. A. Bryant and N. Simon, Dreams of the dead among Cambodian refugees: Frequency, phenomenology, and relationship to complicated grief and posttraumatic stress disorder. *Death Studies*, 37(8) (2013), 750–67.

60. D. E. Hinton, S. Peou, S. Joshi, A. Nickerson and N. M. Simon, Normal grief and complicated bereavement among traumatized Cambodian refugees: Cultural context and the central role of dreams of the dead. *Culture, Medicine and Psychiatry*, 37(3) (2013), 427–64.

61. M. Eisenbruch, From post-traumatic stress disorder to cultural bereavement: Diagnosis of southeast Asian refugees. *Social Science and Medicine*, 33(6) (1991), 673–80.

62. D. E. Hinton, A. L. Hinton, V. Pich, J. R. Loeum and M. H. Pollack, Nightmares among Cambodian refugees: The breaching of concentric ontological security. *Culture, Medicine and Psychiatry*, 33(2) (2009), 219–65.

63. A. Ventriglio and D. Bhugra, Frozen bereavement. *The International Journal of Social Psychiatry*, 63(4) (2017), 285–6.

64. J. Ballard, E. Wieling and C. Solheim, *Immigrant and Refugee Families: Global Perspectives on Displacement and Resettlement Experiences* (Minneapolis,

MN: University of Minnesota Libraries Publishing, 2016).

65. V. Hernandez, (2013). Painful search for Argentina's disappeared. BBC News (updated March 24, 2013). www.bbc.co.uk /news/world-latin-america-21884147

66. S. J. Stotz, T. Elbert, V. Muller and M. Schauer, The relationship between trauma, shame, and guilt: Findings from a community-based study of refugee minors in Germany. *European Journal of Psychotraumatology*, 6 (2015), 25863.

67. M. Eisenbruch, The cultural bereavement interview: A new clinical research approach for refugees. *The Psychiatric Clinics of North America*, 13(4) (1990), 715–35.

68. M. Beiser and F. Hou, Predictors of positive mental health among refugees: Results from Canada's General Social Survey. *Transcultural Psychiatry*, 54(5–6) (2017), 675–95.

69. W. H. Sack, C. Him and D. Dickason, Twelve-year follow-up study of Khmer youths who suffered massive war trauma as children. *Journal of the American Academy of Child and Adolescent Psychiatry*, 38(9) (1999), 1173–9.

70. M. Beiser and K. A. Wickrama, Trauma, time and mental health: A study of temporal reintegration and depressive disorder among Southeast Asian refugees. *Psychological Medicine*, 34(5) (2004), 899–910.

71. M. Beiser and I. Hyman, Refugees' time perspective and mental health. *The American Journal of Psychiatry*, 154(7) (1997), 996–1002.

72. S. Goosen, A. E. Kunst, K. Stronks, I. E. van Oostrum, D. G. Uitenbroek and A. J. Kerkhof, Suicide death and hospital-treated suicidal behaviour in asylum seekers in the Netherlands: A national registry-based study. *BMC Public Health*, 11 (2011), 484.

73. J. Cohen, Safe in our hands? A study of suicide and self-harm in asylum seekers. *Journal of Forensic and Legal Medicine*, 15 (4) (2008), 235–44.

74. A. K. Hagaman, T. I. Sivilli, T. Ao, C. Blanton, H. Ellis, B. Lopes Cardozo et al., An investigation into suicides among Bhutanese refugees resettled in the United States between 2008 and 2011. *Journal of Immigrant and Minority Health*, 18(4) (2016), 819–27.

75. E. Montgomery, Refugee children from the Middle East. *Scandinavian Journal of Social Medicine Supplementum*, 54 (1998), 1–152.

76. K. Almqvist and M. Brandell-Forsberg, Iranian refugee children in Sweden: Effects of organized violence and forced migration on preschool children. *The American Journal of Orthopsychiatry*, 65(2) (1995), 225–37.

77. V. Lecompte, D. Miconi and C. Rousseau, Challenges related to migration and child attachment: A pilot study with South Asian immigrant mother-child dyads. *Attachment & Human Development*, 20(2) (2017), 1–15.

78. N. T. Dalgaard, B. K. Todd, S. I. Daniel and E. Montgomery, The transmission of trauma in refugee families: Associations between intra-family trauma communication style, children's attachment security and psychosocial adjustment. *Attachment & Human Development*, 18(1) (2016), 69–89.

79. D. Bar-On, J. Eland, R. J. Kleber, R. Krell, Y. Moore, A. Sagi et al., Multigenerational perspectives on coping with the Holocaust experience: An attachment perspective for understanding the developmental sequelae of trauma across generations. *International Journal of Behavioral Development*, 22(2) (1998), 315–38.

80. T. Bean, I. Derluyn, E. Eurelings-Bontekoe, E. Broekaert and P. Spinhoven, Comparing psychological distress, traumatic stress reactions, and experiences of unaccompanied refugee minors with experiences of adolescents accompanied by parents. *The Journal of Nervous and Mental Disease*, 195(4) (2007), 288–97.

81. S. Woodhouse, S. Ayers and A. P. Field, The relationship between adult attachment style and post-traumatic stress symptoms: A meta-analysis. *Journal of Anxiety Disorders*, 35 (2015), 103–17.

82. D. Silove, S. Momartin, C. Marnane, Z. Steel and V. Manicavasagar, Adult separation anxiety disorder among war-affected Bosnian refugees: Comorbidity with PTSD and associations with dimensions of trauma. *Journal of Traumatic Stress*, 23(1) (2010), 169–72.

83. K. Almqvist and M. Brandell-Forsberg, Refugee children in Sweden: Post-traumatic stress disorder in Iranian preschool children exposed to organized violence. *Child Abuse & Neglect*, 21(4) (1997), 351–66.

84. S. Eruyar, J. Maltby and P. Vostanis, Mental health problems of Syrian refugee children: The role of parental factors. *European Child & Adolescent Psychiatry*, 27(4) (2018), 401–9.

85. A. A. Thabet, A. Abu Tawahina, E. El Sarraj and P. Vostanis, Exposure to war trauma and PTSD among parents and children in the Gaza strip. *European Child & Adolescent Psychiatry*, 17(4) (2008), 191–9.

86. A. A. Thabet, A. N. Ibraheem, R. Shivram, E. A. Winter and P Vostanis, Parenting support and PTSD in children of a war zone. *The International Journal of Social Psychiatry*, 55(3) (2009), 226–37.

87. E. van Ee, M. Sleijpen, R. J. Kleber and M. J. Jongmans, Father-involvement in a refugee sample: Relations between posttraumatic stress and caregiving. *Family Process*, 52(4) (2013), 723–35.

88. W. H. Sack, G. N. Clarke, R. Kinney, G. Belestos, C. Him and J. Seeley, The Khmer Adolescent Project. II: Functional capacities in two generations of Cambodian refugees. *The Journal of Nervous and Mental Disease*, 183(3) (1995), 177–81.

89. G. Morgan, S. Melluish and A. Welham, Exploring the relationship between postmigratory stressors and mental health for asylum seekers and refused asylum seekers in the UK. *Transcultural Psychiatry*, 54(5–6) (2017), 653–74.

90. K. Zwi, S. Mares, D. Nathanson, A. K. Tay and D. Silove, The impact of detention on the social-emotional wellbeing of children seeking asylum: A comparison with community-based children. *European*

Child & Adolescent Psychiatry, 27(4) (2017), 411–22.

91. R. Kronick, C. Rousseau and J. Cleveland, Refugee children's sandplay narratives in immigration detention in Canada. *European Child & Adolescent Psychiatry*, 27(4) (2017), 423–37.

92. S. Mares, Fifteen years of detaining children who seek asylum in Australia: Evidence and consequences. *Australasian Psychiatry*, 24(1) (2016), 11–14.

93. S. J. Puthoopparambil, M. Bjerneld and C. Kallestal, Quality of life among immigrants in Swedish immigration detention centres: A cross-sectional questionnaire study. *Global Health Action*, 8(1) (2015), 28321. DOI:http://10.3402/gha.v8.28321

94. P. Sen, J. Arugnanaseelan, E. Connell, C. Katona, A. A. Khan, P. Moran et al., Mental health morbidity among people subject to immigration detention in the UK: A feasibility study. *Epidemiology and Psychiatric Sciences*, 27(6) (2017), 1–10.

95. H. C. Gallagher, J. Richardson, D. Forbes, L. Harms, L. Gibbs, N. Alkemade et al., Mental health following separation in a disaster: The role of attachment. *Journal of Traumatic Stress*, 29(1) (2016), 56–64.

96. M. Hodes, D. Jagdev, N. Chandra and A. Cunniff, Risk and resilience for psychological distress amongst unaccompanied asylum seeking adolescents. *Journal of Child Psychology and Psychiatry, and Allied Disciplines*, 49 (7) (2008), 723–32.

97. I. Bronstein, P. Montgomery and S. Dobrowolski, PTSD in asylum-seeking male adolescents from Afghanistan. *Journal of Traumatic Stress*, 25(5) (2012), 551–7.

98. M. Jakobsen, M. A. Meyer DeMott, T. Wentzel-Larsen and T. Heir, The impact of the asylum process on mental health: A longitudinal study of unaccompanied refugee minors in Norway. *BMJ Open*, 7(6) (2017), e015157.

99. N. P. Field, S. Muong and V. Sochanvimean, Parental styles in the intergenerational transmission of trauma stemming from the Khmer Rouge regime in Cambodia. *The American Journal of Orthopsychiatry*, 83(4) (2013), 483–94.

100. B. Bezo and S. Maggi, Living in 'survival mode': Intergenerational transmission of trauma from the Holodomor genocide of 1932–1933 in Ukraine. *Social Science & Medicine*, 2015(134) (1982), 87–94.

101. A. H. Zohar, L. Giladi and T. Givati, Holocaust exposure and disordered eating: A study of multi-generational transmission. *European Eating Disorders Review*, 15(1) (2007), 50–7.

102. R. Yehuda, N. P. Daskalakis, L. M. Bierer, H. N. Bader, T. Klengel, F. Holsboer et al., Holocaust exposure induced intergenerational effects on FKBP5 methylation. *Biological Psychiatry*, 80(5) (2016), 372–80.

103. R. Yehuda, N P. Daskalakis, A. Lehrner, F. Desarnaud, H. N. Bader, I. Makotkine et al., Influences of maternal and paternal PTSD on epigenetic regulation of the glucocorticoid receptor gene in Holocaust survivor offspring. *The American Journal of Psychiatry*, 171(8) (2014), 872–80.

104. A. Lehrner, L. M. Bierer, V. Passarelli, L. C. Pratchett, J. D. Flory, H. N. Bader et al., Maternal PTSD associates with greater glucocorticoid sensitivity in offspring of Holocaust survivors. *Psychoneuroendocrinology*, 40 (2014), 213–20.

105. S. Ekblad and J. M. Jaranson, Psychosocial rehabilitation. In J. P. Wilson and B. Drozdek, eds., *Broken Spirits* (New York: Brunner-Routledge, 2004), pp. 609–36.

106. A. M. Wright, A. Dhalimi, M. A. Lumley, H. Jamil, N. Pole, J. E. Arnetz et al., Unemployment in Iraqi refugees: The interaction of pre and post-displacement trauma. *Scandinavian Journal of Psychology*, 57(6) (2016), 564–70.

107. M. Tousignant, E. Habimana, C. Biron, C. Malo, E. Sidoli-LeBlanc and N. Bendris, The Quebec Adolescent

Refugee Project: Psychopathology and family variables in a sample from 35 nations. *Journal of the American Academy of Child and Adolescent Psychiatry*, 38(11) (1999), 1426–32.

108. A. Caspi, T. E. Moffitt, J. Morgan, M. Rutter, A. Taylor, L. Arseneault et al., Maternal expressed emotion predicts children's antisocial behavior problems: Using monozygotic-twin differences to identify environmental effects on behavioral development. *Developmental Psychology*, 40(2) (2004), 149–61.

109. J. Kim-Cohen, T. E. Moffitt, A. Taylor, S. J. Pawlby and A. Caspi, Maternal depression and children's antisocial behavior: Nature and nurture effects. *Archives of General Psychiatry*, 62(2) (2005), 173–81.

110. J. R. Mazza, J. Lambert, M. V. Zunzunegui, R. E. Tremblay, M. Boivin and S. M. Cote, Early adolescence behavior problems and timing of poverty during childhood: A comparison of lifecourse models. *Social Science & Medicine (1982)*, 177 (2017), 35–42.

111. J. D. Smith, T. J. Dishion, D. S. Shaw, M. N. Wilson, C. C. Winter and G. R. Patterson, Coercive family process and early-onset conduct problems from age 2 to school entry. *Development and Psychopathology*, 26(4 Pt 1) (2014), 917–32.

112. M. McGoldrick, J. Giordano and N. Garcia-Preto, eds., *Ethnicity and Family Therapy*, 3rd ed. (New York: Guilford Press, 2006).

113. J. W. Berry, A psychology of immigration. *Journal of Social Issues*, 57(3) (2001), 615–31.

114. J. W. Berry, Refugee adaptation in settlement countries: An overview with an emphasis on primary prevention. In F. L. Ahearn and J. L. Athey, eds., *Refugee Children* (Baltimore, MA: Johns Hopkins University Press, 1991), pp. 20–38.

115. S. Bhatia and A. Ram, Rethinking 'acculturation' in relation to diasporic cultures and postcolonial identities. *Human Development*, 44(1) (2001), 1–18.

116. E. H. Telzer, Expanding the acculturation gap-distress model: An integrative review of research. *Human Development*, 53(6) (2010), 313–40.

117. J. Walter and J. Bala, Where meanings, sorrow, and hope have a resident permit: Treatment of families and children. In J. P. Wilson and B. Drozdek, eds., *Broken Spirits* (New York: Brunner-Routledge, 2004), pp. 487–519.

118. M. C. Kastrup, Mental health consequences of war: Gender specific issues. *World Psychiatry*, 5(1) (2006), 33–4.

119. D. Hussain and B. Bhushan, Posttraumatic stress and growth among Tibetan refugees: The mediating role of cognitive-emotional regulation strategies. *Journal of Clinical Psychology*, 67(7) (2011), 720–35.

120. S. Powell, R. Rosner, W. Butollo, R. G. Tedeschi and L. G. Calhoun, Posttraumatic growth after war: A study with former refugees and displaced people in Sarajevo. *Journal of Clinical Psychology*, 59(1) (2003), 71–83.

121. M. Sleijpen, J. Haagen, T. Mooren and R. J. Kleber, Growing from experience: An exploratory study of posttraumatic growth in adolescent refugees. *European Journal of Psychotraumatology*, 7(S1) (2016), 28698.

Transgenerational Trauma Transmission in Refugee Families
The Role of Traumatic Suffering, Attachment Representations, and Parental Caregiving

Nina Thorup Dalgaard, Marie Høgh Thøgersen, and Karin Riber

The transgenerational transmission of trauma refers to the transmission of traumatic suffering and related mental health problems from traumatized parents to their offspring. This process was initially documented in a rich body of clinical studies with offspring of Holocaust survivors. Later, in a series of meta-analyses of 32 samples involving 4,418 participants, it was concluded that, in nonclinical samples, there was no evidence for the influence of the parents' traumatic Holocaust experiences on their children, and that secondary traumatization only emerged in clinical samples [1].

More recently, psychosocial refugee studies developed an interest in exploring transgenerational trauma transmission in displaced families. Refugee families' complex histories of traumatization and chronic distress generate questions on the extent to which parental traumatic suffering may affect their children's adaptation. Indeed, the refugee experience consists of a prolonged period of accumulating and interacting stressors during pre-migration, flight, and post-migration [2]. In refugee research, these stressors may operate as a circle of disruptive and intertwined processes of traumatization, acculturation, uprooting, and marginality [3], putting refugees at risk of developing mental health disorders. PTSD, depression, and anxiety disorders in particular are prototypical patterns of distress in refugee children and adults [4, 5]. For refugee families, these increased levels of suffering generate questions about the role of transgenerational trauma transmission in understanding refugee family relationships and wellbeing in parents and children.

From this perspective, studies have explored potential patterns of trauma transmission in refugee families. In a study of children of Vietnamese refugees using the Strengths and Difficulties Questionnaire (SDQ), Vaage et al. [6] found that children of refugee parents born in Norway had significantly lower Total Difficulties scores than their Norwegian peers; however, children's Total Difficulties scores were positively associated with a paternal diagnosis of PTSD [6]. Daud et al. [7] compared 15 refugee families from Lebanon and Iraq, where parents had been subjected to torture, with a matched control group of 15 nontraumatized refugee families where the parents did not have a history of direct torture. This study found that children of tortured parents had more symptoms of anxiety, depression, posttraumatic stress, attention deficits, and behavioral disorders compared with the control group. In sum, this evidence suggests that, although parental trauma is not automatically associated with psychopathology in children, within clinical populations a parental trauma history and subsequent PTSD symptoms can influence children negatively and may lead to their development of psychological distress. Yet the mechanisms by which the transmission is mediated are yet to be determined. Consistent with the broader literature on trauma transmission [1, 8], refugee studies have hypothesized and explored two central mechanisms mediating the transmission of traumatic suffering in parent-child relationships: parental–trauma-related mental health problems [9, 10] and parental disrupted attachment representations [11–13]. Insecure or unresolved parental attachment representations may be associated with decreased parental availability and disrupted caregiving ability. These insecure or unresolved parental attachment representations may precede traumatic life events or occur as a result of these, or they may develop in response to co-occurring trauma and attachment–related disruptive life events [8], suggesting complex intersections between parental traumatic suffering, attachment representations, and parental caregiving in the context of exile.

In this chapter, we review the emerging literature on the complex interactions between parental PTSD, attachment representations, and parental caregiving in understanding processes of transgenerational trauma transmission in refugee families. First, we review literature on parental posttraumatic suffering and its association with parental caregiving behavior and present studies that have explored these dynamics in refugee samples. Second, we discuss how attachment studies have highlighted the role of attachment representations and related disrupted parental behavior in understanding transgenerational trauma transmission, and we review studies documenting attachment representations in refugee families. In order to reflect on potential clinical implications of both perspectives of parental–trauma-related psychopathology and attachment representations, we explore the role of parental traumatic suffering, attachment representations, and their complex interactions in shaping parental caregiving in two case analyses and conclude by discussing core themes in clinical work addressing transgenerational trauma transmission through the lens of parental posttraumatic suffering, disrupted attachment representations, and related caregiving behaviors.

Parental PTSD and Caregiving

Parental traumatic responses may undermine the capacity for sensitive and responsive caregiving. Parents suffering from traumatic distress have been shown to experience more parenting distress and have been observed showing less sensitive and responsive parenting behaviors, including increased avoidance and hostile and controlling behavior [14–16]. A large number of studies suggest that exposure to maternal psychopathology during early development may have a substantial impact on child self-regulation and emotional and psychosocial development [17–20], with parental symptoms of PTSD having a profound negative impact on child self-regulation and emotional and psychosocial development [8, 21–25]. In a study of 52 low-income mother-infant dyads with ethnic/racial minority backgrounds in the United States, Enlow et al. [26] examined the associations between maternal PTSD symptoms and infant emotional regulation. Maternal PTSD symptoms were significantly associated with infant symptoms of externalizing, internalizing, and dysregulation. In sum, a consistent body of findings documents how parental trauma and subsequent PTSD symptoms may interfere with parental interaction and emotional involvement, causing risks for child developmental outcomes.

Parental posttraumatic suffering may have an impact on caregiving capacities through symptoms of withdrawal, hyperarousal, or intrusion [27]. Emotional withdrawal related to PTSD may invoke decreased emotional availability. Furthermore, parental symptoms of arousal or intrusion may be related to the development of aggression, while parental fearful functioning may be related to overprotective caregiving and traumatic expectations in coping with children's explorative behaviors [28].

In refugee samples, evidence has been generated on this potential impact of parental PTSD on parenting capacities in exile. Van Ee et al. [10] documented the association between higher levels of maternal posttraumatic stress symptoms and increased insensitive, unstructured, or hostile parent-child interactions in a sample with 49 refugee mothers and their children (aged 18–42 months). Furthermore, van Ee et al. [9] showed how refugee parents' symptoms of avoidance and numbness were associated with insensitive parenting behavior in a study based on 68 refugee parent-child dyads. These studies indicate that refugee parents suffering from PTSD may develop parental behaviors that oscillate between aggressive parenting behaviors and withdrawal, which may compromise their ability to develop their child's affect regulation. In their study of 80 male refugees and their young children (aged 18–42 months), van Ee et al. [29] documented that paternal posttraumatic stress symptoms negatively affected the fathers' perceptions of their children and the actual quality of father-child interactions on dimensions of sensitivity, structuring, and hostility.

Parental Insecure and Disorganized Attachment Representations Associated with Parental Caregiving

Within attachment theory and research, parental disrupted attachment representations have been hypothesized and empirically explored as a second mediating mechanism in the transgenerational transmission of trauma.

Attachment representations or internal working models refer to the individual's internalized experiences of attachment relationships [30]. Through the child's interactions with the primary caregiver, and based on the caregiver's responses to the child's need to establish a secure base, relational representations or internalized models of self and others in relationship are established in the parent-infant dyad and are hypothesized to be relatively stable throughout the life course. This representational model constitutes an individual's attachment representations of past and present attachment experiences, modeling behavior and expectations in present relationships. In adults, attachment representations are defined as cognitive, affective, and behavioral mental models that involve affect-regulating strategies and that unfold in close relationships [31]. Adult attachment representations can be assessed and classified based on the adult speaker's narrative style in the Adult Attachment Interview (AAI), and the interview transcripts can be assigned to three organized categories: secure-autonomous, insecure-dismissing, and insecure-preoccupied. Furthermore, a fourth category, the unresolved-disorganized attachment classification, reflects unresolved attachment-related experiences of loss, abuse, and trauma, and can be added to the three main classifications.

Within attachment research, associations between parental attachment representations, parental sensitive caregiving behavior, and child attachment security are documented [32]. In this body of research, studies have focused on the interaction between parental traumatic life experiences and attachment representations. Here, evidence documents how traumatic life experiences may cause disruptions in parental attachment representations. Equally, parental insecure or unresolved attachment status may render the individual more vulnerable to the development of posttraumatic symptoms in response to traumatic life experiences [33]. Importantly, parental insecure and/or unresolved attachment status may be related to disruptions in parental interaction and caregiving behavior. Main and Hesse [34] proposed the concept of "frightened or frightening behavior" to describe the impact of unresolved parental attachment status on caregiving behavior. Unresolved loss or failure to complete the mourning process following trauma or loss may lead to the continuing existence of multiple disintegrated and conflicting representational models. The failure to form an organized attachment representation is then thought to cause the parent to behave in a contradictory or disrupted manner when engaging with the child. Hesse and Main [35] suggest that frightened or frightening parental behavior is often guided by parental fright, and it may take three different forms: *threatening behavior, frightening behavior,* and *dissociative behavior,* reflecting the evolutionary-based behavioral fright responses of fight, flight, or freeze. When parents display frightened or frightening behavior it places the child in an insolvable dilemma of "fright without a solution" [35]: The parent becomes a source of both fear and comfort.

The concept of frightened or frightening behavior has been proposed as one of the factors playing an important role in the genesis of infant disorganized attachment status, placing children at increased risk of a range of externalizing symptoms and psychopathology [41]. In a study based on a nonclinical, middleclass sample consisting of 85 mothers and their children, Schuengel et al. [36] tested the hypothesized link between parental unresolved loss, frightened and frightening parental behavior, and disorganized attachment relationships. The study found that secure mothers with unresolved loss displayed less frightening behaviors than insecure mothers, and likewise that unresolved loss in secure mothers did not predict infant disorganized attachment. However, the study also found that frightening parental behavior predicted infant disorganized attachment irrespective of maternal attachment security. This supports the notion of secure parental attachment as a protective mechanism and the proposed link between compromised parental caregiving and infant disorganized attachment regardless of parental attachment status.

Recently, refugee scholars have applied this theoretical framework in studies with refugee families in exile. Almqvist and Broberg [11] and De Haene et al. [37] introduced the attachment perspective in psychosocial refugee studies and hypothesized about the potential impact of forced displacement on parental attachment and caregiving behaviors.

Almqvist and Broberg [11] discuss three clinical cases of refugee mother-child dyads who had fled to Sweden from war and sexual violence, and they hypothesize how mothers' damaged representations of self as caregiver and their inability to deactivate their children's activated attachment systems may invoke the development of a disorganized attachment status in young refugee children.

As part of an explorative, qualitative multiple case study in a non-clinical sample of seven refugee families resettled in Belgium, De Haene et al. [37] aimed at a further empirical exploration of this initial hypothesis and conducted an assessment of parental attachment representation in 11 refugee parents through the administration of the Adult Attachment Interview (AAI), assisted by an interpreter. This explorative study generated preliminary evidence of the potential impact of migration-specific life events on unresolved and insecure adult attachment narratives. Parental attachment narratives indicated the role of external, extreme, disruptive life experiences in precipitating unresolved (in 10 participants) and insecure (in 7 participants) discourse in refugee parents. Both unresolved and fearfully preoccupied parental narratives concerning pre-migration traumatic life events and dismissing discourse of restricted attention to emotional closeness in a context of ongoing separation provided an understanding of how devastating external life experiences encroach on parental attachment representations. They also highlighted the representational processes involved in the potential disruption of parental caregiving capacities during forced migration.

In a clinical study of 43 adult male and female refugees in Denmark referred for PTSD treatment, Riber [13] furthered this evidence through the assessment of attachment representations in refugees (using the Adult Attachment Interview). The study found that 67% of the participants were classified as having unresolved-disorganized attachment representations. The majority of participants had insecure attachment patterns; 39% were classified as Dismissing, 42% were classified as Preoccupied, and only 14% were classified as Secure-Autonomous. These findings support the link between trauma and disrupted attachment representations in adult refugees.

In a study of 30 refugee families from the Middle East, consisting of traumatized parents and an exile-born child living in Denmark, Dalgaard et al. [38] administered the Attachment and Traumatization Story Task [39] to a nontraumatized child between the age of four and nine in each family. The study found that approximately two-thirds of the children could be classified as having an insecure attachment style, and the study further found an association between children's psychosocial adjustment as measured by the Strengths and Difficulties Questionnaire and attachment security, with secure attachment predicting lower symptom scores. Furthermore, the study included a measure of intrafamily trauma communication based on qualitative analyses of interview material and observations during home visits. Intrafamily trauma communication was divided into four categories: silencing, open disclosure, modulated disclosure, and unfiltered speech. The unfiltered speech category refers to a style of family communication where there seems to be an incongruence between what the parents believe they are communicating and what the children are experiencing in everyday life. The study found an association between child attachment style and intrafamily trauma communication, in which Unfiltered Speech was associated with an insecure attachment classification of the child.

Van Ee et al. [9] documented how the disruption of attachment representations may interact with posttraumatic symptomatic functioning in refugee parents in shaping the impact of trauma and exile on parental caregiving behavior. In a study with 53 refugee parents, findings indicate that when refugee parents cannot draw on secure attachment representations, high levels of PTSD symptoms increase the risk of insensitive parenting. Importantly, this study shows the significance of the intersection of posttraumatic suffering and attachment representations in understanding the impact of refugee trauma on parental sensitivity and caregiving behavior.

Case Reflections on Transgenerational Trauma Transmission

In this section, we explore how the understanding of refugee parent-child relationships may be enriched if parental posttraumatic suffering and disrupted attachment representations are theoretically considered as mediating mechanisms in the transgenerational transmission of refugee trauma. Reflecting on two cases, attachment quality, parental posttraumatic functioning, attachment representations, and caregiving behaviors are addressed, indicating how complex interactions shape affective and behavioral patterns in family relationships. We introduce two cases[1] and delineate the differential dynamics at stake when past parental trauma is or is not compounded by ongoing, current stressors in exile.

When Past Parental Trauma Impacts the Current Child-Parent Relationship

The Ahmadi family consists of both parents and their two sons, aged five and six. The mother, Nahda, lost her first husband in the war in their home country in the Middle East before she fled to Denmark. The father, Reza, experienced political persecution, imprisonment, and torture, and both parents suffer from severe PTSD symptoms. Both parents have vocational training from their countries of origin, and they are currently pursuing further education in Denmark. The couple met in the asylum center in Denmark and fell in love. Despite initial protests from both families, they married and became parents of two sons, both born in Denmark after the parents received permanent resident status. The parents are in close contact with their extended family in their country of origin, and they are currently planning a family vacation. As part of the study, Nahda filled out the Attachment Style Questionnaire [42] and the eldest son, aged six, participated in the administration of the Attachment and Traumatization Story Task (ATST), which is a narrative doll-play procedure measuring attachment security in children [43]. Within the test situation, he showed severe symptoms of anxiety and refused to be separated from his mother, so the ATST had to be completed with his mother sitting in a corner of the room. Results revealed that the mother scored low on the confidence scale measuring attachment security (24 out of 48) and high on the 2 dimensions of attachment insecurity: Avoidance (Discomfort with Closeness and Relationships as Secondary) (82 out of 102) and Ambivalence (Need for Approval and Preoccupation with Relationships) (62 out of 90). Similarly, the son was classified in the insecure-avoidant category and scored very low on the continuous measure of attachment security (13 out of 35).

Nahda describes how she is still mourning the traumatic loss of her first husband, even though she also describes her current marriage as a happy one. Nahda describes how both her and her husband's families in their home country are doing relatively well and she describes feeling hopeful about the family's future in Denmark. Nahda describes how she loves her two sons but says that becoming a mother has increased her symptoms of anxiety. Nahda describes excessive worrying about the wellbeing of her sons which has lasted ever since they were born:

> I worry about my children all the time, ever since they were born, I couldn't believe that nothing was wrong with them, even though everyone told me they were fine and when they are in school, I can't help thinking about what might happen to them, and I worry that maybe they are affected by the things which have happened to their father and I, or what

---

[1] The following case material stems from a study carried out as part of the first author's PhD dissertation, "The transgenerational transmission of refugee trauma: How a parental trauma history may affect children without a history of trauma exposure" (Copenhagen: University of Copenhagen, 2016). Informed content was obtained from the parents prior to the families' participation in the study. In order to ensure anonymity, names and other identifying information have been changed.

> might happen to them in the future, I never feel relaxed when they are out of my sight, both me and my husband have to take anxiety medication, so we don't have a lot of energy, and so it is a struggle, because they are only a year apart, like twins, and they want to do so many things like going to the playground or to Tivoli or visiting their friends, and I worry that we can't afford it or that something bad might happen to them if they do go …

Nahda describes how her eldest son recently developed symptoms of psychosocial maladjustment, such as selective mutism and separation anxiety. He had to repeat a year in school and has been referred to the school psychologist, because his teachers are worried about him.

> It was really really difficult, for an entire week I had to be there with him all day every day and he cried until he got used to it, but he is not like his brother, my younger son is much more sociable and loves playing with other children, he [eldest son] isolates himself and doesn't know how to make contact with other children.

As can be seen from the interview excerpt, the son displays severe symptoms of anxiety, mirroring his mother's fearful functioning, potentially indicative of the core patterns of transgenerational trauma transmission in which the parents' posttraumatic symptoms affect child wellbeing, both directly and through the impairment of parental caregiving ability. The clinical material suggests the presence of insecure, anxious attachment representations and the potential role of the impact of maternal unresolved loss and insecure attachment representations [30].

When Past and Ongoing Trauma Impacts the Current Child-Parent Relationship

The Khaled family, consisting of father, mother, and four children, escaped their home country in the Middle East and resettled in Denmark, where the family's two youngest children were born. Preflight, the mother, Zeinab, was imprisoned and witnessed her father and brothers being tortured. Zeinab suffers from symptoms of PTSD, anxiety, and depression and has been referred for treatment at a psychiatric outpatient clinic. Zeinab has primary school education and is on social welfare. The father, Omar, has equally been imprisoned and tortured in the family's country of origin, and in Denmark he has been granted early retirement on the grounds of suffering from PTSD and a physical health condition. The family is very isolated in Denmark, but the parents are in close contact with their extended family in their home country, who are described as being very poor. The mother reports that her husband is physically abusive towards both her and the children, and that the spousal abuse and marital problems have existed since the very beginning of their marriage. As part of the study, Zeinab filled out the Attachment Style Questionnaire [42] and the youngest son, who is eight years old, participated in the administration of the Attachment and Traumatization Story Task, which measures attachment security in children [43]. The results revealed that the mother scored very low on the confidence scale measuring attachment security (20 out of 48) and very high on the 2 dimensions of attachment insecurity: Avoidance (Discomfort with Closeness and Relationships as Secondary) (76 out of 102) and Ambivalence (Need for Approval and Preoccupation with Relationships) (74 out of 90). Similarly, the son was classified in the insecure-avoidant category and scored very low on the continuous measure of attachment security (12 out of 35).

Zeinab describes having a difficult relationship with her children. According to Zeinab, all her children have difficulties forming interpersonal relationships, and all children's developmental trajectories showed signs of psychosocial maladjustments such as enuresis, separation anxiety, generalized anxiety, and conduct problems:

> I have had so many difficulties with [youngest child] . . . in the nursery, for the first six months he cried, all four of my children, they are not very social, they have difficulties adjusting to or becoming part of anything social and they have a hard time bonding with the other children. Like I said, in the nursery he cried for six months and then he only formed an attachment with a single one of the care assistants, and if she wasn't there one day, then that day he would cry the entire day, and also in kindergarten, it was the same thing; he also only formed an attachment with one kindergarten teacher, and again, if he wasn't there, the one that he was attached to, then he screamed that he wanted to go home . . . and in school, the first two grades he would cry every morning.

Zeinab describes feeling incompetent and inadequate as a parent and describes her children in a very negative tone, mirroring findings regarding the impact of maternal depression and PTSD on parental perceptions of their children [44]. Within the interview excerpt it can be seen how Zeinab doesn't seem to reflect on the feelings of her son but focuses on how his behavior was hard for her to manage. Although she says that the children's behavioral and emotional problems may have been brought on by their father's violent behavior and her own use of corporal punishment, she does not seem to dwell on the psychological and emotional impact of this abuse on the children. This may be interpreted as a result of a generally compromised ability for reflective functioning or it may be interpreted as a temporary breakdown of the reflective functioning abilities as the narration of these memories activate Zeinab's own arousal and distress. Furthermore, Zeinab seems to have projected her own hostile feelings towards her husband onto her oldest children, whom she says resemble their father:

> [E]specially the eldest two, they have all the negative character traits of their father, because we hadn't learned how one raises children, and we didn't know how one raises a child. The eldest he used to have these temper tantrums, it wasn't epilepsy but it almost looked like it, and there was four years of suffering with him, when the tiniest thing happened he broke down and cried, but then we came here, and he was treated, and they said that the lack of oxygen may have affected his brain, and he has been treated for 12 years, but he has been subjected to severe physical violence by his father, he has had a lot of difficulties in his life, but he has just finished high school, but it took a lot of pressure and a big effort. [. . .] but so now we know that hitting children is against the law, so regarding this we have learned something, but there was a lot of suffering for us with the two eldest, and those symptoms that they had, they were anxious and had a feeling that something was wrong, and both the eldest suffered from incontinence, I mean they peed in their pants and it is true, he [father] was very harsh, but at the same time he does love them, and as he says, we have to endure a lot of things, because living in a foreign country is tough, but we have to endure for the sake of the children.

As can be seen, the mother's account is characterized by incoherence, time leaps, and emotional ambiguity, simultaneously expressing affection and hostility towards her children. At the cognitive level she is able to see that their behavioral and emotional problems may be understood as a consequence of harsh parenting, but at the emotional level she doesn't seem to empathize with her children, although she underlines that she and her husband have now learned that physical punishment of children is illegal in Denmark and says that the termination of the violence against her children has had a positive impact on their behavior.

At the family level, Zeinab describes her family as very dysfunctional, and she reports how a spousal history of physical violence towards her is currently continuing in resettlement:

> We [husband and I] have never had a childhood. When I opened my eyes for the very first time, there was a war between [home country] and [neighboring country], and I saw what happened to my brothers, and they came and took my father away and we witnessed how they tortured him, and then we were thrown in prison. After I finished high school, you know I had only just finished, had only just experienced being happy, when a new war broke out, and while there was a war I started this education, not university, but a two-year college degree, but then I was forced to marry this man, I mean my husband, and my husband he had been a prisoner of war, he was imprisoned in [neighboring country] for five years, and it is like, I thought that once I married then problems would disappear, but that is not how it went, because he had been a prisoner of war. From the day we were married he started beating me up, and I didn't dare tell anyone, so I never told anyone, that I was being beaten.
>
> Yes . . . we had only been married for four months and then we were expelled, and it was like a prison, we were expelled until the Americans came, and then they took us to these camps in the desert, and there was nothing, for instance there were no toilets and showers, the toilet was a hole in the ground, and my father said, "Okay, you can come back to live with us," and so I felt that I had to choose between my father and my husband, and both options would be hard, so that is why I chose to stay with my husband, and with his physical abuse, and it is like I have gotten used to his violence.

Perhaps as a result of this ongoing abuse, Zeinab describes having bizarre conversations with her youngest son, which may also be interpreted as a verbal form of *frightening* and *frightened* parental behavior:

> When I am in pain, then I tell him [youngest son], "I'm dying" . . . from this pain I mean, then he says that even if you die, then I still have [name of older sister], and it is actually a relief to me that he says this. [. . .] Yes she is very loving towards him and she always takes him for walks.

As can be seen from the excerpt, the family is characterized by sibling parenting and parent/ child role reversal. The mother relies on her older children to take care of the youngest, and again she seems incapable of reflecting on the impact of having a mother who regularly says that she is in such pain that she might die:

> Interviewer: Mm yes, so when you have been feeling really bad with stomachaches and things like that, is that then something that the kids ask about?
> Zeinab: Well, then it is my daughter who answers [the second youngest child explains to the youngest] and it is she who helps me out with the practicalities, and when he asks then she answers, because I am sick, but we don't involve them in the psychological matters.

Here there seems to be an incongruence between what the children experience in everyday life and the awareness that Zeinab has of the children's experiences [38, 45]. Throughout the interview, Zeinab describes episodes in which the children have overheard adults recounting their psychologically traumatizing experiences from the past, yet she claims that the children aren't aware of her psychological and emotional pain. This finding illustrates the link between attachment representations and family communication. Zeinab reports an unfiltered style of communication and seems to lack the ability to empathize with her children when reflecting on the impact of her own individual problems as well as the impact of the conflictual parental relationship and intrafamily communication on the children. Note that in this case the children witness ongoing conjugal violence, and the effects of transgenerational versus present traumas are difficult to distinguish.

Towards Clinical Practice

Although the capacity for developmental change diminishes with age, change continues throughout the life cycle so that changes for better or for worse are always possible. It is this continuing potential for change that means that at no time of life is a person invulnerable to every possible adversity and also at no time of life is a person impermeable to favorable influence. It is this persisting potential for change that gives opportunity for effective therapy

J. Bowlby, Clinical Applications of Attachment: A Secure Base [40]

In order to support refugee families in coping with the sequalae of trauma, attachment representations and their interaction with posttraumatic suffering offer a clinically useful way of understanding the problems faced by traumatized refugee parents who struggle to care for their children. Working with refugee family therapy in the context of potential transgenerational trauma transmission poses a series of complex challenges on the level of the parent, the child, and the family system. Trauma triggers the attachment system and inhibits exploration, and, as a consequence, mentalization is undermined in most people who have experienced trauma, including refugees [33]. According to Allen [46], "feeling alone in the midst of unbearable painful emotion" lies at the core of attachment trauma. It evokes intense emotional distress and results in long-term adverse impacts on the ability to develop and maintain secure attachment relationships. Furthermore, it disrupts the possibility of finding comfort in other relationships, including psychotherapy relationships. As documented in this review, adults' life experiences of multiple complex trauma (war trauma, child abuse, and attachment trauma) may invoke trauma-related psychiatric symptomatology, which will have an impact on affect-regulation and mentalizing capacity. Furthermore, complex and cumulative trauma throughout the life course may influence the adult's individual attachment system and parental caregiving capacities as well as the family system and hence the child. With respect to refugee families where parents suffer from trauma-related mental health problems, it is important to remember that these parents' attachment patterns are not only activated when facing distress or danger [47]. Refugee parents' mental models of attachment are also activated under the more common conditions of illness and anxiety, which, in turn, will affect their caregiving behavior. Thus, in contexts of resettlement, cumulative daily stressors may play an equally important role in triggering attachment-related trauma and posttraumatic reactions.

Consequently, psychological intervention may be called for at the level of the traumatized parent (individual trauma therapy that targets the sequelae of trauma) and at the level of the family (family therapy that supports change towards attachment security and the development of parental mentalization), as well as at the level of the child. In some refugee families, secure attachment representations may serve as a key emotional buffer against hardship, and in other families, designing interventions targeted at repairing and restructuring insecure or disorganized attachment relationships may be seen as the most important therapeutic goal.

In clinical work with refugee families, it seems important to take cultural expressions of meaning and practices of normative parent-child relationships into account. Though different attachment studies of infants and adults point out universal behavioral and narrative structures with respect to caregiving practices and experiences, local ways of expressing attachment interactions and the meaning of safety within child-parent relationships may be embedded cultural phenomena that differ in behavioral patterns and narrative construction. For example, Riber [13] argued that Arabic refugee adults' choices of adjectives for describing their attachment relationships seemed to draw on another set of culture-specific metaphors than those typically seen in Western contexts. Semantic expressions around the emotional quality of the relation with caregivers – for example, 'like a mountain,' 'respect,' 'injustice,' 'patience,' 'my crown, my vein, my blood' – were argued to be cultural variations on the attachment narratives that could or couldn't be supported by narrative behaviors. Thus, it is important to explore and comprehend refugee families' behavioral and narrative understandings and expressions of security within caregiving relationships.

Conclusion

As can be seen from the present review, the attachment paradigm offers a theoretically and clinically meaningful explanatory framework for understanding the transgenerational transmission of trauma within refugee families. Clinically, the review suggests that refugee family care for traumatized families should aim to support sensitivity and responsiveness in parents, foster parental emotional availability, and mobilize parental ability to shape or restore "secure base" and "safe haven" caregiving behaviors and parental reflective functioning, even in the face of cumulative stressors in exile. Supporting the restructuring of attachment relationships and representations may be a key mechanism of positive change for both children and adults. When representations are conceptualized as dynamic phenomena, working on attachment representations develops a nonpathologizing approach that may support refugee parents and children to reconstruct safety in the face of violence and exile.

References

1. M. Ijzendoorn, M. Bakermans-Kranenburg and A. Sagi-Schwartz, Are children of Holocaust survivors less well-adapted? A meta-analytic investigation of secondary traumatization. *Journal of Traumatic Stress*, 16(5) (2003), 459–69.

2. S. L. Lustig, M. Kia-Keating, W. G. Knight, P. Geltman, H. Ellis, J. D. Kinzie et al., Review of child and adolescent refugee mental health. *Journal of the American Academy of Child & Adolescent Psychiatry*, 43(1) (2004), 24–36.

3. L. De Haene, H. Grietens and K. Verschueren, From symptom to context: A review of the literature on refugee children's mental health. *Hellenic Journal of Psychology*, 4(1) (2007), 233–56.

4. M. Fazel, J. Wheeler and J. Danesh, Prevalence of serious mental disorder in 7000 refugees resettled in western countries: A systematic review. *The Lancet*, 365(9467) (2005), 1309–14.

5. E. Montgomery, Trauma, exile and mental health in young refugees. *Acta Psychiatrica Scandinavica*, 124(s440) (2011), 1–46.

6. A. Vaage, P. Thomsen, C. Rousseau, T. Wentzel-Larsen, T. Ta and E. Hauff, Paternal predictors of the mental health of children of Vietnamese refugees. *Child and*

Adolescent Psychiatry and Mental Health, 5 (1) (2011), 2.

7. A. Daud, E. Skoglund and P. A. Rydelius, Children in families of torture victims: Transgenerational transmission of parents' traumatic experiences to their children. *International Journal of Social Welfare*, 14(1) (2005), 23–32.

8. J. E. Lambert, J. Holzer and A. Hasbun, Association between parents' PTSD severity and children's psychological distress: A meta-analysis. *Journal of Traumatic Stress*, 27(1) (2014), 9–17.

9. E. van Ee, R. J. Kleber, M. J. Jongmans, T. T. Mooren and D. Out, Parental PTSD, adverse parenting and child attachment in a refugee sample. *Attachment & Human Development*, 18 (3) (2016), 273–91.

10. E. van Ee, R. J. Kleber and T. Mooren, War trauma lingers on: Associations between maternal posttraumatic stress disorder, parent–child interaction, and child development. *Infant Mental Health Journal*, 33(5) (2012), 459–68.

11. K. Almqvist and A. G. Broberg, Young children traumatized by organized violence together with their mothers: The critical effects of damaged internal representations. *Attachment & Human Development*, 5(4) (2003), 367–80.

12. L. De Haene, H. Grietens and K. Verschueren, Attachment and Traumatisation Story Task (ATST): A migration- and trauma-specific adaptation of the Attachment Story Completion Task by Verschueren and Marcoen (1994) for use with 4- to 9-year-old refugee and asylum-seeking children. Research report (Leuven: K. U. Leuven, 2010).

13. K. Riber, Attachment organization in Arabic-speaking refugees with post traumatic stress disorder. *Attachment & Human Development*, 18(2) (2016), 154–75.

14. J. Despars, C. Peter, A. Borghini, B. Pierrehumbert, S. Habersaat, C. Müller-Nix et al., Impact of a cleft lip and/or palate on maternal stress and attachment representations. *The Cleft Palate-Craniofacial Journal*, 48(4) (2011), 419–24.

15. S. McDonald, P. Slade, H. Spiby and J. Iles, Post-traumatic stress symptoms, parenting stress and mother-child relationships following childbirth and at 2 years postpartum. *Journal of Psychosomatic Obstetrics & Gynecology*, 32(3) (2011), 141–6.

16. D. S. Schechter, E. Willheim, C. Hinojosa, K. Scholfield-Kleinman, J. B. Turner, J. McCaw et al., Subjective and objective measures of parent-child relationship dysfunction, child separation distress, and joint attention. *Psychiatry: Interpersonal and Biological Processes*, 73(2) (2010), 130–44.

17. S. R. Brand and P. A. Brennan, Impact of antenatal and postpartum maternal mental illness: How are the children? *Clinical Obstetrics and Gynecology*, 52(3) (2009), 441–55.

18. S. Brummelte and L. A. Galea, Depression during pregnancy and postpartum: Contribution of stress and ovarian hormones. *Progress in Neuro-Psychopharmacology and Biological Psychiatry*, 34(5) (2010), 766–76.

19. E. P. Davis, N. Snidman, P. D. Wadhwa, L. M. Glynn, C. D. Schetter and C. A. Sandman, Prenatal maternal anxiety and depression predict negative behavioral reactivity in infancy. *Infancy*, 6(3) (2004), 319–31.

20. T. Field, Prenatal depression effects on early development: A review. *Infant Behavior and Development*, 34(1) (2011), 1–14.

21. M. B. Enlow, A. Kullowatz, J. Staudenmayer, J. Spasojevic, T. Ritz and R. J. Wright, Associations of maternal lifetime trauma and perinatal traumatic stress symptoms with infant cardiorespiratory reactivity to psychological challenge. *Psychosomatic Medicine*, 71(6) (2009), 607.

22. S. R. Brand, S. M. Engel, R. L. Canfield and R. Yehuda, The effect of maternal PTSD following in utero trauma exposure on behavior and temperament in the 9-month-old infant. *Annals of the New York Academy of Sciences*, 1071(1) (2006), 454–8.

23. C. M. Chemtob, Y. Nomura, K. Rajendran, R. Yehuda, D. Schwartz and R. Abramovitz, Impact of maternal posttraumatic stress disorder and depression following exposure to the September 11 attacks on preschool children's behavior. *Child Development*, 81(4) (2010), 1129–41.

24. M. Kaitz, M. Levy, R. Ebstein, S. V. Faraone and D. Mankuta, The intergenerational effects of trauma from terror: A real possibility. *Infant Mental Health Journal*, 30(2) (2009), 158–79.

25. E. van Ee, R. J. Kleber and T. Mooren, War trauma lingers on: Associations between maternal posttraumatic stress disorder, parent–child interaction, and child development. *Infant Mental Health Journal*, (2012), 141–6.

26. M. B. Enlow, R. L. Kitts, E. Blood, A. Bizarro, M. Hofmeister and R. J. Wright, Maternal posttraumatic stress symptoms and infant emotional reactivity and emotion regulation. *Infant Behavior and Development*, 34(4) (2011), 487–503.

27. A. F. Lieberman, Traumatic stress and quality of attachment: Reality and internalization in disorders of infant mental health. *Infant Mental Health Journal*, 25(4) (2004), 336–51.

28. J. Walter, Where meanings, sorrow, and hope have a resident permit. In J. P. Wilson and B. Drozdek, eds., *Broken Spirits: The Treatment of Traumatized Asylum-Seekers, Refugees, War and Torture Victims* (New York: Brunner-Routledge, 2004), pp. 487–519.

29. E. van Ee, M. Sleijpen, R. J. Kleber and M. J. Jongmans, Father-involvement in a refugee sample: Relations between posttraumatic stress and caregiving. *Family Process*, 52(4) (2013), 723–35.

30. I. Bretherton and K. A. Munholland, Internal working models in attachment relationships: Elaborating a central construct in attachment theory. In J. Cassidy and P. R. Shaver, eds., *Handbook of Attachment: Theory, Research, and Clinical Applications* (New York: Guilford Press, 2008), pp. 102–27.

31. C. George, N. Kaplan and M. Main, *Adult Attachment Interview Protocol* (unpublished manuscript) (Berkeley, CA: University of California, 1985). Accessed on September 26, 2019 at www.psychology.sunysb.edu/attachment/measures/content/aai_interview.pdf.

32. E. Hesse, The Adult Attachment Interview: Protocol, method of analysis, and empirical studies. In J. Cassidy and P. R. Shaver, eds., *Handbook of Attachment: Theory, Research, and Clinical Applications* (New York: Guilford Press, 2008), pp. 552–98.

33. K. Riber, *Attachment, Complex Trauma, and Psychotherapy: A Clinical Study of the Significance of Attachment in Adult Arabic-Speaking Refugees with PTSD* (Copenhagen: University of Copenhagen, 2015).

34. M. Main and E. Hesse, Parents' unresolved traumatic experiences are related to infant disorganized attachment status: Is frightened and/or frightening parental behavior the linking mechanism? In M. T. Greenberg, D. Cicchetti and E. M. Cummings, eds., *Attachment in the Preschool Years: Theory, Research, and Intervention*, the John D. and Catherine T. MacArthur Foundation Series on Mental Health and Development (Chicago, IL: University of Chicago Press, 1990), pp. 161–82.

35. E. Hesse and M. Main, Frightened, threatening, and dissociative parental behavior in low-risk samples: Description, discussion, and interpretations. *Development and Psychopathology*, 18(02) (2006), 309–43.

36. C. Schuengel, M. J. Bakermans-Kranenburg and M. H. van IJzendoorn, Frightening maternal behavior linking unresolved loss and disorganized infant attachment. *Journal of Consulting and Clinical Psychology*, 67(1) (1999), 54.

37. L. De Haene, H. Grietens and K. Verschueren, Adult attachment in the context of refugee traumatisation: The impact of organized violence and forced separation on parental states of mind regarding attachment. *Attachment*

& *Human Development*, 12(3) (2010), 249–64.

38. N. T. Dalgaard, B. K. Todd, S. I. Daniel and E. Montgomery, The transmission of trauma in refugee families: Associations between intra-family trauma communication style, children's attachment security and psychosocial adjustment. *Attachment & Human Development*, 18(1) (2016), 69–89.

39. L. De Haene, N. T. Dalgaard, E. Montgomery, H. Grietens and K. Verschueren, Attachment narratives in refugee children: Interrater reliability and qualitative analysis in pilot findings from a two-site study. *Journal of Traumatic Stress*, 26(3) (2013), 413–17.

40. J. Bowlby, *Clinical Applications of Attachment: A Secure Base* (London: Routledge, 1988), p. 85.

41. N. T. Dalgaard, *The Transgenerational Transmission of Refugee Trauma: How a Parental Trauma History May Affect Children without a History of Trauma Exposure* (Copenhagen: University of Copenhagen, 2016).

42. J. A. Feeney and P. Noller, *Adult Attachment* (London: Sage, 1996).

43. L. De Haene, K. Verschueren and H. Grietens, *Attachment Security in Refugee Children: The Development of a Migration-Specific Narrative Attachment Measure* (Leuven: K. U. Leuven, 2009).

44. J. Davies, P. Slade, I. Wright and P. Stewart, Posttraumatic stress symptoms following childbirth and mothers' perceptions of their infants. *Infant Mental Health Journal*, 29(6) (2008), 537–54.

45. E. Montgomery, Tortured families: A coordinated management of meaning analysis. *Family Process*, 43(3) (2004), 349–71.

46. J. G. Allen, *Mentalizing in the Development and Treatment of Attachment Trauma* (London: Routledge, 2013).

47. M. Mikulincer and V. Florian, The relationship between adult attachment styles and emotional and cognitive reactions to stressful events. In J. A. Simpson and W. S. Rholes, eds., *Attachment Theory and Close Relationships* (New York: Guilford Press, 1998), pp. 143–65.

Pre- and Post-migration Trauma and Adversity
Sources of Resilience and Family Coping among West African Refugee Families

Aïcha Cissé, Lucia De Haene, Eva Keatley, and Andrew Rasmussen

Trauma, Adversity, and Resilience

There is a broad consensus in scholarly literature that refugee families' mental wellbeing is impacted by both pre- and post-migration adversity [1–3]. Significant stressors, ranging from war trauma, persecution, and prolonged exposure to political and civil unrest to the often chronic absolute poverty that pervades such contexts, form the push factors for migration. The immigration process itself involves a number of migration-specific stressors, starting with the potential for flight-related stressors such as deprivation, detention, exploitation, and human trafficking. Shortly after their arrival in the host country, refugees may face difficulty finding initial housing and employment, the threat of deportation, and the general liminality of initial resettlement contexts [4]. Once settled, refugees face yet another array of potential stressors related to acculturation, parent-child acculturation dissonance, downward shifts in social status and de-skilling [5], loss of extended family and community support systems [6], relative poverty [7, 8], discrimination, and/or social isolation. In addition to causing distress themselves, post-migration stressors may aggravate the effect of pre-migration stressors and impede wellbeing in the host country [9, 10].

The cumulative-effects model contends that early adverse experiences have a long-term impact on wellbeing and functioning to the extent that these effects are reinforced or maintained by later adverse experiences [11]. Similarly, the stress-sensitization model stipulates that exposure to adversities earlier in life reduces an individual's threshold for negative reactions to subsequent stress later in life [12]. Empirical evidence suggests that, even in the absence of childhood adversity, trauma and prolonged exposure to adversity can lead to psychopathology (e.g., PTSD) or to psychological and emotional distress significant enough to impair social functioning [13]. At the family level, the negative impacts of adversity on family members have been linked to disrupted family functioning. Studies have shown that, for parents exposed to trauma, parenting may be challenging because traumatic experiences may lead to overwhelming depressive and anxiety symptoms, which in turn may lead to less effective parenting, frustration with or worry about their inability to protect their children, and diminished ability to be sensitive to their children's needs [14, 15]. Although limited, the literature on refugee parents' relationships with their children mirrors such findings [16].

Although exposure to trauma has been empirically shown to negatively affect mental health, the majority of people who are exposed to trauma do not develop clinically significant mental health problems [13, 17]. A growing body of research has shifted the traditional focus from negative outcomes to resilience. Resilience reflects the ability to maintain a stable equilibrium, consisting of the maintenance of relatively stable levels of psychological functioning following exposure to trauma or adversity [18]. Resilience is more than the simple absence of psychopathology; it refers to psychological wellbeing and healthy functioning across behavioral, cognitive, emotional, and interpersonal domains. Various models have been proposed to explain the processes through which resilience occurs at the individual level. The homeostasis resilience interactive model [18] proposes that environmental-systemic factors at the individual (e.g., coping strategies), microsystem (e.g., social support from community members), and macrosystem (e.g., schools and religious institutions) levels build upon each other to comprise multidimensional stabilizing environments. Similarly, Harvey's ecological model of trauma and trauma recovery [19] contends that "psychological attributes of human beings are best understood in the ecological context of human community" (p. 4). Individual responses to trauma are explained in light of the cultures, values, behaviors, skills, and meanings of adversity that "human communities cultivate in their members" (p. 4). Echoing the homeostasis model, Harvey [19] proposes that resilience is the result of complex interactions between individual and interpersonal factors, cultural understandings, types of trauma, and surrounding environmental factors. Other models of resilience that use family as their unit of analysis have found links between effective parenting practices, healthy family relations, and greater post-trauma resilience in both parents and children [20–24].

In research involving refugee families, examining families' efforts to manage and cope with migration and pre- and post-migration trauma and adversities entails a close analysis of individual- and family-level protective factors, spousal dynamics, parenting styles, ethnocultural identifications, and interactions with pre- and post-migration sociopolitical contexts. Moreover, native and host countries' sociocultural norms and frames of reference regarding mental health may shape the meaning-making of trauma and other adverse experiences, which in turn may influence the individual- and family-level coping strategies involved in resilience processes. Indeed, although post-traumatic psychopathological responses have been observed cross-culturally [25], variations were found in types of responses and conceptualization of trauma [27–31]. Because trauma is a Western construct [26, 27], its conceptualization (e.g., ICD and DSM criteria for PTSD) may not reflect non-Western frames of reference for understanding, defining (e.g., local idioms of distress), coping with, and healing trauma [17, 27–31]. In this regard, research shows that many non-Western communities have relatively well-established frameworks for explaining and addressing post-traumatic responses [28–31]. Working with refugee families entails being aware of and understanding diverse culture-specific trauma-related frameworks.

A Narrative Inquiry on Coping with Pre- and Post-migration Stressors in Refugee Families

In this chapter, we report on a study of family migration narratives of West African refugee families in order to identify patterns of culturally shaped and familial sources of resilience. In pursuing these aims, we focused on participants' lived experiences of pre- and post-migration stressors and the construction of strategies to cope with their impacts within family relationships. Our goal was to develop an in-depth understanding of how the impacts of these stressors were shaped and negotiated within family contexts. To this end, our findings are meant to reflect how participants ascribed meaning to their life experiences and how the processes of meaning-making were shaped within their relational and sociocultural contexts. The study was embedded within a narrative inquiry methodology.

Narrative inquiry distinguishes itself by its focus on experiences as related by participants [32]. Narrative research contends that individuals live and understand their lives in the form of life stories, in which events are connected from past to present [33]. Individual life stories are embedded within particular family, cultural, and sociopolitical contexts intersecting with life experiences and the meanings that people make of them [32]. These stories represent their experiential meaning-making; that is, how they connect and integrate experiences based on both individual and environmental factors. Importantly, narrative researchers distinguish narrative truth from historical truth in that they focus on constructed accounts of experiences, not factual records; the focus is on how people experience and understand life events [32].

Method

Participants

In order to recruit West African refugees with a diverse history of exposure to pre- and post-migration stressors, participants were recruited in cooperation with a mental health clinic serving asylum seekers and several community-based organizations (CBOs) in New York City. Our sample consisted of 16 West African immigrants between the ages of 33 and 61 (M = 42.62) in 8 families. Four families were recruited at the clinic and four through community contacts (i.e., through an Imam and during a health fair held at a CBO).

The number of children per family varied from 2 to 9 (M = 4.75), with ages ranging from 1 to 28. All participants were Muslim and identified as Fulani (n = 12), Mandingo (n = 3), or Sousou (n = 1). Participants were from Guinea (n = 4), Sierra Leone (n = 6), Mauritania (n = 2), Côte d'Ivoire (n = 2), and Liberia (n = 2). All participants reported that they migrated involuntarily (i.e., forced migrants). At the time of the interviews, participants had lived in the USA for between 2 and 19 years (M = 11.13), with residency statuses ranging from undocumented (n = 1), withholding of removal (n = 4), temporary protected status (n = 2), asylee (n = 6), permanent residence (n = 2), and citizenship (n = 1). Participants' educational histories varied from college degree (n = 2), some years of college (n = 1), high school degree (n = 3), 4 to 11 years of formal schooling (n = 3), Koranic schooling only (n = 2), to no schooling at all (n = 5). Ten participants spoke English at or above functional level, while six did not. All but two participants were employed at the time of the interviews.

Procedure

Data collection Data were collected through the administration of two subsequent in-depth, semistructured interviews with each participant family. A first interview procedure consisted of joint parental interviews with both spousal partners, followed within a few weeks by individual parent interviews with each of the spouses. First, joint parental interviews aimed at the construction of pre- and post-migration narratives reflecting the joint meaning-making of pre- and post-migration lived experiences as a couple and as a family (e.g., parenting in exile, coping with separation and reunification). These joint parental interviews aimed at developing the migration narrative as lived by family members: The term "family migration narrative" thus refers to the retrospective account of what happened to different family members and not to the result of some empirical procedure in which all family members were included in data collection. Next, individual parent interviews focused on an in-depth exploration of parental meaning-making of family relationships in exile, addressing relational processes of narrative transmission, family communication on loss and traumatic histories, parental authority, transgenerational and transnational relation-ships, and family roles in relation to migration history and exile. Between interviews, narratives were arranged on timelines, and in second (individual parent) interviews, participants were asked to (1) confirm these timelines and (2) use them to reflect on family functioning over time and on the potential impacts of pre- and post-migration experiences. Interviews were administered using a semistructured interview guide. In total, twenty-four 90-minute in-depth qualitative interviews were administered; inter-views were conducted in English, French (by fluent interviewers), or Fulani (with interpreters).

Data analysis We sought to use a holistic, content-focused approach in order to examine participants' narratives. In line with Schleiermacher's idea of the hermeneutic circle [32], sections of narratives were interpreted in relation to the other sections. Particular attention was given to cultural, social, political, and historical factors mediating the meaning-making of lived experiences. Findings are organized consistent with our aims: narrative content followed by the domains in which we identified sources of resilience.

Reflexivity The first author is of West African descent. As someone who grew up with an African immigrant father who sought political asylum in Europe before she was born, she had a personal interest in attempting to understand the plight of other members of the African diaspora. Besides knowledge she acquired growing up in an African immigrant community and then being an immigrant in the USA, she also learned about African culture on the ground, as she regularly travels to Guinea and other African countries. Coauthors were informed by extensive clinical, research, and community experience with West African immigrants in the USA and Europe.

Sources of Resilience and Family Coping with Pre- and Post-migration Adversity

Refugee Family Narratives: Pre- and Post-migration Experiences

Although participants' degree of agency in the decision to emigrate from home countries varied, all reported that they were forced to migrate because of harsh and sometimes unbearable living conditions. Of the 16 participants, 9 reported experiencing some form of pre-migration trauma, including persecution (e.g., arrest, imprisonment, torture), wit-nessing and being a victim of armed conflict, captivity, forced labor, and sexual violence. Although participants shared detailed information about other pre- and post-migration adversities, those who mentioned potentially traumatic events (often in the form of brief fragmented accounts) did not want to share detailed information about these events. A 36-year-old Guinean woman explained, "I want to forget about that; I got a new life … so

I don't want to get back on that"; a 40-year-old Guinean man said, "I want to bury that; it's the past."

All participants reported pre-migration exposure to chronic adversity, such as concentrated poverty, unemployment, political instability, insecurity, and limited access to healthcare, education, and basic utilities. All reported experiencing common post-migration adversity: financial hardship, difficulty finding employment, discrimination in the workplace (e.g., lower-paying jobs), liminal immigrant status, and housing-related issues. Participants all reported that the most difficult post-migration period consisted of the initial months after arrival. Because none had work permits and some did not speak English, most participants started off with some form of informal employment (e.g., selling goods on the street, hair braiding), and some eventually found more stable employment (e.g., taxi driver, home health aide). All participants also reported housing difficulties, such as living in small and overcrowded apartments. Yet another reported difficulty was obtaining legal immigrant status.

All participants reported that they relied on the help, support, and advice of other Africans (family, friends, or acquaintances) already settled in the USA. Some also reported that they simply found out where African neighborhoods were located and went there to seek help. For example, upon his arrival in New York, one Sierra Leonean participant went to an area where he was told a lot of Africans resided. Once there, he met a Senegalese man who, although they had never met before, provided him with housing, lent him money, and advised him on how to get settled. In a similar vein, a Guinean woman reported that she went to an African hair salon to socialize and ask for advice on how to find employment. Although she had no former experience as a hairdresser, the women working at the salon offered her a temporary job until she found more permanent employment, and they informed her about how to get healthcare.

Another difficulty experienced by most participants was separation from family members left behind in home countries. Seven out of the eight couples faced spousal separation due to migration, with husbands usually preceding wives (except in one case). Length of separation was 18 months to 5 years. All but one participant family reported separation from at least one child due to migration. Separation from children during migration was ubiquitous for men, but also reported by four of the eight women, who resorted to child fostering by family members in the home country until they were able to have their children join them. Except in cases where participants did not know the whereabouts of their children and spouses for some period of time, most expressed that separation was difficult yet surmountable because they knew it was only temporary. Overall, separation from family members was reported as having had little or no impact on spousal and parent-child relations.

Because it was more long term and often permanent, separation from extended family members reflected a more significant source of grief and sense of loss. All participants expressed that they missed not only their relatives but also the collectivist aspects of extended family networks. For many, the loss of extended family structures was identified as the most-missed aspect of West African culture. However, participants reported being in close contact with family members back home. Men who had occupied the role of head of the extended family in their home country reported that they kept their position even after migrating, and thus were regularly solicited when important family decisions had to be made. Participants reported having financial responsibilities in their home countries, mostly in the form of sending remittances to family members in need. Although participants reported that balancing remittance obligations with the high cost of living in the USA was a considerable source of stress, they expressed that these obligations were an important aspect of family life and responsibilities.

Although all participants reported that settling in the USA was a difficult process, each family eventually found living arrangements as well as sufficient employment to provide for their children and meet remittance obligations. At the time of the interviews, all but two participants were employed. Overall, participants viewed coming to the USA as a significant achievement, whether personally or in terms of providing better opportunities for children. This constituted an important aspect of participants' rationale for migrating, as illustrated by a 42-year-old Sierra Leonean man's comment that "If we can't do it, our children will do it one day." In a similar vein, a 43-year-old Sierra Leonean man made the following comment, "I'm like, retiring right now little by little from my ambitions ... now I'm focusing personally on how my kids can go to college." Participants' narratives suggested that life achievement is not viewed only in terms of career success. A 50-year-old Mauritanian father reported, "For us Africans, to live, build a family, and the children you raise, that's a man's objective." In this sense, although these participants might not have fulfilled their professional goals and aspirations to the fullest, they appear to consider getting married, having a family for which one provides, and insuring a better future for one's children as a form of personal success and achievement.

Several participants reported disillusionment about life in the USA. A few of them also expressed regrets about having settled outside their home countries, where they might have had better professional careers than in the USA. Difficulties getting accustomed to the stressful aspects of the American work-oriented lifestyle were also reported. Nevertheless, no participant reported that they planned to move back to their home country and make a life there. Those who reported that they hoped to one day move back to their home country emphasized that they would do so only if the political and socioeconomic situation improved. It is worth noting that most participants reported that they would prefer to live in their home countries if the current situation changed, that is, if there was no corruption, political instability, insecurity, and poverty, along with better access to education, healthcare, and basic resources.

For participants who experienced trauma, post-migration adversity was often contextualized with respect to pre-migration adversity. In general, post-migration adversities were regarded as less extreme in degree than pre-migration ones. First, compared to a host country like the USA, the standard of living in the majority of West African nations is extremely low. Illustratively, a 35-year-old woman from Sierra Leone reported that a major difference between the USA and her home country was that in the USA, "when you work you make money ... in my country you don't have any hope ... there's no job, there's no business." Second, for individuals who experienced trauma in the context of war, civil conflict, or political unrest, post-migration adversities were regarded as benign in comparison to pre-migration traumatic experiences and related living conditions. For example, one family from Sierra Leone witnessed the killing of family and community members and then they were separated for five years, during which the mother and youngest child were captured by paramilitary forces and forced to work. After two (of the five) years in a refugee camp, the husband learned that they were not dead, and they were reunited in the USA, where he had sought asylum. In New York, gangs at school harassed the son, and later the father and son were assaulted at home. This resulted in the son being hospitalized, legal action against the perpetrators, and the family being moved to a shelter for temporary protection. Throughout the narrative, both spouses compared the stress in response to post-migration adversity favorably to that resulting from the pre-migration trauma. Post-migration events, such as gang violence, were considered benign in comparison to situations experienced pre-migration, such as when one cannot turn to the police or the justice system for help and protection. In the wife's words, "in our country they attack everybody … innocent, no innocent, it's attack … this [gang violence] was no issue for my son." It is worth noting that although violence experienced or witnessed in the USA may be considered as being of a lesser extent, hence less impactful, than pre-migration traumatic events and situations, it is likely that at least in some cases community violence may act as a reminder of pre-migration threat. In support of this, a participant living in a high-crime neighborhood in New York reported that hearing gunshots at night reminded her of war in her home country.

Except in reference to children and parenting, only two participants made explicit mentions of difficulties that could be linked to acculturation. These two participants discussed post-migration difficulties generally experienced by immigrants in abstract terms: discrimination against foreigners; xenophobia. All participants reported that living in the USA did not affect their sense of identity or impact their personality in major ways. Overall, participants expressed that they considered themselves Africans and lived and acted according to African culture and values as much as life in the USA allowed for it. Apart from professional interactions, since their arrival most participants had evolved almost exclusively within African immigrant communities, either of their own ethnic group or other African ethnic groups. All participants reported that they socialized mostly along ethnic lines, such as having only African friends or going to social gatherings attended by other Africans only. Participants did not express a wish to integrate into mainstream American culture other than professionally or academically. This did not appear to be experienced as social isolation or as a source of distress, as integration into mainstream American culture did not appear to be considered a necessity other than for practical aspects, such as employment, healthcare, and children's education. When participants expressed frustration related to being an immigrant in the USA, they referred primarily to difficulties related to finding decent employment or discrimination within work settings (e.g., having to accept lower salaries than their American counterparts).

When asked to discuss their current lives, beside the post-migration adversities mentioned earlier, participants also reported many positive aspects of their lives in the USA. Most reported being relatively content to live in a country where one can work and make enough money to provide for one's family in the USA and back home. Moreover, participants reported feeling grateful for being safe, free, and having their basic needs met. While more than half the participants did not have any formal schooling, living in the USA was viewed as an opportunity to improve the status of their families, since their children were getting a better education that would translate into opportunities for the future. As put by the Sierra Leonean participant whose family story was recounted earlier, emigrating to the USA meant not only feeling safe and free, but also feeling hopeful for the future. Once he had brought his wife and children to the USA, he stopped constantly worrying and started thinking about "building a life".

Lastly, religiosity was a salient theme in participants' narratives. When asked about how he dealt with adversities, a 43-year-old Sierra Leonean man explained that "In my religion, we have a duty to hope … so I never lose hope." Most participants repeatedly thanked God for their fortunes (e.g., being alive, being safe, having made it to the USA). Additionally, being a member of a religious community seemed to safeguard against social isolation, as evidenced in the following exchange between an interviewer and a 57-year-old Liberian man:

> Interviewer: 'Do you have a good support group of friends and family . . . or do you feel very alone?'
> Participant: 'No, no, I'm not, we're not alone . . . the people we have, meet at the mosque together, we learn together, we pray together . . . live together.'

Cultural Continuity and Change in Spousal Relations

Our study was particularly concerned with the impact of migration on relations between spouses. Whereas in an initial statement most participants reported little to no change in the nature of their relationships with their spouses (e.g., "no," "only a little bit," "not very much," "no big differences"), their narratives reflected a couple of relevant post-migration gender role shifts. The few who explicitly reported changes in the nature of their relationships reported that living in the USA had resulted in more freedom as a couple and stronger bonds with their spouses because of distance from extended family. The 50-year-old Mauritanian man explained: "In Africa, households are large . . . because there is the brother, half-brother, cousin, aunt, and so on; there is everybody, so conflicts become more acute." For this participant, African couples living in the USA have more freedom because there is less influence of the family. Decreased involvement of extended family members may also result in having to rely and depend on spouses more, whether emotionally, financially, or logistically. A 49-year-old Sierra Leonean man reported, "Here, you are alone, so you are much closer and you understand each other." Additionally, struggling together to surmount pre- and post-migration adversities was also reported as having strengthened spousal relationships.

The most pervasive shifts in family- and household-related behaviors concerned traditional gender norms related to financing. As reported by participants, in many African societies most women do not work and are responsible for taking care of children and housework, whereas men are responsible for providing financially for the family. Although it is not uncommon for women to work in Africa, their earnings are for them to buy small things for themselves or their children. Among participants, all husbands worked in their home countries, while only one wife worked. Once in the USA, all wives eventually worked part or full time.

All but two couples reported that they currently shared household financial responsibilities. In one Guinean couple, only the husband did not work in the USA, and this was due to physical disability, so his wife was the sole provider. When asked about whether this impacted his role as a spouse or father, he responded that it did not because his wife gave him her earnings for him to act as if these were his own. This suggests that, in this couple's case, cultural norms shaped the paternal position around economic provisions, as exemplified in the following comment by the 42-year-old Sierra Leonean participant: "In our tradition, if you are married, it means you are capable of doing stuff for your family. If you can't do anything for them, it's a disgrace for you; it's a disgrace for your family." This participant recounted how, even in the face of his wife's employment and his ongoing struggles to ensure financial income for his family both in the USA and in his home country, his wife continued to preserve his paternal role: "If I bring ten dollar, she will accept it. She'll take it to be a million. She knows that, yes, my husband is doing something he usually do before when we're back home." In this case, while factually performing cultural changes in gender role division pertaining to financial responsibilities, the wife is promoting cultural continuity in gender role division by symbolically restoring the paternal role of economic provision. In contrast, a 39-year-old man from Ivory Coast complained that, in line with traditional norms, his wife did not share her earnings with him but expected him to share his with her. Although he appeared to be in favor of the American way of sharing financial responsibilities for the household, he nonetheless accepted his wife's ways in order to avoid spousal conflict.

In terms of non-financial decisions, all couples reported that both spouses were involved in decision-making and that, when a decision had to be made, it was discussed and addressed together as a couple. Only two participants – both men – reported that making decisions together constituted a difference from pre-migration gender roles. One participant attributed this difference to the fact that, in his home country, husbands usually consulted elder family members instead of wives concerning such issues. Another participant mentioned that, since he and his wife had immigrated to the USA, he had come to respect and seek her opinion more than before. He related this directly to sharing more responsibilities, as life in the USA entailed relying and counting on each other more than back home. Most couples reported that husband-wife disagreements were dealt with through discussion, not conflict. Two instances of overt spousal conflict were reported. One couple and one man divorced from his first wife reported past post-migration spousal conflict. In both cases, conflict was related to polygamy, specifically the first wife not accepting the second marriage. Note that although two participants reported having second wives in home countries, post-migration none reported ever living in the same home with more than one wife.

Overall, participants' narratives reflected collaborative spousal relationships within somewhat adapted but still traditional gender roles. The 50-year-old Mauritanian commented, "It's with reason that one builds a family . . . if you want to have a family for a long time, you must follow reason, not the heart." In this sense, it appears that spousal harmony was considered in terms of the fulfilment of culturally prescribed roles. This aspect of African culture was omnipresent in participants' narratives, as all reported that building and providing for a family was a core life aspiration.

Tradition and Flexibility in Parenting and Parent-Child Relations

Similar to reports of spousal relations, all participants reported that their parenting style had not changed much post-migration, nor was it influenced by American culture. Both female and male participants reported that they had control over their children, who were reported to be obedient, polite, and respectful of adult authority. Although most participants reported no instances of parent-child conflict or problems, a few complained that American norms contradict African parenting norms concerning corporal punishment. There were no explicit reports of the practice, but some felt that American laws prevented them from raising their children as they saw fit, and they worried that this could have negative consequences on their children's overall upbringing. In any case, these participants reported refraining from using corporal punishment because of fear that their children could call the police or child welfare authorities.

Several participants explained that they understood parenting before becoming parents because of collective parenting practices within extended families and communities. One 43-year-old Mauritanian woman explained:

> We don't have to learn this . . . we don't question ourselves as much as Westerners . . . for us, being a parent comes naturally because, in Africa, even if you're not a father or a mother you often live with family; there are nieces, there are nephews, we have authority over these children, we raise them . . . so the idea of one's responsibility to raise one's child is already within ourselves; it's natural . . . automatic.

In a similar vein, her husband, the 50-year-old Mauritanian, appeared surprised when asked whether being separated from his children for seven months had impacted his role as a father: "Me? No! It's a question of mindset; even if they're not here, you are the father; there is no rupture." Echoing this comment, when narrating his reunification with his two-year-old daughter after almost two years of separation, a 49-year-old Sierra Leonean man reported that, after some initial distance, "everything started going back to natural, to a natural place."

Another fundamental aspect of traditional African parenting in participants' narratives concerned parents' lived experience of responsibility to instill their cultural values in their children. All participants reported that they spoke their native language at home and that this was related to values. The 50-year-old Mauritanian man:

> Language is the vehicle of values . . . When you are in your home country, you know that your child is going to evolve in a society that is yours and will define himself, his identity is preserved, which is not the case here.

His worry as a parent was that his children would "lose what is most essential, their roots." Other participants also reported this type of concern and mentioned that they wanted to prevent their children from being negatively influenced by American culture and by disreputable youths from their neighborhood or school. Several participants were critical of American family dynamics, which were perceived as reflecting either neglect or children being treated "as kings." Additionally, all participants reported being practising Muslims whose values were at times at odds with secular American ones. In this regard, they expressed that promoting Muslim principles, such as premarital celibacy, abstention from alcohol and other drugs, and reverence for elders were effective in keeping children "on the right path." Most participants reported that their children had attended Koranic school on a weekly basis at some point post-migration, and several parents mentioned that they prayed most prayers together as a family. The 50-year-old Mauritanian man mentioned that, in his opinion, family crises often result from "a lack of spiritual connection" between parents and children.

Another manner in which participants reported keeping their children from falling prey to negative influences was by monitoring them closely. All participants reported that, regardless of their age, their children were not permitted to "hang out outside" or "with kids from the neighborhood." On school days, children were expected to come straight home from school. Extracurricular activities without trusted adult supervision were not allowed. In some cases, the only friends that parents tolerated were African youths living in the same buildings. Participants often lamented the lack of collective monitoring in the USA. As the 43-year-old Mauritanian woman explained: "In Africa we don't say that one person raises a child, it's the village that raises the child." That is, in Africa parents can count on the fact that, when children are outside, community members will look after them and discipline them if necessary. Because of a perceived lack of community supervision in US neighborhoods, participants appeared to monitor their children more closely than they would in their home country. Note that living in poor neighborhoods with high crime rates may also account for participants' general sentiment of unsafety and the resulting need for increased child monitoring. Some parents also expressed concerns about not being able to dedicate enough time to their children's proper upbringing due to work schedules. Concerned that their adolescent son was not doing well and misbehaved at school, one family decided to send him back to Ivory Coast so that he could be raised "properly ... the African way" by family members and then come back to the USA to pursue higher education.

Overall, participants reported that their children were well adjusted both at home and at school. Except in one case, participants reported no instances of parent-child conflict, nor did they report psychological, emotional, or behavioral disturbances in their children. Participants all reported receiving positive feedback from teachers informing them that their children exhibited good behavior and performed well academically. Even the children who came to the USA not speaking English adjusted relatively quickly. No child was reported to have repeated a class or received special education services. Although almost half the participants did not get formal schooling growing up, all reported that making sure that their children did well in school was one of the most important aspects of their role as parents. Furthermore, children's academic achievements were viewed as a personal success for parents, as illustrated by the Sierra Leonean man's comment that "if we can't do it, our children will do it one day." Here, the participant was referring to the fact that, although he did not fulfill his hopes for a successful career, his consolation was that his children would do so, indicating how refugee children's educational trajectories may operate as vehicles of hope in parental migration histories.

One last element that emerged from participants' narratives is that all those who experienced trauma in their home country reported adhering to a silencing or avoidant pattern of trauma-communication within parent-child relationships. Here, parents accounted for this communicative pattern on the grounds of the rationale that they did not want their children to have negative views of their home countries, potentially as a way to instill cultural connectedness in children. Relatedly, participants expressed their emphasis on sharing stories about the positive aspects of their home countries and cultures. For example, the 50-year-old Mauritanian man reported that

> Talking about your experiences to your children is a negative thing to do ... if you tell her, she will hate all of Mauritania, everything that is there; she will never go back there ... so it's a question of image.

A 36-year-old Guinean woman reported:

> I really don't want tell these things my kids because I do not want to preach hatred or anger. If I tell them about what happened, they could get pretty angry and it could lead into revenge ... I don't want them to have hatred in them ... because if you do something to someone's mother or father, it becomes like a grudge and it builds up.

These quotations suggest that avoiding instilling anger or revenge in children is not only related to preserving a positive image of the family's home country but may also reflect an attempt to avoid the repetition of violence in children's future trajectories.

Discussion

Multilevel Sources of Resilience and Coping within Family Relationships

In order to identify, explain, and understand the various sources of resilience and coping strategies reflected in our findings, we propose a multidimensional approach. Drawing from the interactive homeostasis [18] and ecological [19] models of resilience, we shift beyond an individualized notion of resilience towards a focus on the dynamics of coping within family and community relationships. Here, resilience is conceptualized as the result of complex interactions between individual and interpersonal processes, cultural understandings and strategies, and the family's broader context and interactions with cultural communities and social institutions.

Participants' migration narratives did not reflect traditional trauma and adversity models contending that individuals who experienced trauma or adversity are more vulnerable to subsequent stressors [11, 12, 34] and are at greater risk for negative individual and family outcomes [7, 8, 14]. Rather than increased spousal conflict, narratives reflected stability, cooperation, and support. Rather than family dysfunction, narratives reflected coherence, cohesion, and nonconflicted parent-child relations. Rather than less effective parenting, narratives reflected consistency, active supervision and monitoring, and control over children's behavior. Rather than depressive or anxiety symptoms causing ineffective parenting, participants exhibited agency in their ability to provide for their children and actively protect them from perceived negative influences.

Interestingly, even participants who were former clients at a mental health clinic did not make specific mentions of past or current psychiatric symptoms. Although past or current psychological symptoms were certainly present in some cases, based on participants' narratives these appear to have had limited impacts on functioning in major life domains such as work, family, or community engagement. While it is possible that the underreporting of symptoms reflected cultural attitudes or stigma related to mental health and symptomatology [35], perhaps the impact of psychological disturbances on functioning is mitigated when these are not a salient aspect of the meaning-making of lived experiences. Similar to what emerged from our participants' narratives, in a group of Rwandan war survivors who scored high on PTSD checklists, a majority were nonetheless interested in activities such as work or play, felt that they were able to do things as well as before the war, felt that their future seemed good, and felt able to protect family or self [27].

Traditional trauma approaches focusing on symptomatology often overlook the fact that the presence of trauma-related symptoms does not necessarily imply impaired capacity to function appropriately in major life domains [27, 36]. Also often ignored is the fact that normative modes of coping with trauma and adversity may differ from one culture to another. Accordingly, Western-designed trauma models may have limited applicability among non-Western populations. It is with these counter-theoretical observations that we present our family resilience framework.

Cultural continuity In most traditional African cultures, life revolves around family. One's primary life goals are, first, to maintain strong family connections and, second, to build a family to fulfill one's role as a good spouse and parent. Familistic cultural values were reflected in participants' continued efforts to promote and preserve healthy family relations in the face of adversities. These efforts towards consistency in parenting and spousal relationships may help preserve family cohesion, which in turn may promote resilience in family members. Research shows that parenting practices may mediate child adjustment following trauma exposure and adversity [20–22]. Similarly, healthy social interactions within families have been linked to better post-trauma adjustment and resilience for both parents and children [20]. Family-level models of resilience propose that interactional processes such as parental coherence, collaboration, competence, and confidence are vital aspects of family-level coping strategies and adaptive outcomes in contexts of trauma and adversity [21, 24].

In our sample, familism was not only reflected in the values espoused by participants but also in remittance responsibilities and child fostering. These transnational behaviors are likely to both reflect and reinforce cultural continuity through practical connections with extended family. Both practices not only support culturally prescribed forms of collective caretaking but may also buffer against the grief over the loss of frequent extended family interactions. Remittance responsibilities allow for continued involvement in one's extended family life and, for some, increased prestige within family systems. Most participants reported having used child fostering – that is, sending children to live with family members in home countries – at some point pre- or post-migration in order to transmit traditional values as well as to provide time to establish financial security in the USA. Child fostering is a culturally prescribed practice not uncommon in immigrant communities worldwide. It helps maintain strong extended family connections and serves multiple protective purposes, such as financial security, discipline, and cultural socialization [37]. Besides promoting cultural continuity, pre-migration exposure to child fostering may have better prepared participants to cope with nuclear family separation during migration. In support of this, except in cases where participants did not know the whereabouts of their children and spouses, it was reported that separation from one's spouse and/or children had little or no impact on spousal or parent-child relations.

We propose that the maintenance of native cultural values and norms that prescribe the coherence of spousal and family relations constitute a source of resilience against the negative impact of pre- and post-migration adversities on family functioning, weaving threads of continuity into life histories affected by loss and exile. Even in the face of considerable external stressors, participants strove to maintain consistency in their spousal and parenting roles. Cultural continuity in the form of parents instilling traditional African family values in their children may serve to buffer against the potentially negative impact of parent-child acculturation dissonance and promote family cohesion and connectedness. Further, cultural continuity in spousal relationships was reflected by adherence to traditional African paternalistic values and norms prescribing gender roles and family household organization, with some adjustments when necessary. Most couples reported little or no influence of the host country or culture on the core nature of their relationship. Cultural continuity in the form of the maintenance of culturally prescribed gender roles within the couple may constitute a buffer against post-migration spousal discord. When gender role shifts are necessary (e.g., division of financial responsibilities), these are negotiated in a way that symbolically preserves culturally prescribed gender roles. Last, parents' strong adherence to traditional African values, as opposed to adopting American ones, may not only buffer against individual acculturative stress but also provide some sense of control while adjusting to radically foreign host country settings.

Although participants strove to maintain cultural continuity at both family and community levels, family relationships reflected some flexibility to US norms in order to accommodate cultural, financial, and legal realities. These adaptations were most obvious when monitoring children and spousal relationships. In most traditional collectivist societies, monitoring and disciplining children occurs at the community level, which is largely absent in most US communities. West African parents' increased monitoring of children can thus be viewed as a strategy to counter this difference. Another shift in parenting consisted in not resorting to corporal punishment, a disciplinary practice considered effective yet abandoned to comply with US child welfare laws. Gender role shifts in financial responsibilities among couples represented another necessary post-migration acculturative adaptation, where two earners are almost always necessary within households. Shifting cultural practices were also evident in the abandonment of polygamous living arrangements to comply with US law. While these changes in family functioning were considered adaptive in that they were necessary to meet the demands of life in the host society, participants emphasized their simultaneous adherence to and reliance upon traditional cultural values and norms.

Collectivism A source of resilience related to cultural continuity was the maintenance of traditional collectivism within community relationships. This was most obvious in participants' narratives immediately following arrival, when many participants reported relying on other African immigrants. Panethnic solidarity is common among members of the African diaspora, and this was reflected in the current narratives in practical terms such as finding housing and financial support for the newly arrived. Negative outcomes related to the impact of individual acculturative processes may not have been reflected in participants' narratives because they were mitigated by the fact that they were immersed in communities where social life revolves around shared African cultural values, norms, and habits.

The collectivism of African immigrant communities stands in sharp contrast with the perceived lack of a sense of community in US society. In this sense, the emphasis on collectivism in immigrant communities may have lessened the cultural shock of individualist American culture. This is not to suggest that participants never faced negative experiences related to acculturation, but rather that such experiences were not experienced as impactful enough to be directly incorporated into the meaning-making of post-migration experiences. It is possible that the negative impact of acculturation is decreased when acculturative experiences are not considered an important aspect of one's lived experiences in host countries. Although perhaps problematic in other domains, a certain degree of cultural isolation may be protective. Note that cultural isolation is not analogous to marginalization. All participants made the informed decision to settle in African immigrant communities. Whether voluntary or not, this type of regrouping along ethnic lines is rather common in the metropolitan USA. Historically, most immigrant groups have regrouped into close-knit communities living in distinct city areas. It is also not uncommon for various conservative groups (e.g., Hasidic Jews) to promote what Berry [38] defined as *separation* (i.e., low host culture but high native culture identification).

Religiosity Also related to cultural continuity is religiosity. For all participants, religion was a core aspect of family and community life, thus promoting cultural continuity. Religious faith was also used to bolster individual wellbeing through meaning-making. Many Muslims hold the belief that God has a plan for everyone and that therefore individuals are not responsible for misfortunes. Positing such an external locus of control for distress may mitigate the impact of adversity, constituting an effective coping mechanism. Religious coping may be especially relevant among disadvantaged or impoverished populations that lack access to mental health services [39]. A growing body of research shows that religious coping, spirituality, and faith-based approaches to dealing with adversity promote resilience by alleviating individual-level distress through ritual, helping to uncover meaning and clarify identity, and improving connections with others through community [39].

Downward comparison All participants experienced chronic pre-migration adversity (e.g., poverty, insecurity, lack of opportunities), and most were exposed to traumatic events (e.g., war, persecution, captivity, sexual violence). However, rather than increasing vulnerability to subsequent adversity, the pre-migration experiences related in participants' narratives seemed to operate as a source for coping with post-migration adversities. Participants' narratives did not reflect the assumption that prior adversities lead to more psychologically impactful adversities (i.e., cumulative effect). Post-migration adversities were often contrasted with pre-migration adversities in countering interviewers' expressions of sympathy. If taken at face value, this suggests that individuals who experience high degrees of pre-migration adversity – from chronic poverty to unreliable justice systems and exposure to trauma – may experience post-migration adversities as relatively mild and surmountable.

An important aspect of pre- and post-migration adversities often overlooked in the empirical literature is the fact that post-migration adversities are often less extreme in degree than pre-migration ones. Compared to a host country like the USA, the standard of living in the majority of West African countries is extremely low. Exposure to chronic adversity may promote the development of effective coping strategies, which in turn may foster a higher capacity for resilience in the face of subsequent exposure to adversity. Although in the current study downward comparison should be contextualized in the differences between West African countries and the USA, the idea that previous exposure to adversity might protect against the effects of later adversity has been noted in the psychological literature [40, 41].

A specific way of coping with losses related to migration consisted of comparing the educational and professional opportunities one had in one's home country with the opportunities that one was able to provide to one's children post-migration in the host country. In this sense, actively making sure that one's children are provided with better educational opportunities may foster resilience in parents, who, instead of dwelling on the fact that they have limited opportunities in terms of personal professional achievements, find solace in the fact that their children have better ones. In support of this, using the same data set as the current study, Roubeni et al. [42] examined the connections between experiences of loss and educational aspirations for children. They proposed that West African parents cope with the loss of hope for successful educational and social trajectories they initially had for themselves by projecting their aspirations onto their children. Relatedly, Walsh [24] proposed that well-functioning families have "an evolutionary sense of time and becoming" (p. 6), and tend to contextualize and normalize distress as a way to enlarge family perspectives on the future.

Limitations

Both a strength and a limitation of narrative inquiry is its emphasis on understanding storytellers' points of view [32] rather than on the theoretical or clinical perspectives of the researchers. As a result, this methodological approach may not generate the type of scientific cause-and-effect data that can readily be translated into evidence-based treatments. A further limitation of the present study is that, by focusing on participants' own perspectives, the researchers did not account for the presence of biases related to social desirability vis-à-vis the research context or broader host society. It is also possible that aspects of participants' narratives reflected the development of an idealized post-migration narrative within the participants' cultural communities, which in turn could have influenced the meaning-making of pre- and post-migration experiences. Our findings concerning resilience and cultural continuity should not be interpreted as minimizing problems associated with forced migration, nor do we wish to give the impression that all family narratives are uniform. Rather, we wish to highlight themes and sources of resilience that emerged across narratives, narratives that are rarely conveyed in the clinical literature on refugees.

Conclusion

We propose that, as sources of resilience, cultural continuity, collectivism, religiosity, adaptive flexibility, and downward comparison constitute sociocultural protective factors that may buffer against the negative impacts of pre- and post-migration trauma and adversity. Clinical research and practice involving refugee populations should identify and attend to these protective factors with the aim of fostering the full range of potential sources of resilience available to individuals and families. Although critical to modern resilience theory, culture-specific sources of resilience have received little empirical attention. In clinical practice, rather than being fostered, culture-specific sources of resilience are often ignored, as most models informing intervention and treatment favor etic approaches to trauma based on a biomedical approach to psychopathology, individualism, and Western diagnostic systems. Identifying potential sociocultural sources of resilience may lead to more culturally sensitive and more effective approaches to psychological healing.

Given the likelihood that they experienced pre-migration trauma or chronic adversity, refugee populations are assumed to be at higher risk for developing mental health problems and related functional impairments. However, in a majority of cases, exposure to trauma or chronic adversity does not lead to psychopathology [13, 36]. Despite this, the primary focus of traditional trauma models and related clinical interventions is to predict, assess for, and treat trauma-related negative psychosocial outcomes. Taken together, these perspectives may lead unseasoned clinicians who work with refugee populations to both overlook resilience processes and overpathologize their clients while ignoring their current stressors, concerns, aspirations [43], and, in particular, unique meaning-making. Therapeutic approaches that involve assessing and promoting sources of resilience are likely to be more effective than those focusing primarily on symptom reduction. Importantly, when working with refugee clients who have strong affiliative values, clinicians should adopt frameworks that assess and promote family- and community-level modes of coping and resilience [24].

As indicated by our findings, sources of resilience may be culturally negotiated. For this reason, certain taken-for-granted therapeutic approaches may be at odds with culturally normative ways of coping with trauma and adversity. For instance, all participants reported that focusing on the present and future while actively avoiding recalls of past trauma-related memories constituted a mode of coping with past trauma. Echoing this finding, it has been reported that both Mozambican and Ethiopian refugees described "active forgetting" as their normative mode of coping with past adversity [27]. This culturally prescribed coping strategy contrasts sharply with the familiar idea in Western psychology that recovery from trauma and adverse events implicates talking about and "working through" past difficulties [27]. Implementing this approach with African refugees seeking mental health services may not only antagonize them but also deprive them of a sense of agency in their own recovery process. When providing mental health services to this population, strength-based approaches that promote wellbeing by meeting clients where they are, whether they want to focus on past or current stressors or both, are likely to be not only more effective but also more empowering. In other words, treating trauma-related mental illness among refugees should emphasize their agency in choosing whether they want treatment to focus on past trauma, current stressors, concerns, and/or aspirations.

To conclude, we urge clinicians and other individuals who work with refugee populations to adopt emic stances with the aim of promoting the utmost respect for both individual meaning-making and sociocultural modes of coping. This is not to be achieved simply through knowledge or "understanding" of culturally diverse paradigms. Rather, as much as possible, these paradigms should be incorporated into clinical and other psychosocial treatments and interventions. When working with non-Western refugee populations, a failure to consider the fact that all cultural traditions have their own frames of reference can potentially lead to unintended harm or further victimization.

References

1. M. Fazel, J. Wheeler and J. Danesh, Prevalence of serious mental disorder in 7000 refugees resettled in western countries: A systematic review. *The Lancet*, 365(9467) (2005), 1309–14.

2. E. Heptinstall, V. Sethna and E. Taylor, PTSD and depression in refugee children. *European Child & Adolescent Psychiatry*, 13(6) (2004) 373–80.

3. R. Schweitzer, F. Melville, Z. Steel and P. Lacherez, Trauma, post-migration living difficulties, and social support as predictors of psychological adjustment in resettled Sudanese refugees. *Australian and New Zealand Journal of Psychiatry*, 40(2) (2006), 179–87.

4. K. Hampshire, G. Porter, K. Kilpatrick, P. Kyei, M. Adjaloo and G. Oppong, Liminal spaces: Changing inter-generational relations among long-term Liberian refugees in Ghana. *Human Organization*, 67 (2008), 25–36.

5. E. H. Telzer, Expanding the acculturation gap-distress model: An integrative review of research. *Human Development*, 53(6) (2010), 313–40.

6. A. Rasmussen, T. Chu, A. M. Akinsulure-Smith and E. Keatley, The social ecology of resolving family conflict among West African immigrants in New York:

A grounded theory approach. *American Journal of Community Psychology*, 52(1–2) (2013), 185–96.

7. R. D. Conger, X. Ge, G. H. Elder Jr., F. O. Lorenz and R. L. Simons, Economic stress, coercive family process, and developmental problems of adolescents. *Child Development*, 65(2) (1994), 541–61.

8. L. Morrison Gutman, V. C. McLoyd and T. Tokoyawa, Financial strain, neighborhood stress, parenting behaviors, and adolescent adjustment in urban African American families. *Journal of Research on Adolescence*, 15(4) (2005), 425–49.

9. B. H. Ellis, H. Z. MacDonald, A. K. Lincoln and H. J. Cabral, Mental health of Somali adolescent refugees: The role of trauma, stress, and perceived discrimination. *Journal of Consulting and Clinical Psychology*, 76(2) (2008), 184.

10. E. Montgomery, Trauma and resilience in young refugees: A 9-year follow-up study. *Development and Psychopathology*, 22(2) (2010) 477–89.

11. D. A. Lloyd and R. J. Turner, Cumulative adversity and posttraumatic stress disorder: Evidence from a diverse community sample of young adults. *American Journal of Orthopsychiatry*, 73(4) (2003), 381–91.

12. K. A. McLaughlin, K. J. Conron, K. C. Koenen and S. E. Gilman, Childhood adversity, adult stressful life events, and risk of past-year psychiatric disorder: A test of the stress sensitization hypothesis in a population-based sample of adults. *Psychological Medicine*, 40(10) (2010), 1647–58.

13. R. McNally, Posttraumatic stress disorder. In P. H. Blaney and T. Millon, eds., *Oxford Textbook of Psychopathology*, 2nd ed. (London: Oxford University Press, 2008), pp. 176–97.

14. K. Appleyard and J. D. Osofsky, Parenting after trauma: Supporting parents and caregivers in the treatment of children impacted by violence. *Infant Mental Health Journal*, 24(2) (2003), 111–25.

15. B. K. Jordan, C. R. Marmar, J. A. Fairbank, W. E. Schlenger, R. A. Kulka, R. L. Hough et al., Problems in families of male Vietnam veterans with posttraumatic stress disorder. *Journal of Consulting and Clinical Psychology*, 60(6) (1992), 916.

16. V. Igreja, The effects of traumatic experiences on the infant–mother relationship in the former war zones of central Mozambique: The case of *madzawde* in Gorongosa. *Infant Mental Health Journal*, 24(5) (2003), 469–94.

17. G. A. Bonanno, Loss, trauma, and human resilience: Have we underestimated the human capacity to thrive after extremely aversive events? *American Psychologist*, 59 (1) (2004), 20.

18. H. Herrman, D. E. Stewart, N. Diaz-Granados, E. L. Berger, B. Jackson and T. Yuen, What is resilience? *The Canadian Journal of Psychiatry*, 56(5) (2011), 258–65.

19. M. R. Harvey, An ecological view of psychological trauma and trauma recovery. *Journal of Traumatic Stress*, 9(1) (1996), 3–23.

20. A. Gewirtz, M. Forgatch and E. Wieling, Parenting practices as potential mechanisms for child adjustment following mass trauma. *Journal of Marital and Family Therapy*, 34(2) (2008), 177–92.

21. J. M. Patterson, Integrating family resilience and family stress theory. *Journal of Marriage and Family*, 64(2) (2002), 349–60.

22. J. M. Patterson, Families experiencing stress: I. The family adjustment and adaptation response model. II. Applying the FAAR model to health-related issues for intervention and research. *Family Systems Medicine*, 6(2) (1988), 202–37.

23. F. Walsh, The concept of family resilience: Crisis and challenge. *Family Process*, 35(3) (1996), 261–81.

24. F. Walsh, Family resilience: A framework for clinical practice. *Family Process*, 42(1) (2003), 1–8.

25. D. E. Hinton and R. Lewis-Fernández, The cross-cultural validity of posttraumatic stress disorder: Implications for DSM-5. *Depression and Anxiety*, 28(9) (2011), 783–801.

26. A. Young, *The Harmony of Illusions: Inventing Post-Traumatic Stress Disorder* (Princeton, NJ: Princeton University Press, 1997).

27. D. Summerfield, A critique of seven assumptions behind psychological trauma programmes in war-affected areas. *Social Science & Medicine*, 48 (1999), 1449–62.

28. E. Watters, *Crazy Like Us: The Globalization of the Western Mind* (New York: Free Press, 2010).

29. C. Abbo, E. S. Okello, S. Ekblad, P. Waako and S. Musisi, Lay concepts of psychosis in Busoga, Eastern Uganda: A pilot study. *World Cultural Psychiatry Research Review*, 3(3) (2008), 132–45.

30. T. S. Betancourt, J. E. Rubin-Smith, W. R. Beardslee, S. N. Stulac, I. Fayida and S. Safren, Understanding locally, culturally, and contextually relevant mental health problems among Rwandan children and adolescents affected by HIV/AIDS. *AIDS Care*, 23(4) (2011), 401–12.

31. H. M. Keys, B. N. Kaiser, B. A. Kohrt, N. M. Khoury and A. R. Brewster, Idioms of distress, ethnopsychology, and the clinical encounter in Haiti's central plateau. *Social Science & Medicine*, 75(3) (2012), 555–64.

32. R. Josselson, Narrative analysis. In K. Charmaz and L. M. McMullen, eds., *Five Ways of Doing Qualitative Analysis:*

Phenomenological Psychology, Grounded Theory, Discourse Analysis, Narrative Research, and Intuitive Inquiry (New York: Guilford Press, 2011).

33. T. R. Sarbin, *The Narrative as a Root Metaphor for Psychology* (New York: Praeger /Greenwood, 1986).

34. K. L. Harkness, A. E. Bruce and M. N. Lumley, The role of childhood abuse and neglect in the sensitization to stressful life events in adolescent depression. *Journal of Abnormal Psychology*, 115(4) (2006), 730.

35. A. M. Kleinman, Depression, somatization and the "new cross-cultural psychiatry". *Social Science & Medicine (1967)*, 11(1) (1977), 3–9.

36. M. G. Wessells, Do no harm: Toward contextually appropriate psychosocial support in international emergencies. *American Psychologist*, 64(8) (2009), 842.

37. C. Coe, Transnational parenting: Child fostering in Ghanaian immigrant families. In R. Capps and M. Fix, eds., *Young Children of Black Immigrants in America: Changing Flows, Changing Faces* (Washington, DC: Migration Policy Institute, 2003) (cited September 13, 2012). www.migrationpolicy.org/research/ CBI-book-ChildrenofBlackImmigrants

38. J. W. Berry, Acculturation as varieties of adaptation. In A. Padilla, ed., *Acculturation: Theory, Models, and Some New Findings* (Boulder, CO: Westview Press, 1980), pp. 9–25.

39. T. Bryant-Davis, A. Belcourt-Dittloff, H. Chung and S. Tillman, The cultural context of trauma recovery: The experiences of ethnic minority women. In J. L. Chin, ed., *Diversity in Mind and in Action* (3 vols.) (Santa Barbara, CA: Praeger/ABC- CLIO, 2009), pp. 127–47.

40. M. Başoğlu, S. Mineka, M. Paker, T. Aker, M. Livanou and Ş. Gök, Psychological preparedness for trauma as a protective factor in survivors of torture. *Psychological Medicine*, 27(6) (1997), 1421–33.

41. L. N. Dooley, G. M. Slavich, P. I. Moreno and J. E. Bower, Strength through adversity: Moderate lifetime stress exposure is associated with psychological resilience in breast cancer survivors. *Stress and Health*, 33(5) (2017), 549–57.

42. S. Roubeni, L. De Haene, E. Keatley, N. Shah and A. Rasmussen, "If we can't do it, our children will do it one day": A qualitative study of West African immigrant parents' losses and educational aspirations for their children. *American Educational Research Journal*, 52(2) (2015), 275–305.

43. K. E. Miller and A. Rasmussen, War exposure, daily stressors, and mental health in conflict and post-conflict settings: Bridging the divide between trauma-focused and psychosocial frameworks. *Social Science & Medicine*, 70 (1) (2010), 7–16.

Chapter 4

Cultural Belonging and Political Mobilization in Refugee Families
An Exploration of the Role of Collective Identifications in Post-trauma Reconstruction within Family Relationships

Ruth Kevers and Peter Rober

Trauma and Post-trauma Reconstruction: Processes at the Intersection of Individual and Collective Meaning

Through its cumulation of disruptive life events, losses, and cultural transitions, the process of forced migration creates a context of chronic distress for refugee children and families [1, 2]. Mass conflict and persecution fundamentally disrupt core psychosocial experiences of security, social connection, justice, identity, and existential meaning. Post-trauma reconstruction therefore centrally revolves around the restoration of these pillars [3]. For example, violent conflict and displacement often disrupt the sense of meaning and continuity within family, social, and cultural relationships, compelling survivors and their communities to revise their worldviews and belief systems. When alienation and fragmentation are too overwhelming, trauma-focused interventions have been developed to assist individuals in restoring safety, meaning, and connection [4].

Importantly, the human rights violations and persecution that characterize organized violence not only target individuals but often operate as collective trauma by primarily destroying social bonds and cultural structures within a community [5–7]. As a result, refugees' predicament revolves around collective themes like social rupture and injustice and not merely around individual experiences. Trauma-related distress and narratives describing this suffering unfold in a particular cultural and sociopolitical context, bearing cultural hallmarks and revealing elements of a collective traumatic history [8, 9]. Hence, in post-trauma suffering and reconstruction, individuals' experiences should be understood as situated within a particular community and cultural history, which was equally affected by collective violence [3, 10, 11].

Acknowledgement: This chapter is adapted from Kevers et al. (2017) [47] with permission from Kurdish Studies. Reference: R. Kevers, P. Rober and L. De Haene, 'The role of collective identifications in family processes of post-trauma reconstruction: An exploratory study with Kurdish refugee families and their diasporic community'. *Kurdish Studies*, 5 (2017), 107–133.

This strong interconnection of individual and collective meaning may lead us to question how collective identifications are at play in individual processes of post-trauma reconstruction. For example, how will somebody who was persecuted because of their religious and cultural affiliation relate to these aspects of collective identity in the aftermath of conflict and forced migration? Will collective identifications be mobilized as resources in restoring continuity, meaning, and connectedness – taking into account that precisely these collective identifications were sometimes the central target of oppression and persecution? In this chapter, we take this explorative question as our point of departure. Drawing upon social identity theory [12–14], we use the notion of *collective identifications* in referring to practices that derive from individuals' connectedness to particular cultural, ethnic, religious, and/or political groups. Concretely, these collective identifications[1] may be expressed through, for example, the adherence to particular religious beliefs or rituals, frequent attendance at community events or political manifestations, or the transmission of cultural or ideological narratives [15, 16]. In particular, the potential role of collective identifications in individual and family processes of post-trauma reconstruction is at the heart of this chapter's interest. Drawing on the findings of a multiple case study with Kurdish refugee families, we analyze how collective identifications are mobilized within family relationships, exploring how the interconnection of individual and collective levels of meaning is at play in Kurdish refugee families' attempts to rebuild continuity, connectedness, and meaning in their personal and familial history of persecution and exile. Before presenting a thematic analysis of empirical data collected throughout research conversations with Kurdish refugee family members, we provide an overview of existing scholarship on the role of collective identifications in processes of post-trauma reconstruction.

Cultural Identification, Political Mobilization, and Post-trauma Reconstruction: A Brief Overview of Existing Scholarly Work

On the one hand, collective identities (such as ethnicity or religious affiliation) are among the contributing causes of conflict worldwide, leading to large-scale forced migration. In refugee settlements and receiving countries, reinforced notions of collective identity may invoke further conflict among refugee populations and between diasporic groups and other communities. For example, a study with young Congolese refugees resettled in neighboring countries documented that their post-flight reinforced notion of 'Congoleseness' created conflict with the original citizens [17]. Hegemonic narratives about conflicts (for example, in school textbooks) may reinforce essentialist views of collective identities and lead to neat ethnic categorizations aligned with guilt on one hand and victimhood on the other hand. For example, in the context of colonial Rwanda, the divisive structure of education consolidated fixed Hutu and Tutsi identities, which eventually contributed to genocidal conflict. Although Rwandan refugees defied this essentialist perception of ethnicity, they were often viewed as genocidaires [18]. As a result, conflicts rooted in such essentialist readings of

---

[1] Inspired by Auger's metasynthesis on cultural continuity [15], we conceptualize collective identifications as dynamic, multiple, subjective, and relational: (a) they are inclined to change (e.g., influenced by the process of acculturation in the host society or a child's developmental stage); (b) they are not restricted to one identity (e.g., someone may connect to both Syrian nationality and Kurdish ethnicity); (c) they are unique to each individual and invested with subjective meanings, feelings, and perceptions; (d) at the same time they are negotiated within families and communities and gain a certain social status within societies.

collective identities may lead to the fragmentation of families and communities across several generations.

On the other hand, a range of studies in different refugee communities explore the role of collective identifications in processes of post-trauma reconstruction. In what follows, we provide an overview of existing scholarship on this topic, including both qualitative and quantitative studies. Indeed, a growing body of research illuminates the different roles that cultural and political identifications can fulfil in individuals and families coping with lived experiences of traumatization and exile, indicating the intricate interconnections between collective and personal dimensions of meaning imbuing collective identifications in life histories of collective violence and exile. In the following brief exploration of this existing body of scholarly work, we first discuss studies that explore the role of collective identifications in individual coping and meaning-making. Second, we briefly address some important findings of quantitative studies that look at the connection of collective identifications with parameters of mental health and wellbeing. Third, we point to previous research that explores the transmission of collective identifications in family relationships, upon which we further elaborate with our own case study.

Studies have repeatedly documented how cultural and political identifications may provide refugees with a means to *transform individual experiences of trauma into solidarity and empathy* in the social-political realm. In general, research shows that refugees' concerns are not restricted to an inward direction or a preoccupation with their individual mental health. Rather, survivors of collective violence frame their memories and hopes for the future on a macro scale of political change, emphasizing the importance of communal bonds, social values, and cultural connectedness [10]. Here, the embeddedness of personal life stories within social, political, and cultural contexts underpins this focus on social justice and community cohesion, as was shown in studies with different refugee communities. For example, Cameroonian asylum seekers' memory work, which involved the intertwining of official historical narratives, shared experiences of political involvement in their home country, and personal memories, was shown to reinforce social bonds within the diasporic community [19]. A study with Tamil refugees in Norway analyzed how cultural-political narratives and symbolism related to heroes and martyrs provided Tamil refugees with a sense of meaning by promoting their engagement in community service [20]. In another study, it was documented how Rwandese genocide survivors who suffered from feelings of survivor guilt restored meaning by engaging in several commemoration projects and voluntary associations, keeping the memory of their communities' plight alive and assisting other refugees [21].

Further examining the association of collective identifications and post-trauma reconstruction, correlational studies have explored the relation between *collective identifications and parameters of individuals' wellbeing*. For example, Taylor and Usborne emphasized the importance of cultural identity clarity for post-trauma reconstruction [22]. Theoretically and empirically, they demonstrated positive relationships between identity clarity, self-concept clarity, and psychological adjustment among an array of cultural groups and concluded that a clearly defined cultural identity may promote psychological wellbeing in communities that have been exposed to collective trauma. In a study with Syrian refugees in Turkey, Smeekes et al. investigated the role of multiple group memberships and identity continuity for mental health and wellbeing [23]. They found that having multiple group identities before migration served as a protective factor for refugees' wellbeing because it allowed for a sense of continuity in the volatile post-migration context. Yet at the same time it was related to higher levels of depression, because multiple group memberships before migration also implied the possibility of increased experiences of loss when these social ties are disrupted. In a study with Southeast Asian refugees in Canada, Beiser and Hou similarly found a more complex relationship between collective identifications and parameters of mental health [24]. Instead of finding a direct (positive or negative) effect of ethnic identity continuity on depressive affect, they found a significant interaction of ethnic identity with the experience of resettlement stressors: Depending on the stressor, ethnic identity either amplified or buffered the effects on depressive affect. One concrete finding was that, faced with discrimination in the host society, participants who were strongly attached to their ethnic heritage experienced greater distress than persons with weaker ethnic identities, on whom experiences of discrimination appeared to have no impact. Another aspect of collective identifications that has been studied in relation to psychosocial wellbeing is the role of ideological commitment. Although findings on the association between strength of political attitude and psychosocial adjustment are mixed [25], some studies point to the protective role of strong ideological commitment in the mental health of children and youth who have experienced political violence [26, 27]. Further exploring the meaning-making processes behind these correlations between collective identifications and parameters of wellbeing, studies indicated how connecting individual recollections of trauma and hardship to a larger collective narrative of the family and the community enables refugees to deal with experiences of discontinuity and disconnection caused by forced displacement [28]. Here, anchorage in tradition may protect refugees in post-conflict situations from chaos and fragmentation in the wake of violence and atrocity [29].

Increasingly, studies have also focused on the *transmission of collective identifications within family relationships.* Previous studies showed that the intrafamily sharing of personal testimonies interwoven with aspects of family and community history may allow parents to provide their children with a sense of stability and continuity in a context of family separation, cultural change, and exile [29, 30]. A study with Palestinian refugees in Lebanon illustrated that intrafamily transmission of heroic exile narratives combined with a strong focus on community belonging played a cohesive role in families, providing psychosocial support to the younger generations [31]. However, at the same time, the intergenerational transmission of homogenous national and political identifications may leave the second generation feeling ambivalent and 'in-between,' as these constructions might be in tension with their own developing articulations of their diasporic identity [32]. Yet refugee parents may also move along the continuum of cultural continuity and change, dealing flexibly with the transmission of cultural identifications and thereby equipping their children with resources for constructing belonging and participation across homeland and diaspora and across different generations [33]. The present chapter connects to this interest in understanding the role of collective identifications in intrafamily processes of coping with collective trauma, loss, and forced migration. In what follows, we develop an explorative analysis of how Kurdish refugees' coping with a history of persecution and trauma is shaped within the collective identifications that are transmitted in the family. In developing this account, we specifically explore the operating and meaning of cultural and political identifications in parent-child relationships through addressing interconnections between the transmission of collective identifications and post-trauma meaning-making and coping between parents and children.

The Transmission of Collective Identifications in Refugee Families: An Exploratory Study

Fieldwork Context and Method

The thematic analysis presented in this chapter is based on fieldwork conducted between March 2015 and June 2016 with Kurdish refugee families from Turkey and their community organizations located in Belgium. Since the foundation of the Turkish republic in 1923, Turkey's Kurds have been through decades of oppression, war, and uprising. From its inception, the Turkish government tried to deprive Kurds of their ethnic identity by prohibiting them from wearing traditional Kurdish clothing in the cities, banishing the use of the Kurdish language in public spaces, including schools, and giving new Turkish names to Kurdish towns and villages [34]. Indeed, for the Kurds, persecution and exclusion practices have always involved strong cultural oppression. Kurdish resistance against these policies throughout the twentieth century culminated in the foundation of the Kurdistan Workers' Party (PKK) in 1978, whose guerrilla fighters became involved in an armed struggle with the Turkish State in the 1980s and 1990s. Uprooting of citizens, destruction of property, and persecution of Kurdish activists and community leaders led to a large influx of political refugees into the Kurdish diaspora across Western Europe [35]. After several temporary ceasefires and insurgency and counter-insurgency operations, a peace process was launched in early 2013, yet it collapsed in 2015. As a result, Turkey formed the backdrop for an escalation of violence involving extended curfews, military operations, and armed clashes throughout the course of our study.

In order to develop a qualitative understanding of the role of collective identifications in familial processes of coping with trauma and exile, this study combined an ethnographic approach at the community level with in-depth interviews with participants from five Kurdish refugee families. In order to gain an emic understanding [36] of processes of collective identifications at the level of the community at stake, data collection at this level involved open-ended interviews with key figures in different Kurdish institutions and associations and participant observation during community events. Kurdish associations in Belgium are numerous and diverse, yet almost all engage in the organization of cultural (e.g., folkloric dance), political (e.g., demonstrations), and educational (e.g., language classes) activities for diasporic Kurds.

Participant Families

After gaining access to and building trust with some of these Kurdish associations, we were assisted by community leaders and key figures to recruit families for participation in our study. The 5 participating families (10 parents; 17 children) came from different Kurdish villages and towns in their home region of Southeast Turkey and applied for asylum in Belgium after persecution triggered by their affiliation with political or activist groups or their ethnic background as Kurds. The families arrived in Belgium between 2000 and 2012. Three families had one child born in exile; all other children (n = 14) were born in Turkey. Almost all family participants had been granted official refugee status except for some fathers whose asylum applications were still pending because of their connection to the PKK. Postponement of decisions in Kurdish asylum cases is part of a diplomatic strategy not to burden EU-Turkey relations, which also involves governmental surveillance of pro-

Kurdish political activities in several European countries and the continued presence of the PKK on the EU terrorist list [37].

Data Collection

After negotiating informed consent during two or three introductory meetings, consecutive in-depth, semistructured interviews were carried out with each of the five participating families. With the aim of analyzing the role of collective identifications in families' meaning-making and coping with lived experiences of persecution and exile, data collection in each family concretely involved one family interview (with both parents and children; mostly spread over two or three sessions) and one parent interview (with both parents) as an integrative part of long-term participant observation during families' daily activities at their homes (e.g., sharing a meal, watching television, playing with the children). Data collection in the participating families turned out to be highly intertwined with ethnographic fieldwork at various community events, given that we regularly, yet mostly inadvertently, ran into family participants at these demonstrations and cultural gatherings. Research conversations with participating families took place at the families' homes and were conducted in close cooperation with professional interpreters who had a Kurdish background and a history of (forced) migration themselves. Interviews with parents and children together aimed to explore families' practices of remembering life preceding migration and their patterns of intrafamily trauma communication [38]. Parent interviews invited the parents' further reflection on the intergenerational transmission of memories related to collective violence and trauma in their family. Prior to commencing the study, approval of the research design was obtained from the university's Ethics Committee.

Data Analysis

Qualitative data analysis of ad verbatim transcripts was conducted in different stages and involved both thematic and dialogic analyses of the interview material [39]. In the context of the current chapter, thematic analysis focused on those codes that were considered particularly relevant in relation to the present research question on collective identifications, involving, for instance, sub-codes on participants' cultural and political meaning-making as well as sub-codes that addressed families' memory practices, given that the latter had been found to contain multiple references to participants' cultural and political identity as Kurds. After scrutinizing all relevant thematic codes, prominent cross-case themes concerning the role of collective identifications in dealing with trauma and exile were identified [40].

The Role of Collective Identifications in Kurdish Refugee Families

In the following sections, interview excerpts illustrate the transmission of cultural and political belonging between parents and children. Thematic analysis documents the intricate interconnectedness of these collective identifications with post-trauma meaning-making and coping in refugee families. In what follows, we subsequently discuss how collective identifications may operate as sources of dealing with cultural bereavement and loss, commemorating trauma, and reversing versus reiterating trauma.

Collective Identifications in Dealing with Loss and Cultural Bereavement

Developing and celebrating elements of collective identifications in the family context appeared to assist participants in soothing the pain of being separated from their homeland and its cultural practices. Although the participating families regularly referred to their home region as a site of trauma where they had endured severe state repression and human rights violations, they especially characterized it as a source of pride, resistance, and social belonging, which they deeply missed and where they hoped to return one day. A mother of two children, who had arrived in Belgium three years prior to the interview, narrated how her grief was related to a persistent longing to go back home:

> It's not easy to adjust to this new life. I keep thinking all the time: 'When will we go and visit our land? When will the time come when we may return for good?'

In parent-child relationships, communication about the homeland often focused on this dream of returning, as explained by one family's father:

> We don't talk about the [difficulties of the] past, but we do look ahead . . . We make plans and fantasize about returning to the homeland, and dream about its gardens, animals, and farmlands and about what we could do there.

In several participating families, parents and children attempted to ease the pain of loss by replicating typical elements of the Kurdish way of life in their new homes. For example, two families reinstalled the traditional practice of pigeon-raising in their host country gardens, and we learned how parents actively engaged their children in this ancient tradition. Pigeon caretaking is a prevalent cultural practice in immigrants from Turkey and has been found to be closely connected to individuals' understandings of their ethnic identity and culture [41]. Therefore, refugee families' involvement in this particular practice of pigeon-keeping may be one of the ways in which they attempted to maintain connections to the homeland by cultivating its cultural customs in the host country. In another family, one son spent much time constructing a wooden chicken coop in the garden, and he told us how his mother wanted him to recreate the atmosphere of life in Kurdistan in order to make life in the host country, far away from their former neighbors, bearable. The mother remained closely in touch with these neighbors in the homeland and even considered it important to have their approval of how she currently furnished her garden and decorated her home. During a family interview, she explained why:

> It is very important [to keep in touch with the neighbors] because we shared what happened in the 1990s. We've been through everything together.

Here, it seems as if the mother, by recreating the homeland environment in and around her new house, also evoked these dark years of armed conflict and persecution that she and her family had endured together with their neighbors. For this mother, the furnishing of her garden was required to be able to feel close to her neighbors, who had played a crucial role in helping her and her family survive the years of war.

Collective identifications also appeared to operate as vehicles of indirect communication about loss and grief in the family, as illustrated by a 12-year-old boy who explained the significance of his saz[2] as follows:

---

[2] The saz (bağlama in Turkish) is a stringed musical instrument often used in Turkish and Kurdish folk music.

> When I play my saz, my mother knows that I'm thinking about my homeland. One time she saw me playing and she told me: 'Soon, we will go back to visit Turkey.' [Silence] I think she wanted to console me.

As seeing her son play the saz encouraged his mother to comfort him or start a conversation about his feelings of missing and grief, this example illustrates how engaging with cultural practices in the family context may equip refugee families with a medium to dwell on lived experiences of loss, homesickness, and cultural bereavement.[3]

In this same family, watching video recordings of traditional Kurdish wedding parties was a recurring family activity. After the son had shared that attending these traditional weddings constituted an important part of their diasporic lives, the mother explained how watching these videotapes reminded her that she was part of a strong community that would carry her through hard times:

> I'm very happy that the Kurdish community is so bound together. We have left so much behind and live in a different country now, yet when Kurds meet among themselves, it's like they are all family. There's a large commitment to each other within our community; you can note that at our cultural festivals and weddings, but also when someone in the community has died: We all get together and support each other. This strong connection makes it easier to be so far away from home.

This example illustrates the driving force of collective belonging. Through its evocation via video images watched in the private context of the family, social connection and trust could be reestablished in the wake of forced displacement from their homeland. However, the right to rely on the commitment and solidarity of other Kurds in the diasporic community for this mother seemed to be dependent on one's efforts to participate in collective agendas, as she made critical remarks about Kurds who were not fully engaged in social engagement within the community:

> Many Kurds who have come here applied for asylum based on the events in our homeland, for example, by referring to family members who have died in the armed struggle. Yet some of them are not doing anything in favor of the Kurds. I always say: 'You're here thanks to our combatants; God will punish you for not doing anything.'

For this mother, conveying her membership of the Kurdish community also seemed to relate to her lived experience of being personally indebted to the Kurdish guerrillas for being able to live freely in the host society, while they had to continue the resistance in dangerous circumstances.

Overall, a strong sense of belonging to a larger collectivity and remaining attached to the homeland seemed to be actively transmitted in all participating families by means of different cultural practices, which served as important sources of dealing with loss and cultural bereavement.

---

[3] The term 'cultural bereavement' was introduced by Eisenbruch, who argued that it should be used to refine the diagnosis of post-traumatic stress disorder in refugees [42]. According to Eisenbruch, cultural bereavement is an existential aspect of the refugee's predicament that involves the loss of social structures, cultural values, and self-identity after abandoning culture and homeland.

Collective Identifications and Commemorating Trauma

Other cases suggested that cultural identifications also played a role in channeling painful memories of collective violence and trauma experienced in the home country. Several respondents mentioned how traditional Kurdish music evoked sad memories related to these personal and collective experiences of trauma, which they considered important not to forget. In fact, some participants were actively involved in learning to sing and play these traditional songs themselves, recording their musical interpretations and sharing these on their social media profiles. Here, songs referring to the revolution made participants dwell on their memories, as a 25-year-old daughter explained:

> We Kurds have a lot of revolutionary songs, and in these days [of escalating violence], those songs are very painful. There are many songs about failed love or about the martyrs. They also make me emotional and sad ... When I listen to those songs, I think about my child-hood, about the good things in life, but not always. Sometimes I think about sad moments. By listening to this music, I relive those memories or those events; they remain fresh in my mind.

In family relationships, collective identifications were mobilized by parents to transmit the family's history of persecution and forced displacement to their children. Here, several parents explained how the transmission of elements of Kurdish cultural and political identity within the family enabled them to remind their children of their Kurdish roots, whose historical oppression had been an important reason why they had migrated to Belgium. This was illustrated by the following quote by a mother of two children who herself had suffered under the discriminatory policies and cultural oppression of the Turkish government and several of whose family members had been killed during armed conflict and ethnic cleansing operations:

> The importance that I attach to the transmission of Kurdish identity does not mean that I'm not well integrated, or that I think my children should not integrate ... We know this country and its laws and regulations; we have a good life here. Yet we also want to tell our children: 'Don't forget who you are; don't forget why you are here.' That is very important; it's a kind of lesson you want to pass on to your children.

Actively reminding her children of their Kurdish roots enabled this mother to make them remember their collective history of marginalization, repressive assimilation, and forced displacement, while at the same time reversing this historical oppression by emphasizing instead of repressing Kurdish identifications in the family context. For this mother, claiming a sense of intergenerational cultural continuity enabled her to preserve dignity and resist assimilation. Indeed, when Kurdishness is not recognized as a legitimate national identity, the transgenerational transmission of Kurdish cultural identification and practices becomes a form of resistance against the denial and oppression of Kurdish ethnic or national identity [33]. In several participating families, this role of collective identification in commemorating traumatization in exile could be found, and Kurdish political and cultural identifications appeared to be symbolized and transmitted by different means. For example, the father of the aforementioned family referred to the symbolic force of the colors of the Kurdish flag:

> These colors are the reason why we are here. They symbolize our honor, our culture, our history . . . Other people might say, 'Those are just the colors green, yellow, and red,' but they mean something else to us.

Earlier in that same interview, the father had explained that these colors reminded him of his first encounter with Kurdish activists and their violent persecution when he was a young boy, recounting how the Kurdish colors operated as markers of memory to how his life had become entwined with this resistance. Yet his personal war-related experiences were no topic of conversation in the family; instead, these widely shared colors seemed to function as silent reminders of the family's close commitment to their community's ongoing struggle.

Research encounters with another family were always succeeded by sharing a large Kurdish meal. Always eager to talk about her homemade recipes, the mother of this family once explained what one of her favorite dishes reminded her of:

> We used to prepare this dish at weddings or town meetings, together with all the mothers, grandmothers, and young girls. When we prepare it here at home, we often reminisce about life in our home region. This dish is closely related to Kurdish culture. When the Kurdish guerrillas secretly visited us at night, we served them these dolmas, their favorite dish.

Spending much time on teaching her daughters how to prepare traditional Kurdish food, this mother not only transmitted typical recipes but also made sure they remembered life in their home region, which involved personal encounters with representatives of the Kurdish armed struggle. This may have helped her children understand themselves as members of a cultural and political community they did not cease to be a part of in exile, as well as serving as a reminder of the meaningful role their family had played in the Kurdish resistance.

Overall, the transmission of cultural practices and other important aspects of Kurdish collective identity in family relationships played an important role in parents' and children's commemoration of their collective and familial history of persecution and displacement. Addressing these personal memories of traumatization in the family context was closely interwoven with cultural and political meaning-making.

Collective Identifications in Reversing versus Reiterating Trauma

The mobilization of cultural and political identifications within families also seemed to operate as a means to preserve or restore belief in the possibility of peaceful coexistence, which in many participants had been damaged as a result of confrontations with man-made violence and atrocity. In some families, the PKK's current framework of anticapitalism, ecologism, democratic confederalism, and women's emancipation permeated parents' and children's daily discourse [43]. In these families, PKK-related symbolism (e.g., pictures of martyrs, scarves traditionally worn by Kurdish guerrilla fighters) was omnipresent in the family home, as was also illustrated by one two-year-old child who always greeted us making a peace sign with her fingers, cheerfully saying 'Apo, Apo,' a frequently used nickname for Abdullah Öcalan. Here, clinging to the optimistic project of the Kurdish movement, which promises the possibility of a more equal world, may have provided families with a positive perspective for the future and a means to continue to believe in the benevolence of humanity despite the oppression and persecution they had endured.

In other families, parents expressed hesitation about bringing their children into contact with the ideology and iconography of the Kurdish movement. One father connected his hesitation to the desire to avoid his children's involvement in a repetition of violence:

> I could show my children images of guerrilla fighters on Kurdish television channels, but if I would do so, I might encourage them in that direction, and they may become soldiers in their thoughts and language by the time they turn 14. I experienced the war myself, and I see how bad war is. I want to keep them away from that; I wish them to have a different life. I don't want them to go through the same feelings or experiences as I did.

Concerned about the possibility that his children would only understand the language of violence, this father explained us that he wanted his children to engage in a different kind of resistance in order to reverse the family's history of trauma. With the purpose of instilling in his children a sense of hope and trust in humanity despite ongoing conflict, he turned to ancient cultural legends and myths as important sources of inspiration:

> When I tell these ancient legends to my children, I can imagine or even feel how people used to live at that time . . . Thousands of years ago, private property did not yet exist; everything was shared by the collective . . . Repression did not yet exist; all people were equal. Those stories and myths hold important lessons for today. That is why I consider it important to tell my children.

Tracing the possibility of a world of peaceful coexistence without oppression in Kurdish mythology and folklore, this father employed cultural identification as a means to transmit moral values of equality and solidarity to his children. Furthermore, he encouraged them to read a lot themselves, considering these attempts to gain extended knowledge and understanding of Kurdish culture and distant history as a means to reverse the deliberate negation of his people's heritage in Turkey.

Relatedly, another father explained that he preferred to transmit cultural identifications clearly separated from his personal history of persecution, as he feared that his children's excessive involvement with the Kurds' history of oppression could possibly hamper fruitful adjustment in the host society:

> We attach considerable importance to the transmission of our cultural habits and practices, but we do not transmit the difficult experiences we have been through because we want to avoid that our children would be concerned about these issues. It's very important that they are integrated here, and if we excessively transmit our history, it will hinder their successful integration.

Children's successful integration into the host society was an important concern for parents and seemed to imply high educational aspirations and expectations of positive intergroup relations. Herein, the transmission of collective identifications, such as elements of PKK ideology combined with aspects of the Kurds' distant history, were employed by parents to nourish their children's belief and involvement in the creation of a better world. A mother of two children, who herself had lost several family members in the armed conflict, explained it as follows:

> We teach our children that people of different color and ethnicity exist. We teach them to be in solidarity with the rest of the world . . . The Kurdish people, the people from Mesopotamia, they have always protected and helped each other when there was a war. Following the Kurdistan Workers' Party, we are convinced that the [nationalist] belief of 'one people, one

community' is not the right way. Rather, we transmit values of respect and solidarity to our children, speaking as Kurds who are descendants from the people of Mesopotamia, where there have always been different colors, religions, and ethnic groups.

The transmission of political ideologies and cultural stories in refugee families appeared to operate as an important source of reversing traumatization by restoring hope for a better future. At the same time, our respondents repeatedly voiced the suffering that was caused by their perception of the deliberate silencing of the Kurdish people's predicament by European institutions. In response to the long-lasting curfews and security operations in Turkey at the end of 2015, one 23-year-old son sent us a text message:

No Turkish or European television channel, no Turkish nor European political party, no European newspaper is paying attention to it. Supposedly it is terrorists that are killed, but unfortunately that is not true. It's a massacre.

Several respondents expressed their sense of the disrespect shown by Belgian institutions through the perceived criminalization of Kurds as potential terrorists [37]. For instance, a father of two adolescents, who was actively engaged in the Kurdish cultural center of the city where he lived, shared his indignation about the unequal treatment of diasporic Turks and Kurds during a parent interview:

Our community associations are put under pressure; they are closely monitored. In our city, there is a large Turkish community, and the municipality's elected representatives don't want to lose their voters. For that reason, they don't treat us equally; they are not impartial. Once, the city council invited all nonprofit associations in town to a meeting. Fifty associations were invited, except us, the Kurdish association: We did not receive an invitation. We are brushed aside and perceived as 'different.'

Within this tense sociopolitical context, participating parents also expressed concerns that their children's strong involvement with their collective identity as Kurds might reiterate trauma by inciting racist sentiments and stirring up intergroup tensions with nationalist Turks, for example in the school setting. They explained that this had influenced the transmission of the collective predicament of the Kurdish people in family relations, which can be illustrated by the following quote from an 18-year-old daughter during a family interview:

When I was younger, I used to tell my classmates that there is a war in Kurdistan, but as I grew older, my parents started to talk to me more often, and they told me I had to be careful with what I said at school; that bad things could happen.

Her father further clarified this during the parent interview:

Of course we talk about our history, about who we are and where we come from, but I don't always tell them about what the Turkish regime did to the Kurds. Why? In order to protect my children: I don't want them to have their minds on politics too soon, and I want to avoid them becoming racists.

These concerns about peaceful coexistence in the host society appeared to impact on participating families' lives in the private contexts of their homes as well, as illustrated by the following excerpt of a dialogue between mother and daughter, taken from one of our interviews:

Mother: Most people in our neighborhood don't know we are real Kurds; if they would know, they would—

Daughter [interrupting her mother]: Yes, they know we are Kurds, but we will never really talk about our political views. For example, in our house you will see objects with traditional designs, but you will never find political symbols. In our previous house, we had a portrait of Abdullah Öcalan and a PKK flag. But in this house, we did not put them, because we don't want a fight.

This family's sons, in contrast, did not want to give in to this implicit censorship and recounted anecdotes of how they had attempted to defend the honor of their family when Turkish neighbors had provoked the situation.

Overall, it seemed that cultural and political identifications allowed parents and children to reverse trauma by retaining a hopeful perspective on social relationships and the future of humanity, despite their history of trauma and exile. At the same time, these same elements of Kurdish identity risked fostering resentment and causing polarization in the host society's current context of negative representations of Kurdish activism and interethnic tensions between Turks and Kurds. This led most participants to carefully consider the public as well as the private expressions of these identifications. Here, participants' experience of again having to worry about the consequences of asserting cultural continuity indicates the possible role of collective identifications in reiterating trauma-induced fear and restraint.

Discussion

This contribution explored how the transmission of collective identifications in refugee families may operate as a vehicle of post-trauma meaning-making and coping within family relationships. Although previous studies increasingly recognize the potential role of collective identifications in post-trauma reconstruction [20, 29], few studies have yet explored how these collective identifications are concretely mobilized in parent-child relationships, taking into account the broader contexts of community and host society. The present study aims to fill this gap by offering a look into the rich variety of practices through which post-trauma coping and meaning-making in Kurdish refugee families is closely connected to the transmission of collective identifications.

A key explorative finding is that there seems to exist a paradoxical tension between the potentially reparative and the perilous role of collective identifications. Despite the important role of collective identifications in families' ways of dealing with loss and cultural bereavement, commemoration of trauma, and reversing their collective and personal history of traumatization, our analysis indicates that these same collective identifications paradoxically turn out to be potential sources of conflict and exclusion, possibly leading to a repetition of previous experiences of marginalization and isolation. In participants' narratives, the coexistence of a supportive and a perilous role of collective identifications is indicated in different ways. For example, it is remarkable how the wish to reverse oppression and assimilation appears to coexist with the fear that pursuing strong collective identifications will hinder fruitful integration into the host society. Concretely, several respondents, both parents and children, related their strong tendency towards cultural continuity (e.g., transmitting Kurdish roots through history, language, or music) to the ongoing struggle of the Kurdish people. Here cultural identifications became instruments of political change, opposing the decades-long negation of Kurdish identity [33, 44]. At the same time, however, several parents conveyed that they were worried that a strong orientation towards collective identifications might lead to new problems in the host society, for example, conflicts with Turkish neighbors or exclusionary practices in schools. Hence, cultural and political identifications also entail the risk of renewed exclusion. Looking for a way out of this paradox, participants told us how they carefully weighed the trade-offs between which collective identifications to transmit and which to withhold (e.g., sharing cultural legends but silencing the history of the armed conflict, or wearing traditional Kurdish clothes but censoring the use of political symbols). Another example of the paradox between reparative and perilous aspects of collective identifications concerns participants' attempts to repair social connectedness in exile. Several respondents told us how they felt indebted to community members (e.g., neighbors who helped them out during wartime, guerrilla fighters who are still involved in the armed struggle) and illustrated how a strong sense of loyalty and collective belonging underpinned (and was strengthened by) their transmission of collective identifications (such as, for example, listening to and singing revolutionary songs). Yet, paradoxically, this strong sense of loyalty also entailed the risk of excluding community members who did not engage as strongly in collective agendas, possibly leading to further fragmentation and alienation within the Kurdish community. This recalls previous research that has emphasized how reinforced notions of collective identity may contribute to the fragmentation of families and communities [17, 18].

In order to understand the full range of meanings underpinning the transmission of collective identifications in refugee families, our exploratory findings indicate the need for a contextual lens that locates the role of these collective identifications within dynamics in refugee families' broader social fabric. Concretely, our study with Kurdish refugee families suggests situating the transmission of cultural and political belonging within the larger social contexts of diasporic community and host society in all three cross-case themes. In the first theme of mobilizing collective identifications in coping with cultural bereavement, participants' narratives about the importance of collective identifications resonated with a strong sense of belonging to and solidarity with their own cultural community. Indeed, intimate family practices of coping with lived experiences of (cultural) loss and grief involved recalling the strong social ties in their homeland, which was subsequently connected to the wish to reinstall these strong connections within the diasporic community of Kurds. In the second theme of commemorating trauma, the transmission of collective identifications allowed families to inscribe their personal history of trauma in the community's collective history of persecution and displacement. Yet refugee families' differential engagement with collective identifications in familial memory practices suggests that the extent to which family members inscribe themselves within the community's collective memory should also be taken into account. What is publicly remembered and forgotten in the diasporic community serves several collective and political interests, and analysis of interview material tentatively indicates how refugees shape the intrafamily exchange of experiences of war and persecution in light of their position in relation to the community's collective plight. For instance, several participating families had members that had been involved in guerrilla activities themselves. Although the transmission of collective identifications conveyed families' ongoing commitment to their community's ongoing struggle, parents sometimes decided to silence personal involvement in community activism and armed resistance. Good reasons behind such decisions could be related to family members' feelings of disillusionment that deviate from the community's collective story that glorifies armed resistance [38, 45]. Also, acculturation demands in the host society for some families resulted in a complex balancing of different loyalties and made parents look for ways to transmit Kurdish identity without hampering children's integration in a host country with other laws and regulations. In the third theme of reversing versus reiterating trauma, the dual collective context of both the diasporic and the broader host community in which cultural and political belonging was transmitted in Kurdish families is particularly evident. In participating families, sharing elements of cultural and political identification was often weighed against possible negative repercussions of this transmission, such as increased tensions with other ethnic communities (i.e., people with a Turkish background) or negative representations of their diasporic community in the host society. Here, a perception of a collective identity invested with negative stereotypes (e.g., Kurds as terrorists) seemed to result in the hesitant transmission of collective identifications in private family contexts. Hence, the transmission of collective identifications should be located within contemporary host society dynamics. Capitalizing on national anxieties, the rise of right-wing populist parties goes hand in hand with coercive assimilation policies towards, in particular, Muslim migrants and refugees, making the public expression of collective identifications increasingly suspicious [46]. There are thus clear barriers, related to larger social dynamics, to the transmission of collective identifications. Therefore, when thinking about the possible role of collective identifications in post-trauma reconstruction, it is important to include the perception of out-group attitudes towards these collective identifications in our reflection [24, 47].

Reflecting on possible clinical implications, this contribution first of all suggests that clinical work with refugee families should involve an explicit interest in cultural, social, and political meanings imbuing refugee family members' lived experiences and interactions. In aiming for such an approach, fully considering the collective identifications that circulate in intimate family practices as potential protective cultural resources in dealing with trauma, loss, and displacement may be an interesting avenue. Here, clinicians may gradually explore, support, and assist in activating these coping strategies in families [48]. Yet at the same time, the current study's findings outline a more complex picture by calling for a further exploration of the paradoxical coexistence of healing and potentially painful aspects of these collective resources. From a contextual perspective, it may be hypothesized that a group's social status in the host society, as well as an individual's perception of out-group attitudes towards the cultural and political groups he/she identifies with, may influence whether the transmission of collective identifications is positively related to processes of reconstruction [24]. Furthermore, it seems pivotal to explore the meaning and position of refugees' collective identifications in pre-migration contexts: was a person's cultural, religious, or ethnic background the central target of oppression, discrimination, and persecution before the flight? In such cases – as was the case for the Kurdish families in our study sample – collective identifications may become politicized, and the underlying risks to the reinforcement or suppression of collective identities in exile (e.g., polarization between and fragmentation within communities) should be taken into account. An important focus for clinicians working with refugee families should therefore be to develop an understanding of the social context in which these collective identifications are employed and to be aware of the potential trade-offs between different individual and collective interests.

This understanding of collective identifications as located within broader social dynamics equally implies an interest in the dynamics of hybridization in family members' collective identifications. In diasporic life, family members will engage in an active, dynamic negotiation of cultural belonging, in which collective identifications may shift across developmental phases and are differentially mobilized within particular social contexts [33]. In the clinical encounter, therapeutic dialogue may invite family members' lived experiences and meaning-making on collective identifications in self and family members. Here, parents and children may find a conversational space to express their experiences of shaping collective and cultural belonging in navigating home, school, peer, and communal fabrics and in relation to family relationships, family migration and traumatic history, developmental transitions, or social dynamics in host society spaces. For example, parents may be invited to account for how their emphasis on preventing their children from expressing strong Kurdish affiliation is imbued by their profound wish not to hinder their integration. Or the therapeutic dialogue may create a joint understanding of how children express loyalty to their parents and their communal history of traumatization by emphasizing certain aspects of collective identification (e.g., language, music). In doing so, the clinical encounter centrally opens a dialogical space where therapist and family members explore how collective identifications are mobilized and negotiated within family relationships and serve as important resources in post-trauma coping and meaning-making.

Conclusion

This contribution shows that post-trauma reconstruction is shaped within the collective identifications that are transmitted in refugee families. These collective identifications can be resources in dealing with loss and cultural bereavement, remembering trauma, and reversing the collective and personal history of traumatization. Our explorative findings thereby support a perspective on post-trauma coping and meaning-making that involves relational, cultural, and political dimensions, developing in interactional contexts of family, community, and society [11]. Future research could further explore the paradox between reparative and perilous aspects of collective identifications in refugee families' practices of post-trauma reconstruction, locating such inquiry within the situatedness of these practices in the larger contexts of the diasporic community and host society.

References

1. L. De Haene, H. Grietens and K. Verschueren, From symptom to context: Review of the literature of refugee children's mental health. *Hellenic Journal of Psychology*, 4(3) (2007), 233–256.

2. J. Walter and J. Bala, Where meanings, sorrow, and hope have a resident permit: Treatment of families and children. In J. P. Wilson and B. Drozdek, eds., *Broken Spirits: The Treatment of Traumatized Asylum Seekers, Refugees, War and Torture Victims* (New York: Brunner-Routledge, 2004), pp. 487–519.

3. D. Silove, The ADAPT model: A conceptual framework for mental health and psychosocial programming in post-conflict settings. *Intervention*, 11(3) (2013), 237–248.

4. J. L. Herman, *Trauma and Recovery: The Aftermath of Violence – From Domestic Abuse to Political Terror* (New York: Basic Books, 1992).

5. I. Derluyn, S. Vindevogel and L. De Haene, Toward a relational understanding of the reintegration and rehabilitation processes of former child soldiers. *Journal of Aggression, Maltreatment & Trauma*, 22(8) (2013), 869–886.

6. I. A. Kira, A. Ahmed, F. Wasim, V. Mahmoud, J. Colrain and D. Rai, Group therapy for refugees and torture survivors: Treatment model innovations. *International Journal of Group Psychotherapy*, 62(1) (2012), 69–88.

7. C. Rousseau, Les réfugiés à notre porte: Violence organisée et souffrance sociale. *Criminologie*, 33(1) (2000), 185–201.

8. R. Beneduce, Traumatic pasts and the historical imagination: Symptoms of loss, postcolonial suffering, and counter-memories

among African migrants. *Transcultural Psychiatry*, 53(3) (2016), 261–285.

9. C. Zarowsky, Writing trauma: Emotion, ethnography, and the politics of suffering among Somali returnees in Ethiopia. *Culture, Medicine & Psychiatry*, 28(2) (2004), 189–209.

10. M. Brough, R. Schweitzer, J. Shakespeare-Finch, L. Vromans and J. King, Unpacking the micro-macro nexus: Narratives of suffering and hope among refugees from Burma recently settled in Australia. *Journal of Refugee Studies*, 26(2) (2013), 207–225.

11. R. Kevers, I. Derluyn, P. Rober and L. De Haene. Remembering collective violence: Broadening the notion of traumatic memory in post-conflict rehabilitation. *Culture, Medicine & Psychiatry*, 40(4) (2016), 620–640.

12. B. Simon, M. Loewy, S. Stürmer, U. Weber, C. Kampmeier, P. Freytag et al., Collective identity and social movement participation. *Journal of Personality and Social Psychology*, 74(3) (1998), 646–658.

13. H. Tajfel, *Human Groups and Social Categories: Studies in Social Psychology* (Cambridge, UK: Cambridge University Press, 1981).

14. J. C. Turner, M. A. Hogg, P. J. Oakes, S. D. Reicher and M. S. Wetherell, *Rediscovering the Social Group: A Self-Categorization Theory* (Oxford: Basil Blackwell, 1987).

15. M. D. Auger, Cultural continuity as a determinant of indigenous peoples' health: A metasynthesis of qualitative research in Canada and the United States. *The International Indigenous Policy Journal*, 7(4) (2016), 3.

16. S. Groen, A. Richters, C. Laban and W. Devillé, Cultural identity among Afghan and Iraqi traumatized refugees: Towards a conceptual framework for mental health care professionals. *Culture, Medicine & Psychiatry*, 42(1) (2018). 69–91.

17. C. R. Clark, *Borders of Everyday Life: Congolese Young People's Political Identification in Contexts of Conflict-Induced Displacement* (HiCN Working Papers No. 38) (Households in Conflict Network, 2008).

18. E. King, Educating for conflict or peace: Challenges and dilemmas in post-conflict Rwanda. *International Journal*, 60(4) (2005), 904–918.

19. E. Pineteh, Memories of home and exile: Narratives of Cameroonian asylum seekers in Johannesburg. *Journal of Intercultural Studies*, 26(4) (2005), 379–399.

20. E. Guribye, Sacrifice as coping: A case study of the cultural-political framing of traumatic experiences among Eelam Tamils in Norway. *Journal of Refugee Studies*, 24(2) (2011), 376–389.

21. E. Bourgeois-Guérin and C. Rousseau, La survie comme don: Réflexions entourant les enjeux de la vie suite au genocide chez des hommes rwandais. *L'Autre*, 15(1) (2014), 55–63.

22. D. M. Taylor and E. Usborne, When I know who 'we' are, I can be 'me': The primary role of cultural identity clarity for psychological well-being. *Transcultural Psychiatry*, 47(1) (2010), 93–111.

23. A. Smeekes, M. Verkuyten, E. Çelebi, C. Acartürk and S. Onkun, Social identity continuity and mental health among Syrian refugees in Turkey. *Social Psychiatry and Psychiatric Epidemiology*, 52(10) (2017). 1317–1324.

24. M. N. Beiser and F. Hou. Ethnic identity, resettlement stress and depressive affect among Southeast Asian refugees in Canada. *Social Science & Medicine*, 63(1) (2006), 137–150.

25. M. Shamai and S. Kimhi, Exposure to threat of war and terror, political attitudes, stress, and life satisfaction among teenagers in Israel. *Journal of Adolescence*, 29(2) (2006), 165–176.

26. P. Kanagaratnam, M. Raundalen and A. Asbjørnsen, Ideological commitment and post-traumatic stress in former Tamil child soldiers. *Scandinavian Journal of Psychology*, 46(6) (2005), 511–520.

27. R. Punamäki, Can ideological commitment protect children's psychosocial well-being

in situations of political violence? *Child Development*, 67(1) (1996), 55–69.

28. R. Ramsden and D. Ridge, 'It was the most beautiful country I have ever seen': The role of Somali narratives in adapting to a new country. *Journal of Refugee Studies*, 26(2) (2013), 226–246.

29. A. Mekki-Berrada and C. Rousseau, Tradition, quête de sens et expériences traumatiques vécues par les réfugiés algériens installés à Montréal. *L'Autre*, 12 (1) (2011), 68–76.

30. K. Bek-Pedersen and E. Montgomery, Narratives of the past and present: Young refugees' construction of a family identity in exile. *Journal of Refugee Studies*, 19(1) (2006), 94–112.

31. J. Chaib and T. Baubet, La transmission du récit et son héritage chez une famille Palestinienne réfugiée à Chatila. *L'Autre*, 16(1) (2015), 17–27.

32. E. Mavroudi, Learning to be Palestinian in Athens: Constructing national identities in diaspora. *Global Networks*, 7(4) (2007), 392–411.

33. U. Erel, Kurdish migrant mothers in London enacting citizenship. *Citizenship Studies*, 17(8) (2013), 970–984.

34. D. McDowall, *A Modern History of the Kurds* (New York: I. B. Tauris & Co Ltd, 2004).

35. M. van Bruinessen, *Transnational Aspects of the Kurdish Question* (Florence: Robert Schuman Centre for Advanced Studies, European University Institute, 2000). https://dspace.library.uu.nl/bitstream/1874/20511/1/bruinessen_00_transnational_aspectsKurds.pdf (accessed January 8, 2019).

36. T. N. Headland, K. L. Pike and M. Harris, *Emics and Etics: The Insider/Outsider Debate* (New York: Sage, 1990).

37. M. Casier, Designated terrorists: The Kurdistan Workers' Party and its struggle to (re)gain political legitimacy. *Mediterranean Politics*, 15(3) (2010), 393–413.

38. R. Kevers, P. Rober, C. Rousseau and L. De Haene, *Silencing or Silent Transmission? An Exploratory Study on Trauma Communication in Kurdish Refugee Families* (manuscript under review, 2016).

39. C. K. Riessman, *Narrative Methods for the Human Sciences* (Thousand Oaks, CA: Sage, 2008).

40. G. W. Ryan and H. R. Bernard, Techniques to identify themes. *Field Methods*, 15(1) (2003), 85–109.

41. C. Jerolmack, Animal practices, ethnicity, and community: The Turkish pigeon handlers of Berlin. *American Sociological Review*, 72(6) (2007), 874–894.

42. M. Eisenbruch, From post-traumatic stress disorder to cultural bereavement: Diagnosis of Southeast Asian refugees. *Social Science & Medicine*, 33(6) (1991), 673–680.

43. G. Yarkin, The ideological transformation of the PKK regarding the political economy of the Kurdish region in Turkey. *Kurdish Studies*, 3(1) (2015), 26–46.

44. J. Keles, The politics of religious and ethnic identity among Kurdish Alevis in the homeland and in diaspora. In K. Omarkhali, ed., *Religious Minorities in Kurdistan: Beyond the Mainstream (Studies in Oriental Religions)* (Wiesbaden: Harrassowitz Verlag, 2014).

45. C. Gunes, Explaining the PKK's mobilization of the Kurds in Turkey: Hegemony, myth and violence. *Ethnopolitics*, 12(3) (2013), 247–267.

46. R. Jaffe-Walter, 'The more we can try to open them up, the better it will be for their integration': Integration and the coercive assimilation of Muslim youth. *Diaspora, Indigenous, and Minority Education*, 11(2) (2017), 63–68.

47. R. Kevers, P. Rober and L. De Haene, The role of collective identifications in family processes of post-trauma reconstruction: An exploratory study with Kurdish refugee families and their diasporic community. *Kurdish Studies*, 5 (2) (2017), 107–133.

48. J. Bala and S. Kramer, Intercultural dimensions in the treatment of traumatized refugee families. *Traumatology*, 16(4) (2010), 153–159.

Forced Separation, Ruptured Kinship and Transnational Family

Ditte Shapiro and Edith Montgomery

Introduction

Family is fundamental to human agency and well-being, while kinship represents the basic social fabric of most societies. Even though family practices and understandings vary across cultures, the notion of family as a unit of parents and children is dominant in western psychological research, international conventions and national policy [1–4]. Forced separation of family members in kinship communities is a central aspect of forced migration because of the widespread killing of civilians, imprisonment and geographical dispersal in war zones and trajectories of flight. Involuntary fragmentation of kinship communities is one of several major disruptions of everyday family life that most refugees experience during flight from war and resettlement in transit and exile countries [1, 2, 5, 6]. Forced migration radically changes the configuration of families and their living conditions, which challenges families to adapt and transform their shared conduct of everyday life in and across local and transnational contexts [2, 7]. Recently, researchers have documented the profound emotional implications of ruptured family ties and established that forced separation represents a major source of distress for refugees re-settling in exile [8, 9]. Involuntary family separation is found to be associated with depression and anxiety in refugee populations [8], while emotional reactions to ruptured ties can have a compounding effect on traumatization following collective violence [5]. Prolonged separation can also be experienced and understood as ambiguous loss, because permanent uncertainty about the safety of family members in war or transit zones makes their physical absence highly present in the everyday lives of refugees in exile [7, 10].

Research has primarily documented the severe mental health consequences of the forced separation of children, parents and spouses, with limited research on involuntary separation from relatives beyond the child-parent relationship. Echoing the dominant focus on the nuclear family unit in much of the western literature, this focus on parent-child separation renders the emotional distress and struggles of refugees related to forced separation from kin invisible to professionals and local citizens in receiving countries. Despite the growing evidence of profound emotional distress following forced separation in refugee populations, personal perspectives of forced migrants on their experiences and the emotional impact of family separation have gained little attention in research [8]. At the same time, scholarly work has shown that concerns related to kin residing in the country of origin are dominant in refugees' everyday life in exile and that reunification with family members is a main priority [1, 2, 7]. These findings indicate the need for empirical studies focusing on transnational ties and the changing everyday life of forced migrants [9].

This chapter explores personal perspectives and local knowledge of Syrian refugee family members in their first one and a half years years of resettlement in Denmark. The analysis offers insights into the lived experience and complex meanings of forced separation during the transition from moving across borders to re-establishing and transforming everyday life in exile [1, 2]. The empirical insight draws on a qualitative study that explores the trajectories of five Syrian families from their escape from armed conflict in retrospect and during their first one and a half years years in exile. The study was based on a practice research approach and inspired by ethnographic methodology [1, 2]. The analysis of this chapter shows that the fragmentation of kinship communities is followed by emotional distress and estranged agency of family members in exile, illustrating how the personal meaning and emotional reactions to involuntary separation are shaped by family practices in the country of origin and socio-political conditions in the host country.

This chapter begins by laying out the theoretical dimensions and methodological basis of the research, followed by a reflection on four main themes in the participants' lived experience of coping with and giving meaning to forced separation in exile. The first theme addresses the fact that forced migration can be followed by ongoing ruptures of kinship communities and living conditions in exile that radically change the composition of refugee families. The second theme focuses on the presence of physically absent relatives, who did not flee the war, in the daily life of Syrian refugees in exile. Experiences of fear, concern and other complex emotional reactions are shaped by the restricted contact with relatives in Syria and social isolation in exile. The third part of the analysis explores the changing conflictuality of daily family life in transnational contexts and how it can be sustained through silence and selective sharing. Finally, a fourth theme documents how refugees in exile are coping with the increased complexity of their family life by transforming their local family practices. In our concluding remarks, we point at the implications of the analysis for policy and rehabilitation practices concerning forced separation from kinship communities.

Theoretical Approach: Complex Everyday Family Living

The chapter draws on subject-theoretical psychology and socio-historical practice theory as part of an ambition to develop a subject-based and dialectical approach to psychological refugee research [1, 2, 11, 12]. Within this analytical perspective, the personal suffering and social struggles following forced migration and separation are situated in historical and political contexts of refugee family practices [13, 14]. The subject-theoretical approach is based on an understanding of human subjectivity as given in the first person [11, 12]. This entails that research on lived experiences and meanings is based on an analysis of multiple personal perspectives on social practice [12, 15]. The analysis draws on a decentred perspective on family life in which family life is conceptualized and explored as social practice [16]. This approach highlights the fact that the reproduction of everyday life by family members is contingent on and shaped by the connections to and separation from other practices [17]. 'Conduct of everyday family life' is a key concept of the analysis that centres on the collective agency of family members in their daily efforts to sustain a shared everyday life by transforming social practices [1, 2, 11, 16, 18]. Family is defined analytically as a conflictual community based on an understanding of conflictuality as a basic feature of human sociality [19]. The different positions of family members, which are related to differences in age, gender, position, responsibility and interests, shape their personal perspective on the shared life [16, 17].

Based on insights into the collective practices of families in Syria, North African countries and asylum centres in Denmark, the notion of relatedness is relevant in analysis of the personal experience and meanings of forced separation [1]. The concept of relatedness is based on numerous ethnographic studies of kinship and represents an understanding of emotional bonds as created and nurtured through shared daily practices rather than a universal and biological given [20, 21]. The exploration of local practices and understandings of relatedness allows for thinking beyond the often-taken-for-granted notion of family as parent-child relationships.

Methodology: Extended Practice Research

The analysis is based on an extended qualitative study that traced the complex trajectories of Syrian families in the process of fleeing armed conflict and sustaining life in North African countries retrospectively and longitudinally from when they applied for asylum through their first year of temporary residence in Denmark [1, 2]. The study found that the co-operation of family members and the possibilities for establishing connections with other refugees and local communities are paramount in the process of adjusting and transforming challenging social-material conditions of everyday life in exile. The study was conducted in the historical context of 2014–15, characterized by an unprecedented number of 65 million forced migrants worldwide, with 1 million seeking safety in Europe [22, 23]. At that time, the war in Syria had caused five million people to flee the country and seven million to be internally displaced [24].

Inspired by the methodology of practice research and ethnographic fieldwork, the first author followed five Syrian families in their everyday life periodically during their first one and a half years as asylum-seeking and refugee families in Denmark [1, 15, 25]. The families were interviewed in co-operation with an Arabic-speaking translator, while participant observation was conducted in asylum centres, temporary housing, local neighbourhoods and schools. The families were randomly selected based on the following criteria: parents with children, who had fled Syria and applied for asylum in Denmark during 2014 and who were housed in two selected asylum centres. The first author approached six families with a translator and an information letter in Arabic. After a dialogue about the study and the current situation of the families respectively, five families agreed to take part in the study.

The study was approved by the Danish Data Protection Agency and conducted according to the 'Ethical Principles of Nordic Psychologists', which implies informed consent of the participants, securing anonymity, and confidentiality [26]. The research process was characterized by recurrent reflections on dilemmas related to studying the lived experience of families in marginal positions [27], for example, on how to access and leave the field in an ethical manner and on the potentially fruitful and harmful implications of taking part in the project as a family. The empirical material consisted of detailed field notes from participant observation and recurrent semi-structured interviews with parents and children. The interviews were transcribed verbatim and analysed thematically. This thematic analysis included a dialectical engagement with field notes, theory and other relevant refugee and migration family research [12].

The participants of the study included 3 married couples, 2 single mothers and 21 children between the ages of 3 and 19 years. The two single mothers had lost their husbands in the armed conflict in Syria. Four of the families were Arabic and one Kurdish. The families came from different regional capitals of Syria and represented the middle class in socio-economic terms [28]. The families had fled Syria in the second part of 2012 while the war formed a direct threat to their lives and after having lost several close relatives [1]. The present analysis is based on the accounts of four women and a male adolescent whose personal perspectives provide insight into the complex phenomena of forced separation following collective violence and forced migration:

> **Fatima** is 42 years old and her husband was killed in the war. She fled to Denmark with her 3 children and her 40-year-old nephew **Ahmed**, his 32-year-old wife **Aisha** and their 4 children. **Mohammed** is 19 years old and the oldest son of Fatima. **Reem** is 37 years old and fled to Denmark with her husband and their 5 children. Thirty-six-year-old **Nour** fled to Denmark with her husband, their 3 children and a 12-year-old nephew. They are all separated from close relatives; parents, siblings, uncles, aunts and cousins who live in encamped areas of Syria.

Lived Experience of Involuntary Separation and Transnational Family Practices

The lived experience of forced separation from close relatives stood out as a central aspect in the qualitative analysis of the everyday lives of Syrian families in exile [1, 2], documenting the frequency and intensity of emotional distress related to involuntary separation that fundamentally impacts the well-being and agency of family members and hereby confirming previous findings on severe emotional distress invoked by forced separation [5, 8, 9]. The centrality of forced separation in the everyday life of refugees is investigated by focusing on the following aspects: continuing ruptures of family ties and isolation in exile, transnational family living and difficult emotions, sustaining transnational family ties through silence and selective sharing, and coping with forced separation by transforming local family practices.

Continuing Ruptures of Family Ties and Isolation in Exile

We know that families are fragmented in war zones due to collective violence such as imprisonment, torture and the disappearance and killings of civilians. In the acute phase of seeking safety and the demanding process of crossing borders illegally, families are separated involuntarily while others disappear, for example, in the pursuit of crossing the Mediterranean Sea. Many refugees witness ongoing war and suffer from the recurrent loss of family members in their country of origin, even after arriving in receiving countries. However, it is less widely acknowledged that forced separation from family members in some cases continues in exile. Refugee communities are involuntarily scattered due to bureaucratic processes, for example, moving asylum-seeking families between asylum centres [29] and geographical dispersal laws based on political intentions to integrate refugees through placement in provincial towns [2–4].

The experience of Fatima is an example of how the disruption of family bonds is continuing in exile [2]. In the process of reaching safety in Europe, Fatima expected to suffer less after arriving in a safe country. When her oldest son Mohammed was 15 years old, he was imprisoned for demonstrating against the regime. Mohammed was tortured and released after four months. Shortly afterwards, a sniper shot Fatima's husband, who is Mohammed's father, on his way home from work. After six months in exile, Fatima said:

> We thought that we would experience less suffering when we came here. We were suffering in Syria and it seems that we are also going to suffer here. It is two different ways of suffering. There I at least had somebody to talk with. That is important.

When Fatima's husband was killed and their neighbourhood was invaded, Fatima fled Syria with her 3 children, her 40-year-old nephew Ahmed, his wife Aisha and their 4 children. Ahmed took on the responsibility for Fatima and her children. In Libya, the extended family shared a collective everyday life under strenuous conditions as illegal immigrants for almost two years. When the civil war broke out in Libya, they survived crossing the Mediterranean Sea together, led by people-traffickers. When they arrived in Denmark, they lived as a kinship community among other Syrian refugees in asylum centres. When the family was granted a temporary residence permit, they were placed in different municipalities in two separate parts of the country [1, 2]. Fatima and her children were separated from Ahmed, Aisha and their four children, to whom they felt closely related after having shared a collective everyday life and surviving the flight from Syria together. The separated families were unable to move closer to each other due to a dispersal law and integration programme in Denmark that obliges refugees to stay in the same municipality for three years [4].

This involuntary separation came as a shock to everyone in the kinship community. Mohammed and his brother suffered greatly from the separation due to the strong sense of relatedness to Ahmed that had grown out of living and working together while Ahmed was supporting them as a father:

> He is like a father to us.

Fatima linked her experience of aggravated suffering following the unexpected separation in exile to the fact that she was conducting an isolated everyday life for the first time in her life. When Fatima got married, she moved from her childhood home to the house of her in-laws. For 15 years she lived as part of an extended family community and shared the care of the children with her husband, mother-in-law, aunts and uncles.

In Denmark, Fatima was housed with her children in a city where they were not welcomed or supported by local communities. As a single mother, having lost her husband and being separated from her in-laws and extended family, Fatima struggled to re-establish and transform her conduct of everyday life in co-operation with her children. Mohammed, who had turned 19, changed his participation in the family based on his new position as the oldest male of the household. He took on new responsibilities, like handling bills and seeking help from neighbours to read official letters from the municipality and other authorities.

Previous studies have established that re-settling in exile entails multiple loss of resources, like network, language, knowledge and money, and coping with daily stressors, like language barriers, poverty, isolation and discrimination [30–32]. Fatima had to deal with these great challenges and the loss of her husband as the only adult in a dramatically altered family configuration. The multiple ruptures demanded that she transformed the daily practices of the fragmented family life and that she adapted her self-understanding after being separated from the geographically scattered kinship community. As exemplified by Fatima's account, she suffered greatly from being isolated as the single mother and sole adult in the household. The emotional distress following her losses and the new demands, changed conditions and isolation made her doubt whether fleeing from Syria had been the right choice. Her current living situation is dominated by fundamental doubts and uncertainty about the future which rest a dilemma. Fatima is aware that returning to Syria would be life-threatening and it would be extremely difficult to provide for her children as a single mother, but at the same time she finds her everyday life in exile strenuous and emotionally unbearable.

This case exemplifies how ruptures of kinship can continue in exile even after the dire process of moving geographically across borders is completed. The analysis illustrates how refugees can suffer from a nexus of prior and present losses in their conduct of everyday life struggling with difficult living conditions in exile [1, 2, 31, 32]. Furthermore, the involuntary separation from kin in exile represents a loss of fundamental social support that might reactivate the stressful emotional reactions related to pre-migration losses, for example, of close family members, which can be traumatic [5].

All of the parents in the five Syrian families described a sense of loneliness after being housed as nuclear families in different local neighbourhoods with temporary residence permits in Denmark [1]. A few studies have documented how forced migration often entails a changed configuration of families into nuclear family households, which reflects the dominant understanding of family as 'parents and children' in resettlement programmes, housing and reunification policies [4, 32]. Forced migration is thus followed by a process of being shaped and housed as a nuclear family, even though many refugees are used to living as part of an extended family community in their country of origin. With the nuclear family as the standard model of western policy, the cultural variations in family practices are overlooked and the emotional distress and practical challenges following family separation is not acknowledged by authorities and professionals.

Aisha's account exemplifies the common cultural practice of collective family living in Syria [33]. When Aisha was separated from Fatima and housed with her own husband Ahmed and their four children, she experienced that the continuing ruptures of kinship ties had radically changed the configuration of the family. She said:

> We are not used to live without other people in the house. [. . .] Suddenly the apartment was so empty. [. . .] If we were in Syria, the whole family would have been around us. Then uncles, aunts and everybody would have been around us. But here we are only my husband and I. So the children have to learn from him or me. If they were in Syria they could have learnt from other members of the family.

Aisha points to the fact that the continuing ruptures of family ties and being housed as a nuclear family mean that they have to conduct their everyday family life with fewer human resources available. In Syria, they shared the care of the children with their parents and siblings as part of a kinship community. The altered family configuration entails that parents and children transform their everyday caring practices in exile.

The experience of Reem represents yet another example of the personal meaning of changed family configuration in the process of forced separation. Reem used to conduct her everyday life in a manner that was tightly knit with the daily routines of her parents and siblings when they lived in a shared building in Syria. She said:

> We saw each other every day. If we didn't, we felt something was missing.

Based on a biological and historically created relatedness, Reem suffered intensely from the involuntary separation from her close relatives after having fled Syria. In the process of re-establishing everyday life in co-operation with her husband and five children in a small Danish town, Reem had not been able to get access to local contexts beyond the language school. As a result of that, she and her children and her husband did not participate in any local communities and therefore did not exchange any informal social support, which they really missed. Reem described how their isolated conduct of everyday life affected her:

> It affects me a lot that I don't have family. I can't describe the feeling. But because I do not have family here . . . I think about it a lot, that I don't have anybody. And will it ever get better? [. . .] Some days I do not feel like getting out of the house. I feel strangled. I am under great pressure.

The separation from her parents and siblings, the social isolation and the fact that her husband suffered from chronic pain, which was very stressful, made Reem feel lonely. Furthermore, Reem stood alone with the primary responsibility for sustaining the daily practices of housekeeping and care of the five children. She was distressed and felt power-less, which challenged her hope of improving her everyday family life in the near future. This example illustrates a nexus of forced separation, local isolation, emotional distress and restricted agency in exile [1, 17]. As illustrated in the previous section, the dynamics in the family related to the nexus of forced separation and lacking social support in exile might also be shaped by potentially traumatic pre-migration loss [5].

Women like Fatima, Aisha, Nour and Reem have no prior experience of living with their children and husbands in separated households without being part of a local kinship community on a daily basis, as they did after being granted refugee status in Denmark. Studies have showed how forcibly migrated families draw on strategies that they developed in their home countries and during transit in camps or neighbouring countries to handle the challenges related to re-establishing life in exile [32]. When family configurations are altered and families are settling in foreign contexts, they have to transform these strategies, for example, by taking part in local communities and building new social networks. The possibilities for refugees to participate in local communities are contingent on, for example, how they are perceived and received by local citizens and the availability of community houses and other local meeting places [1, 4]. The availability of social support is of paramount importance for refugees who are struggling to cope with forced separation from their kinship community and other losses related to forced migration in the complex process of re-establishing and transforming their conduct of everyday life in exile.

Transnational Family Living following Forced Migration and Separation

Geographical separation does not prevent family members from sharing everyday life and exchanging care at a distance [21, 34, 35]. Separation, whether it is voluntary or involuntary, pushes family members to conduct transnational everyday lives that are mediated by information technology in order to maintain their emotional relatedness despite the physical absence. The analytical focus on transnational family life captures the exchanges across borders and the complex processes by which relatives retain and develop a sense of community despite being geographically fragmented [21, 34]. Research that focuses on the transnational orientation of forced migrants and the personal meaning of restricted contact with relatives in the country of origin is limited [36, 37]. The following analysis illustrates how the ongoing war in Syria and the harsh conditions of the everyday lives of relatives in encamped areas represent technologically mediated contexts in the everyday life of exiled families. This transnational family living entails experiences of daily fear and serious concerns for the well-being of family members who live in war zones.

Reem, who fled to Denmark with her husband and five children, exemplifies this point. On a daily basis, Reem feared for the safety of her parents, her siblings and their children, who lived in an encamped neighbourhood in Syria.

> I think a lot about my family in Syria. As soon as something happens, I think: 'What if something happens to them?' It takes up a lot of my attention and energy. I cannot help thinking about how they are doing in Syria.

The constant stream of news about the escalating armed conflict mediated by information technology aggravated Reem's constant grave worry and fear of losing family members.

As another example we turn to Nour, who at the time had lived in Denmark with her husband and four children for one year. She described an intense fear of receiving information about more deaths in her family. This emotional reaction to anticipated loss made her resent answering the phone.

> I really appreciate that my children and husband are here with me. It means a lot. [. . .] But sometimes I walk around for a whole day in fear of an unexpected call. Sometimes I don't feel like answering the phone because I fear what they are going to tell me. [. . .] Not long ago when the neighborhood was encamped, they could not buy food or other basic things to survive. Some were sick and they could not get the treatment that they needed. There are a lot of things that I worry about all day. Sometimes I cannot do the things that I ought to do because of the worries.

Nour's account illustrates that the fear of family members being killed in Syria and getting caught up in imagining worst-case scenarios can be paralyzing and restrict the agency of family members in exile.

Just like Reem's husband, Nour suffered from chronic pain, which is especially common among traumatized refugees [38]. The pain often hindered her participation in the language school which is an obligatory part of the three-year integration programme she was enrolled in [4]. Because of the chronic pain, Nour conducted an everyday life that was even more isolated from local contexts than her husband and children who were attending language school. The analysis of Nour's and Reem's experiences highlights how the interaction between social isolation and chronic pain in the household shapes the personal meaning and emotional impact of forced separation from relatives in Syria. These intense experiences of fear and uncertainty about the life of relatives shows how the armed conflict and the geographically absent family members are highly present in the everyday life of families in exile [7].

Due to the ongoing nature of the armed conflict in Syria and other countries, the fear of losing family members is often verified by checking information about new casualties as part of family interactions [1]. During a 2-day visit to Fatima and her 3 children, she and her 19-year-old son Mohammed shared anecdotes about continually receiving WhatsApp messages and calls with news about relatives who had been killed in the war. Mohammed had recently lost his best friend and a peer cousin, who were both killed. Fatima recounts how she cried in the street on her way to the language school after receiving yet another call. They received these alarming news while they were pursuing their everyday life in physically safe exile contexts.

These examples illustrate how forced migrants in exile have to deal with continuing loss, which can be a central aspect of their complex everyday lives in and across local and transnational contexts. Their experiences of ongoing and multiple losses of relatives are often invisible to local citizens and professionals when the home countries are not perceived as a present context in the everyday life of refugees who conduct a transnational family life [37].

The Syrian family members in exile were not able to sustain a close contact with their relatives in Syria because the Internet connection was often cut off in the encamped neighbourhoods. During a conversation with Fatima and her son Mohammed, the painful experience of being separated from close relatives was addressed. Fatima showed a photograph on her mobile phone of her ageing mother in black clothes and conveyed:

> There is nothing I can do. [...] I cannot recognize my mother because she has grown old. [...] We cannot talk with them. For three months I haven't talked with them. [...] I wish that I could hear my mother's voice. [...] I cried a lot when I saw my mother's photograph.

Fatima's longing for contact with her mother can be understood as an expression of emotional relatedness between an adult daughter and an ageing mother. The three-year-long involuntary separation of Fatima and her mother can also be understood as an example of ambiguous loss, because of the emotional presence of the physically absent mother and the uncertainty about whether the separation represents an irreversible loss [7, 10]. The sense of powerlessness that Fatima expresses in relation to the separation from her mother might be compounded by the dramatically changed living situation and prior and continuing loss in exile, which all together can represent a reiteration of pre-migration traumatic loss.

Sustaining Transnational Family Ties: Silence and Selective Sharing

Sustaining a shared family life by co-creating a transnational conduct of everyday family life may be challenging and changes the dynamics of separated kinship communities. When families are able to sustain their connection and exchange care transnationally through social media, family members who live in exile experience a great contrast. The divergence between living in physically safe contexts of exile and the profound struggles and distress of their relatives who are living in encamped areas evokes difficult emotional reactions [9]. This point is exemplified by the experiences of Fatima. The great divergence between the harsh living conditions of her relatives in Syria and herself were causing her complex emotions.

> It is some strange feelings [...] I am sad. Here I am well, and they are there [...] It is hard to witness their situation. I tell them that I am well and happy. They are not well, which makes me sad. [...] We know their situation and would like to help. But we cannot help them. So that makes us even more sad.

Witnessing the suffering of her family made Fatima sad and aggravated the sense of powerlessness related to being unable to help her family [8]. These emotional reactions were also intermingled with restricted agency, social isolation and suffering following the forced separation from extended family in exile.

Aisha's account represents another example of how the restricted contact is causing complex emotional responses and changing the dynamic in transnational family communities. Like many Syrian refugees in exile, Aisha was only able to talk with her family every 2–3 months due to the restricted Internet connection in the besieged area where her parents and siblings lived. She described how she handled the contrast between her living conditions in exile and the life-threatening situation that her family was facing in Syria.

> I don't tell them much about what happens in our life. [. . .] I don't tell them what we eat. [. . .] We can have fruit while they cannot. [. . .] Once during Ramadan my brother asked me to turn on the camera when we had dinner. [. . .] I just wanted to show him a small part of our dinner, so I showed him olives and yoghurt. And he said, 'Oh, you can have olives and yoghurt. If only I could have that I would make a party.' And he did not see all the other dishes that I had made. It makes me sad that my family are starving.

Aisha's navigation of the increased complexity of the emerging transitional family community illustrates how sustaining transnational family ties involves changed dynamics and considerations in the kinship communities. Aisha tried to take care of her brother by refraining from sharing information or showing him how much food she could provide for her children and husband. She tried to cope with the altered dynamics in the family community and the related sense of guilt by transforming her participation in the mutual exchange of care by being selective and silent about certain aspects of her everyday life in exile.

Fatima described how she managed the fragmented contact with her relatives in Syria by participating in similar ways as Aisha did. When Fatima on rare occasions was able to talk with her family in Syria, she abstained from sharing information about the emotional distress and powerlessness that she experienced following the involuntary separation, social isolation and serious concerns about her relatives. Fatima refrained from sharing information about her emotional reactions to her radically altered everyday life even though she was longing to experience mutual care. Like Aisha, Fatima was selective and silent about central aspects of her life in exile. Fatima intended not to burden her relatives and trouble them with the emotional distress, powerlessness and doubts about the future that characterized her living situation. But the silence about her experience of emotional distress hindered Fatima in exchanging care and thus receiving emotional support from her relatives.

A study of transnational family ties among Sudanese refugees describes the way in which transnational everyday living demands that relatives negotiate tensions related to the interplay of concerns for family in the homeland and striving to build a life in exile [9]. Migration research on transnational family life highlight that the maintenance of contact and connections with relatives across borders are conflictual, just as in family life in geographical proximity [34]. The present analysis shows how the fundamental conflictuality of care practices in family communities is aggravated when families are involuntarily separated and that transnational family living introduces new concerns and increased complexity to family life. The analysis shows how family members in exile are navigating the divergence in living conditions and the related sense of guilt by being selective and silent. These social practices reflect the conflictuality of transnational family life. Furthermore, as expressions of connectedness to kin, these complex practices may prevent family members from engaging in practices of mutual care and solidarity, which might exacerbate the fragmentation of kinship ties following forced separation.

Coping with Forced Separation by Transforming Family Practices

The emotional distress related to involuntary separation from relatives and social isolation in exile make some parents prioritize shared practices in the new household. Based on participant observation and interviews with parents and children, shared dinners were found to represent practices of joy, sharing school experiences and mutual support in coping with the difficult living conditions of exile [1]. Nour and her husband Tarek tried to compensate for the changed configuration of the family due to the separation from their kinship community and lacking local network by transforming their shared family practices in the house.

> We have to create joy and cosiness at home, because our children lack what we had in Syria. We were part of a big family and went to a lot of parties. We gathered and were invited to weddings, engagements and birthdays. We experienced happiness in the company of other people. Here our children are far away from all that. They only have us. So it is our duty to create joy and make sure that they are happy and well.

Based on their past experience of joy and connectedness from participating in celebrations as part of a big kinship community in Syria, Nour and her husband transformed and shaped the social practices of celebrating birthdays and Eid with their children in the exiled household. They perceived the shared practices as vital practices of social support and care for their children in a situation where they found it difficult to access local communities and build local networks.

As a consequence of being isolated from local communities, families conduct their everyday life in isolated ways, thereby social isolation and limited access to social resources might produce an inexpedient centring on the relations of the family members living in the same household [17]. Conducting isolated everyday lives put pressure on the relations of the emerging nuclear families that seems to represent a fragile arrangement of family life when it is isolated from local contexts [1, 36]. In the case of Nour and the other Syrian families, the isolated nature of their present everyday life was undesirable, and all of the parents expressed a wish and a longing to be part of local communities and build new connections. The families suffered from missing the joy related to the shared everyday family life as part of an extended kinship community.

The encounter between refugees and local citizens in exile can be complex due to the language barriers, diverse understandings of neighbourhood and family practices, and prejudices [1, 39, 40]. As a contrasting example to the widespread isolation of refugees in exile [30–32], we turn to Aisha. After a year in Denmark, concern for close relatives in Syria was taking up less of her attention in the complex everyday life that she was conducting in co-operation with her husband Ahmed and their four children. When they moved to the designated municipality after being separated from Fatima and her children, Aisha worried about her family in Syria 'all the time', as she said. After six months in the new neighbourhood, the family conducted a rich everyday family life in and across local arenas. The parents and four children were participating in several different local contexts, such as kindergarten, school, afterschool club, language school and a community house. When the issue of concern for family members in Syria was addressed, Aisha said:

> I don't always think about it. But of course they are always in my consciousness. But we are also busy with our own life.

Aisha and her husband Ahmed highlighted that their introduction, on their first day in the municipality, to the community house that served as a meeting place for refugees and local volunteers was crucial for their opportunities to expand their conduct of everyday life. In the beginning, they visited the community house on a daily basis and participated in diverse social practices which provided them with the social and practical resources that are paramount for re-settling families in exile [30, 31]. The family built a new social network of Syrian refugees, neighbours and volunteers. Their participation in multiple local contexts where the parents and children were met with interest and support enabled them to develop a sense of belonging to the local neighbourhood.

This example illustrates how fear concerning the safety of relatives in war zones is a central aspect of the daily lives of refugee families but one which is changeable when the conduct of everyday family life is expanded through participation in multiple local contexts [1, 17]. Whether a family is isolated locally or met with access to local communities and social support plays a vital role in the experience of emotional distress following forced separation.

Forced Separation, Ruptured Kinship and Transnational Family Life

Prior studies have shown that involuntary separation from family members is a key aspect of forced migration, invoking pervasive distress in the everyday lives of refugees [5]. But research that explores the personal perspectives of refugees and how the impact of family separation is played out in everyday life is limited [8]. By taking the uprooted everyday life of forced displaced families as the point of departure, the analysis explores the personal meanings and lived emotional responses to forced separation in transnational family living, situated in a nexus of destructive historical events and local conditions of everyday life in exile. The analysis provides new insight into the phenomenon of forced separation by tracing the emotional effects of frag-mented kinship beyond the parent-child relationship. The findings point to an under-standing of the personal meaning and emotional impact of forced separation as shaped by practices of relatedness created in collective everyday lives prior to collec-tive violence and the disruption of kinship communities.

The analysis shows that ruptures of family ties continue in exile due to frequent re-locations between asylum centres and geographical dispersal of refugees. Moreover, refu-gees who have fled countries torn by continuing armed conflict must endure ongoing experiences of loss because family members are at risk and sometimes killed due to collective violence in the home country. The understanding of ruptures of family ties as ongoing processes of loss and separation adds to the growing evidence of daily stressors in the everyday lives of refugees as multiple, recurrent and continuing into re settlement [1, 30]. This finding points to a process-based understanding of how disruptions and living conditions undermine the mental health of refugees, which adds complexity to the understanding of increased emotional distress in refugee populations. Thus, the analysis both builds on and contributes to the paradigmatic shift from understanding the sequelae of forced migration as characterized by trauma and vulnerability to focusing on the complex interplay of past and present loss, disruptions, ruptures of family ties and collective agency in changing contexts [7, 8, 30].

Prior research have explored the present absence of family members who are living at a geographical distance [7]. This analysis confirms that forced separation can unfold as a daily present absence of relatives who are trapped in war zones, which is mediated by information technology, fear, uncertainty and open-endedness. By highlighting a paradox between on one hand being exposed to the atrocities of war at a geographical distance through social media and on the other hand experiencing restricted possibilities for staying in touch with relatives, it illustrates how forced separation is a major source of emotional distress. Restricted contact hinders family members from relating actively to the separation by sharing emotional reactions and exchanging care with kin abroad through social media. Refugees in exile are navigating the major differences in living conditions by being selective and silent about aspects of their everyday life in exile, such as meals and emotional distress, and thereby take care of their relatives by not exposing them to their relative wealth and hardship in exile. This illustrates how mutual care practices can be increasingly complex and potentially hinder engagement in practices of solidarity with relatives, which can reinforce the fragmentation of separated kin communities across borders. The discovery that a fundamental sense of powerlessness is related to forced separation from family members who live in encamped areas and war zones confirms the findings of prior research [8]. In addition, the analysis shows that restricted agency related to social isolation in exile seems to aggravate the sense of powerlessness and hopelessness following the involuntary separation and daily fear of suffering more losses of close relatives.

The analysis confirms and adds to existing knowledge by highlighting the emotional and practical aspects of sustaining and transforming everyday family lives that are dramatically altered by forced migration and separation from kinship communities. The emotional distress related to family separation is intertwined with and aggravated by difficult living conditions in exile, such as social isolation. Understanding the emotional reactions to forced separation as an aspect of a changing everyday life in exile invites us to change the dire impact of fragmented kinship by ensuring that refugees have access to supportive and helpful local communities. Through participation in social contexts, displaced and ruptured families can become part of local communities and build a sense of local belonging that potentially mitigates the emotional distress related to forced separation.

Implications for Policy and Practice

Even though most western countries have ratified international conventions on the right to family life and reunification following forced migration, current policies and practices are increasing the risk of being separated and prolonging the separation of family members [4, 8]. In 2016, the Danish government introduced a new protection status for refugees in the Aliens Act, which postpones the right to reunification with spouse and children for three years [41]. The right to reunification of children and parents is threatened, while suffering related to being separated from extended family based on family practices that are more diverse than the standard model of the nuclear family is not reflected in international conventions and national policies. Insight into the grave emotional impact of forced separation underscores the urgency of policy-makers and professionals to take the variation of family practices in refugee populations into account. This chapter provides insight into the altered constellation and complexity of transnational family life that challenges families to transform their daily practices of care in new contexts. This points to the importance of basing social services, interdisciplinary interventions and community support on nuanced understandings of the complex processes of practical challenges and emotional distress in the transnational everyday lives of refugee families [30, 42].

By addressing the challenging social-material conditions that refugees are struggling with and prevent continuing disruptions of social ties in exile, the aggravation of emotional distress related to collective violence and separation can be reduced. If the geographical placement of refugees in exile was based on a more diverse understanding of family than the ethnocentric nuclear family model, efforts of refugee families to cope with forced displacement by co-operating in extended transnational family communities could be supported. By placing new refugees in close proximity to diverse, welcoming communities in exile, receiving countries can support separated families in building new mediating and bridging social networks. The analysis underscores the importance for separated families of being welcomed by members of local communities and representatives of social services, who are guiding new citizens in gaining access to relevant local communities. Being able to participate in and contribute to social practices of support in local communities is crucial for fragmented refugee families, who are often struggling to re-establish and develop their conduct of everyday life in exile. Welcoming local communities can represent a mirror of kinship and operate as vital extended family networks for fragmented families following forced migration.

References

1. D. K. Shapiro, *Familieliv på flugt: Syriske familiers oplevelser af brud og genskabelse af hverdagsliv* (Roskilde: Institut for Mennesker og Teknologi, Roskilde University, 2017).

2. D. K. Shapiro, Disrupted refugee family life: Collective agency and conflictual care. In G. B. Sullivan, J. Cresswell, B. Ellis, M. Morgan and E. Schraube, eds., *Resistance and Renewal in Theoretical Psychology* (Concord: Captus Press, 2017).

3. K. F. Olwig, 'Integration': Migrants and Refugees between Scandinavian Welfare Societies and Family Relations. *Journal of Ethnicity and Migration Studies*, 37(2) (2011), 179–96. www.tandfonline.com/doi/abs/10.1080/136918 3X.2010.521327

4. B. R. Larsen, Becoming part of welfare Scandinavia: Integration through the spatial dispersal of newly arrived refugees. *Journal of Ethnicity and Migration Studies*, (37)(2) 2010, 333–50.

5. C. Rousseau, A. Mekki-Berrada and S. Moreau, Trauma and extended separation from family among Latin American and African refugees in Montreal. *Psychiatry Interpersonal & Biological Process*, 64(1) 2001, 40–59. http://guilfordjournals.com/doi/10.1521/psyc.64.1.40.18238

6. B. Mcdonald-Wilmsen and S. M. Gifford, (2009), *New Issues in Refugee Research: Refugee Resettlement, Family Separation and Australia's Humanitarian Programme* (research paper no. 178).

7. C. Rousseau, M.-C. Rufagari, D. Bagilishya and T. Measham, Remaking family life: Strategies for re-establishing continuity among Congolese refugees during the family reunification process. *Social Science and Medicine*, 59(5) (2004), 1095–108. www.sciencedirect.com.ep.fjernadgang.kb.dk/science/article/pii/S0277953603006993?via%3Dihub

8. A. Miller, J. M. Hess, D. Bybee and J. R. Goodkind, Understanding the mental health consequences of family separation for refugees: Implications for policy and practice. *American Journal of Orthopsychiatry*, 88(1) (2017), 26–37. http://doi.apa.org/getdoi.cfm?doi=10.1037/ort0000272

9. S.-L. Lim, 'Loss of Connections Is Death'. *Journal of Cross Cultural Psychology*, 40(6) (2009), 1028–40. http://journals.sagepub.com/doi/10.1177/0022022109346955

10. P. Boss, Ambiguous loss theory: Challenges for scholars and practitioners. *Family Relations*, 56(2) (2007), 105–11.

11. O. Dreier, Conduct of everyday life: Implications for critical psychology. In S. Højholt, ed., *Psychology and the Conduct of Everyday Life* (New York: Routledge, 2016), pp. 15–33.

12. E. Schraube, Why theory matters: Analytical strategies of critical psychology. *Estudos de Psicologia (Campinas)*, 32(3) (2015), 533–45. www.scielo.br/scielo.php? script=sci_arttext&pid=S0103-166X2015000300533&lng=en&tlng=en

13. C. Højholt, Situated inequality and the conduct of life. In S. Højholt, ed., *Psychology and the Conduct of Everyday Life* (New York: Routledge, 2016), pp. 145–63.

14. D. C. Holland and J. Lave, History in person: An introduction. In D. C. Holland and J. Lave, eds., *History in Person: Enduring Struggles, Contentious Practice, Intimate Identities* (Santa Fe, NM: School of American Research Press, 2001), pp. 3–36.

15. C. Højholt and D. Kousholt, Participant observations of children's communities Exploring subjective aspects of social practice. *Qualitative Research in Psychology*, 11(3) (2014), 316–34. www .tandfonline.com/doi/full/10.1080/147808 87.2014.908989

16. D. Kousholt, Researching family through the everyday lives of children across home and day care in Denmark. *Ethos*, 39(1) (2011), 98–114. http://doi.wiley.com/10 .1111/j.1548–1352.2010.01173.x

17. O. Dreier, *Psychotherapy in Everyday Life* (New York: Cambridge University Press, 2008), p. 333.

18. K. Holzkamp, Conduct of everyday life as a basic concept of critical psychology. In E. Schraube and C. Højholt, eds., *Psychology and the Conduct of Everyday Life* (New York: Routledge, 2016), pp. 65–98.

19. C. Højholt and E. Schraube, Introduction: Toward a psychology of everyday living. In S. Højholt, ed., *Psychology and the Conduct of Everyday Life* (New York: Routledge, 2015), pp. 1–14.

20. J. Carsten, Cultures of relatedness. In J. Carsten, ed., *Cultures of Relatedness: New Approaches to the Study of Kinship*

(Cambridge, UK: Cambridge University Press, 2000), pp. 1–36.

21. J. C. Long, Diasporic families: Cultures of relatedness in migration. *Annals of the American Association of Geographers*, 104 (2) (2014), 243–52. www.tandfonline.com/ doi/abs/10.1080/00045608.2013.857545

22. United Nations High Commisioner for Refugees, (2015), Worldwide displacement hits all time high war persecution increase. www.unhcr.org/new/latest/2015/6/5581938 96/worldwide-displacement-hits-all-time-high-war-persecution-increase

23. T. Gammeltoft-Hansen, *Hvordan løser vi flygtningekrisen?* (How do we solve the refugee crisis?) (Viborg: Informations Forlag Moderne ideer, 2016).

24. United Nations High Commisioner for Refugees, (2017). Syria emergency. www .unhcr.org/syria-emergency.html

25. A. M. Jefferson and L. Huniche, (Re) Searching for persons in practice: Field-based methods for critical psychological practice research. *Qualitative Research in Psychology*, 6(1–2) (2009), 12–27. www.tandfonline.com/doi/ abs/10.1080/14780880902896507

26. S. Brinkmann, The ethics of working with everyday life materials. In S. Brinkmann, *Qualitative Inquiry in Everyday Life* (Los Angeles, CA: Sage, 2012).

27. M. Guillemin and L. Gillam, Ethics, reflexivity, and 'ethically important moments' in research. *Qualitative Inquiry*, 10(2) (2004), 261–80.

28. S. Gallagher, *Contemporary Issues in the Middle East: Making Do in Damascus: Navigating a Generation of Change in Family and Work* (Syracuse, NY: Syracuse University Press, 2012).

29. S. S. Nielsen, M. Norredam, K. L. Christiansen, C. Obel, J. Hilden and A. Krasnik, Mental health among children seeking asylum in Denmark: The effect of length of stay and number of relocations: a cross-sectional study. *BMC Public Health*, 8 (1) (2008), 1–9. http://dx.doi.org/10.1186 /1471–2458-8-293

30. K. E. Miller and A. Rasmussen, The mental health of civilians displaced by armed

conflict: an ecological model of refugee distress. *Epidemiology & Psychiatric Science*, 26(2) (2016), 129–38. www.cambridge.org/core/product/identifier/S2045796016000172/type/journal_article

31. A. S. Betancourt, B. S. Ito, G. M. Lilienthal, N. Agalab and H. Ellis, We left one war and came to another: Resource loss, acculturative stress, and caregiver–child relationships in Somali refugee families. *Cultural Diversity and Ethnic Minority Psychology*, 21(1) (2015), 114–25. http://doi.apa.org/getdoi.cfm?doi=10.1037/a0037538

32. S. M. Weine, E. Levin, L. Hakizimana and G. Dahnweih, How prior social ecologies shape family resilience amongst refugees in US resettlement. In M. Ungar, ed., *The Social Ecology of Resilience: A Handbook of Theory and Practice* (New York: Springer, 2011), pp. 309–23.

33. K. Hadfield, A. Ostrowski and M. Ungar, What can we expect of the mental health and well-being of Syrian refugee children and adolescents in Canada? *Canadian Psychology/Psychologie canadienne*, 58(2) (2017), 194–201. http://doi.apa.org/getdoi.cfm?doi=10.1037/cap0000102

34. L. Baldassar and L. Merla, Introduction: Transnational family caregiving through the lens of circulation. In L. Baldassar and L. Merla, eds., *Transnational Families, Migration and the Circulation of Care: Understanding Mobility and Absence in Family Life* (London: Routledge, 2013), pp. 3–24.

35. S. Weine, N. Muzurovic, Y. Kulauzovic, S. Besic, A. Lezic, A. Mujagic et al., Family consequences of refugee trauma. *Family Process*, 43(2) (2004), 147–60. www.ncbi.nlm.nih.gov/pubmed/15603500

36. S. Weine, Family roles in refugee youth resettlement from a prevention perspective. *Child and Adolescent Psychiatric Clinics of North America*, 17 (3)(2008), 515–32, vii–viii. www.sciencedirect.com/science/article/pii/S1056499308000205

37. O. B. Guribye, Life in exile before and after a crisis in the country of origin. In G. Overland, E. Guribye and B. N. J. Lie, eds., *Nordic Work with Traumatized Refugees: Do We Really Care?* (Cambridge, UK: Cambridge University Press, 2014), pp. 88–101.

38. U. Harlacher, L. Nordin and P. Polatin, Torture survivors' symptom load compared to chronic pain and psychiatric in-patients. *Torture*, 26(2) (2016), 74–84. www.ncbi.nlm.nih.gov/pubmed/27858781

39. E. Montgomery and A. Foldspang, Discrimination, mental problems and social adaptation in young refugees. *European Journal of Public Health*, 18(2) (2007), 156–61. https://academic.oup.com/eurpub/article-lookup/doi/10.1093/eurpub/ckm073

40. B. R. Larsen, Drawing back the curtains: The role of domestic space in the social inclusion and exclusion of refugees in rural Denmark. *Social Analysis*, 55(2) (2011), 142–58. https://search-proquest-com.ep.fjernadgang.kb.dk/docview/892574439/fulltextPDF/C0FE9AF0980F4B49PQ/1?accountid=13607

41. M. C. Bendixen, (2017), Family reunification for refugees. Refugees.dk. http://refugees.dk/en/facts/legislation-and-definitions/family-reunification-for-refugees/

42. T. Measham, J. Guzder, C. Rousseau, L. Pacione, M. Blais-McPherson and L. Nadeau, Refugee children and their families: Supporting psychological well-being and positive adaptation following migration. *Current Problems in Paediatric Adolescent Health Care*, 44(7) (2014), 208–15. http://linkinghub.elsevier.com/retrieve/pii/S1538544214000303

Chapter

6

Family Relationships and Intra-family Expectations in Unaccompanied Young Refugees

Ilse Derluyn and Winny Ang

Unaccompanied Refugee Minors

Worldwide, about 60 million people are currently forcibly displaced [1], of which more than half are children under 18, with a considerable group of them being separated from their parents, guardians or previous caregivers [1]. These "unaccompanied refugee minors" (URMs) are a relatively new group in migration policy. While young people have always migrated, including when separated from their family, this group of unaccompanied refugee minors has mainly been 'discovered' or 'labeled' as a separate group by policy makers since the late 1980s. Official definitions of this group mainly rely on three distinctive elements: being unaccompanied/separated, being a minor and being a refugee/migrant/foreigner.

First, being *unaccompanied* is interpreted in diverse ways: While some, rather strict, definitions refer to the absence of biological/legal parents or legal guardians, other definitions more broadly refer to minors not accompanied by or separated from their legal or previous caregivers [2]. These interpretations are important, as they can imply whether or not a child will become separated from an adult who is indeed a previous caregiver but not the legal parent or guardian [3], or, in contrast, whether sufficient attention will be paid to the early detection of possible abusive situations such as human trafficking [4, 5]. Most unaccompanied young refugees lived with their family before they left home [6], while (some) family members stayed behind in their home country or a third country. Others had already been separated from their families for a long time before their migration journey actually started. Moreover, a supposedly increasing group of unaccompanied youth get separated from their family along the way: They flee their country of origin together with (some) family members, yet get separated during the journey, often being unaware for a long time, or even for ever, whether their parents and/or siblings are still alive. This particular situation of URMs who get separated or orphaned along the migration journey is, of course, evoking particular challenges for their wellbeing and further development. Additionally, for some unaccompanied children, their familial separation is only intended to be temporary, given that they expect to be reunited after a considerable period of time, through procedures of family reunification in the country of arrival, for example. Yet often this separation lasts (much) longer than expected, and the entire process, including the reunification, poses particular challenges for the wellbeing of the child, the parents and eventually the other siblings.

Second, being a *minor* is typically defined as being a child or an adolescent younger than 18 years old [3]. This age limit is not unproblematic [4]: Several countries, including those where UMRs originate from, apply other age limits for adulthood (e.g., 16 or 21 years), and age limits as such do not always correspond with the cultural idea of transition to majority or with individual development processes [3]. In addition, this age limit implies that governments aim to verify the age of those who claim to be under 18 years old, using medical tests (e.g., X-rays of teeth, collarbones or wrists) and/or psychosocial screening measures [2, 8]. Despite being widely applied, the 'objectivity' of these age assessment methods is seriously questioned [9, 10], and their impact on the young refugees' emotional wellbeing is substantial [7]. Most unaccompanied young refugees are between 15 and 18 years old, although there is a considerable group of young children under the age of 10 [11].

Third, being a refugee is interpreted in diverse ways depending on the specific context of where a minor is fleeing from and migrating to. The countries of origin of unaccompanied refugee minors are very diverse and their migration motives are heterogeneous, as studies indicate that adolescents leave their homelands and families for myriad reasons, such as war and collective violence, intra-familial problems, trafficking, economic hardship and poverty [2, 8, 12]. While only a limited proportion of them will be granted recognition as 'refugees' under the Geneva Convention (if they apply) [3], we choose to label them all as 'refugees' given that research has indicated how most of them have felt forced to leave their countries and thus do not regard their departure as a 'voluntary' decision [12]. They felt forced in relation to their migration motives, whereby also intra-familial violence or lack of economic opportunities are considered as circumstances necessitating and justifying the decision to leave and migrate. The decision to leave and its effectuation often come relatively fast, and we have indications that the decision to migrate was often made and even imposed by others, such as family or community members, also indicating the 'forced' character of their migration [13, 14]. Yet we also see here considerable variety, as there are also some young-sters who make the decision to leave entirely on their own, without consulting anyone, and for others, the decision is made after mutual and shared consultation. This process of decision-making can impact young refugees' wellbeing, especially when the decision to leave the country is entirely made by others, particularly parents, and imposed onto the child: The youngster's missing of and longing for their family then can contrast strongly with the (sometimes growing) feelings of being sent away and rejected by the same family members. At the same time they often do not feel entitled to complain, given their 'better' and 'safer' situation in the new country.

Given that URMs are considered as a particularly vulnerable group within the refugee population, because they are migrating as minors and not supported or protected by their parents or guardians, the International Convention on Children's Rights, with its almost worldwide ratification, has inscribed specific standards to protect these young refugees [11, 15]. As a consequence, most countries and organizations involved in the reception and care of refugees and migrants have created specific protection measures for URMs, such as giving them temporary residence documents, organizing specific/separate reception facilities and creating legal guardianship systems [15, 16]. While undoubtedly this group of children and young people does have specific care needs that are often very different from those of other groups of young people in need of support, it remains rather surprising that these separated care and reception structures – in line with the very 'homogenizing' definition of a URM – seem to consider unaccompanied young refugees as one homogenous group, starting from the idea that all of them have more or less the same needs. Indeed, seen from the legal definition, they are quite easy to identify as a homogenous group [3], and all of them have left their home country and gone through a migration process, yet when looking more closely, we can easily see that these children and adolescents are very different in terms of countries of origin, age, gender, migration motives, projects and expectations, in familial contexts and educational and socioeconomic backgrounds, in experiences before and during the flight, in coping strategies and in ways of expressing emotional distress.

Mental Health Problems in Unaccompanied Young Refugees

Migration, and forced migration in particular, impacts refugee children's psychological wellbeing. Elevated levels of 'internalizing' mental health problems, such as symptoms of post-traumatic stress, depression and anxiety, and of 'externalizing' behavioral problems, such as substance use and aggressive behavior, have been widely documented in young refugees and migrants [6, 17, 18]. Yet unaccompanied young refugees consistently show even more emotional problems, and in some studies more than half of the participants report having severe to very severe levels of psychological symptoms [19–22]. These levels of psychological problems vary considerably in similar study groups, necessitating the identification of possible risk factors that can lead to increased levels of emotional problems.

In a first wave of refugee studies, lots of attention has been paid to the psychological impact of traumatizing experiences that took place in the refugee's country of origin [23], such as war-related violence, torture or sexual violence [24, 25]. Additionally, increasing attention is paid to the often very difficult experiences during the migration journey of these young people, such as abuse and mistreatment by smugglers and border authorities, acts of racism in transit countries, harsh living conditions in transit camps and detention centers, and life-threatening events, such as almost drowning in the Mediterranean or walking for days in the Sahara desert [4, 26–29]. Unaccompanied children are at particularly high risk of experiencing difficult events before or during the flight, given that the absence of parental protection leads to increased exposure to such traumatizing events and thus to elevated risks of developing psychological problems [30–32]. Some studies hereby have indicated that the *number* of traumatic experiences has a stronger impact on URMs' psychological wellbeing than the *type* of trauma they went through [20]. This points to a kind of *cumulative impact* of trauma, with a higher number of traumatic experiences leading to an increasingly negative mental health impact [33].

In a second wave of studies, and as a critique of the dominant trauma-related focus in the first wave [34–36], scholars highlighted the impact of post-migration experiences and living conditions in host countries onto refugees' psychological wellbeing. Here, a range of factors that possibly have an impact on refugee minors' psychological wellbeing have been identified, including daily material stressors (e.g., limited housing facilities, lack of financial resources), daily social stressors (e.g., limited social networks, exposure to acts of racism and discrimination, acculturative stress) and the lack of access to professional support, in particular psychological care [17, 18, 37]. Quantitative studies with unaccompanied young refugees have illustrated the huge emotional impact of several daily (material and social) stressors [17, 18, 38], while qualitative accounts have emphasized the psychological burden of particular stressors, such as the lack of (permanent) residence documents, constrained housing facilities and limited access to schooling [39–42].

The interesting, and seemingly counterintuitive, finding in several cross-sectional studies is that the psychological wellbeing of URMs is not associated with the length of time they have resided in the host country, which also points to the persistent impact of the pre-flight and/or post-arrival experiences [19, 20]. Additionally, the longitudinal study by Vervliet et al. [17] on unaccompanied refugee adolescents in Belgium clearly documents the long-term strong impact of both past trauma and daily (material and social) stressors on youngsters' psychological wellbeing. In resettlement, there is strong evidence that the daily stressors that these young peoples are confronted with in the host country pervasively impact unaccompanied minors' wellbeing, illustrating how the current reception and care structures in host countries are causing important stressors: Large-scale reception centers create, for example, a lack of privacy, experiences of violence and abuse, limited possibilities for interaction with the staff and deep feelings of being bored; evaluations of semi-independent living arrangements indicate that minors experience insufficient housing and income, a limited social network and related loneliness, and huge responsibilities for organizing their current lives [18, 39].

> I am dying here [in the asylum center]. Here you cannot be really happy. You cannot for heart smile. I am so tired. I want to leave, live alone in our house. I need bigger room. I have little room, no good. Water is coming from the wall; it's too cold. They give me nothing. It's not good for the baby here. (Yugoslavian mother, 17 years old [40])

This clearly raises important challenges in how we approach and care for this group of young refugees, including the way we approach them as children within a broader context of familial and social relationships [43, 44].

Overall, it is clear that for young unaccompanied refugees, cumulative stressors are lived in a context of being separated from their parents and related lack of parental support. This raises important questions, as minors have to engage in dealing with loss, traumatizing experiences and choices to be made without the support, advice and affection of their parents, cut off from the wider network of relationships in which they have grown up. Social support is generally considered to be a highly important protective factor when dealing with challenges, reducing the detrimental effect of stress on health and wellbeing [45]. Relationships we maintain with other individuals, whether close and longstanding or ordinary and brief, are among the most important features of life [46]. Social support is defined as the perception or experience that one is loved and cared for, esteemed and valued, and part of a social network of mutual assistance and obligations [47]. While different sources of social support have been documented as important variables in a positive acculturation process and healthy adaptation among URMs [46], surprisingly, little is known about how family dynamics and parental relationships, once living separately in the host country, may play a role in these young people's mental health.

Family Relationships of Unaccompanied Refugee Minors

In this section, we first reflect on the concept of 'family relationships', hereby also consider-ing cultural notions of family interactions. Second, we explore the complex strategies of URMs for maintaining long-distance family relationships.

In understanding the role of family relationships in URMs' wellbeing in exile or their coping with the impact of ongoing separation from family members, it is important to explore cultural meanings and patterns of performing family relation-ships. Theories about the parent-child relationship, such as attachment theory, predict that parent-child separation invokes negative child outcomes. Such frames of reference are limited by the fact that they are developed within a Western framework. Family relationships are defined not only by gender and socioeconomic background but also by cultural values underlying intergenerational obligations, responsibilities and filial duty [50]. Filial responsibility and duty refers to the sense of obligation experienced by adult children to meet their older parents' physical and emotional needs [51]. Filial obligations are socially shared and reflect the culture in which people live. Professionals have to be aware of these complex family and cultural dynamics. Notions of family life and culture thus intervene in how professionals perceive clients from diverse backgrounds and how their needs are addressed [52]. There is a need for a cultural perspective, exploring how psychosocial outcomes may be affected by sociocultural contexts within the country of origin [53] or addressing specific cultural meanings and parameters of attachment security in the particular context of migration [54].

A limited body of studies documents strategies for maintaining relationships in exile. A study in Norway [55] highlights the crucial role that family and peer networks may play in a positive acculturation process and mental health, even across long distances and national borders. These networks serve different and important purposes in the acculturation process of the URMs. Social media enhances migrants' capacity to maintain family contacts over long distances and has an influence on the dynamics of how URMs can stay in touch with their family and friends. Social media is not only a 'new' communication channel in migration networks: It actively transforms the nature of these networks and thereby facilitates migration [56]. Regular online communication via platforms like Viber, Skype and Facebook is used in addition to cell phones. You can have face-to-face contact on a daily basis. The role of social media in bonding social capital is mainly rooted in the migrants' need to receive emotional support, overcome feelings of loneliness and monitor friends and family back home. Social media provides migrants with new forms of interaction with both home and host societies [57]. Some scholars have argued that social media may decelerate the integration process into the host society, as newcomers become less dependent upon finding friends and developing social connections in their host society [58]. In contrast, research has provided strong evidence that maintaining social relationships in the home country can help migrants overcome adjustment challenges instead of producing social segregation in the new society [59].

Nevertheless, it is an ongoing challenge for URMs to create and maintain social support networks in their home country for several reasons. First, access to the Internet on both sides is sometimes precarious, especially in the home country. Even in the host country, it can be difficult and costly to get access to the Internet. Second, even when communication with family provides a sense of comfort and normalcy for refugees, it can also introduce vicarious trauma and new stress. Using social media on a regular basis could mean being in touch with the home country almost 24 hours a day.

> Yousif is a 15-year-old refugee from Iraq. He has an ambiguous relationship with social media: On one hand it is a source of information; on the other hand it is too painful to see the news of every attack. Through Facebook he almost immediately knows if someone close to him has died. The internet connection of his family in Iraq is also very poor, which frustrates and worries him, especially when he knows there has been an attack. Even though social media makes it really easy to interact with others, it is an entirely different way of communicating. During these conversations, he gets overwhelmed by the feeling of missing his family even more. He cannot see his parents in real life, hold them or do typical things from day-to-day life with them, like having dinner with them.

It is also a challenge for him to keep social media from controlling his life. In the assisted living group, they are trying to find a way to prevent Yousif from using his smartphone until late at night because it disturbs his sleep. But he's also ambivalent on this subject: Watching YouTube videos also puts his mind at ease; it distracts him and helps him fall asleep.

Maintaining close relationships can be challenging for unaccompanied minors because their relationship with their parents may become estranged and distant. There is a lack of daily shared experiences with family members which used to be the case in the homeland prior to immigration [49]. Interestingly, there is some evidence that mothers (more than fathers) try to maintain regular contact with their children, attempting to maintain 'emotional intimacy from a distance' [60]. Furthermore, adolescents may avoid sharing the problems they face in the host country, not finding a space to open up to their family members in the home country about their daily struggles. Often, adolescents wish to transmit a positive representation of their current situation or refrain from discussing the complexities of cultural adaptation, depriving them of the possibility of support from their family in these stressful circumstances.

Cultural Adaptation and Trajectories of Resettlement: Transnational Family Expectations

In this section, we explore in a detailed way possible ambivalences in maintaining family relationships, and we address how this may intersect with unaccompanied minors' trajectories of adaptation and integration in their settlement process.

Living With and Without the Family

With the exception of studies of the so-called "lost boys of Sudan" [61], little attention has been paid to the role of family ties in the post-resettlement adaptation of URMs. Family members abroad may represent a crucial source of emotional support in terms of URMs' perceptions of belonging and being valued and loved [45]. Furthermore, having contact with the family abroad creates a certain cultural continuity that may provide the children with a sense of a bridge between the past and the present that sustains identity and facilitates further development of their heritage culture [62]. The youngsters who have contact with their families abroad perceive high levels of support from them, in spite of barriers to physical contact and direct communication [55].

At the same time, ongoing contact with family members is a reminder of the dangerous living conditions that loved ones continue to deal with. The young refugees feel worried and unsettled because of their serious concerns about the safety, welfare and health of family members who stayed behind in their home countries. Such concerns are considered by URMs to significantly hinder their ability to resettle and establish themselves in their newly adopted countries [63]. As such, support from these networks is diminished. Accordingly, emotional support that might have been previously available cannot be obtained as easily anymore. This means a change in the qualitative value of distant relationships.

Looking into the complex dynamics of parental expectations and loyalties, there are changes in family roles. The URMs are often sent away with a certain 'task' – with expectations imposed by parents, family members or others – such as sending money back home or obtaining a diploma or a high-skilled job [2]. The pursuit of higher education is a key goal for many refugee children, youth and their parents resettling in Western countries [64].

Once they have arrived in the destination country, minors realize that fulfilling these expectations will be extremely hard: Making money is not as easy as it was made out to be [2]. They feel the pressure to send remittances to their family and become their family's breadwinner. Yet learning a new language in a new educational system without direct family support is challenging, and gaining a diploma may be an impossible goal, while education may play an important role in the adjustment and resettlement process of the URMs. On the other hand, aspirations are also dynamic in nature [12]. URMs express a changed pattern of aspirations compared to those pre-departure, depending on a range of factors: the migration journey, the stories of peers, the arrival in the host country, etc. [12].

Another often unrealistic image and continuous hope is family reunification within a short period of time. The issue of family reunification and concerns about the family left behind are among the most critical determinants in the refugee resettlement process [65]. When families separate, they often expect to reunite soon. However, the reunification of the entire family often takes years, especially when confronted with financial hurdles and complicated immigration regulations [49]. Although parents may maintain contact during the separation period through all kinds of communication tools, these separation/ reunification processes involve difficult psychological experiences for the children, both during the separation phase and after reunification [66]. It appears that for many migrant youth, irrespective of their culture of origin, separation causes anxiety that may create at least a temporary challenge to family relationships and development [49]. More research is required to look into the long-term effects of familial separations and identify the risk and protective factors herein. Still, youth display remarkable resilience in the face of the adversities of family separation. Even if reunification is a joyful and important step in the lives of URMs and their families, it is clear that the reunification process can be complicated and thus sometimes requires professional support.

Another stress factor can be the 'constructed' stories of the URMs, meaning that parts of their stories are created in such a way that these stories may increase the chances of obtaining a residence permit [67]. For many children, breaking with their story is unthinkable, because they have been urged by parents, family members or people-traffickers not to tell the truth: They may indeed remain convinced that this story will give them the best chance. Nevertheless, keeping up the story can create enormous stress [2].

Overall, URMs have to deal with often unrealistic expectations and pressure in a framework of ongoing uncertainties.

Anila is an adolescent struggling every day to cope with the uncertainties of her life. She is a 16-year-old girl from Albania. She fled with her whole family to Belgium, but she lost her parents on the journey. She is living in Belgium now with her two younger brothers in a group home for unaccompanied minors. Anila's situation is complex. Anila and her brothers arrived as unaccompanied minors, but immigration services had doubts about their story. Anila says she has lost contact with her parents and that she is not aware of their current location. Immigration authorities again didn't believe her, since they found interactions with her parents on social media. Anila and her brothers obtained a temporary residence permit. When they turn 18, they will probably have to leave the country. This is a very stressful situation for Anila, especially because she is the eldest and she is very concerned about what will happen to her brothers when she is expelled from the country. Anila does not seem to be angry but rather sad and concerned. Anila has reached out for help and has been referred to a therapist. The therapist is not trying to find out the truth about the migration story but is mainly trying to follow her rhythm in what she wants to share. A few sessions are required to establish trust.

She is very reluctant to reveal her migration story in detail. There are no concrete solutions in the therapy, but talking about these issues is sometimes helpful. Pointing out the powerlessness and putting it into context helps Anila deal with these uncertainties. She is trying to live from day to day and believes that one way or another a view of the future will unfold. Anila is a very resilient person. She has an active, typical 'adolescent' life in Belgium; she keeps her focus on the future. She studies hard in school and participates in a youth association. These are important steps, but it remains an unstable equilibrium bearing all these contradictions of an uncertain future. Anila's emotions are changeable and the degree to which she can cope with these tensions varies.

Negotiating a New Life

The differences between the experiences of URMs and those of young people settled in their own families are exacerbated because these young people have to negotiate changes in cultural contexts, language and social expectations at the same time as they are adjusting to changes within themselves and in their close relationships [68]. Their life circumstances are much more difficult given the need to manage and find ways through these multiple challenges without parental support. During adolescence and young adulthood, youth engage in ongoing negotiation with their parents to develop autonomy and independence. Research suggests that young migrants without adult support, and especially those facing the possibility of deportation, experience significant difficulties in the transition to adulthood [69].

The struggle of URMs to find a balance in their 'new life' can impair them from adjusting to the new host country. Despite the strength of transnational kinship bonds, parents and adolescents are not developing in tandem. The youngsters are often concerned that their parents will be unhappy if they adopt too much of the host countries' culture [64]. Yet new social relationships and friendship ties are at the same time very important to help refugee youth to connect to resources. While host culture competence is often associated with being successful in school or work and integrating into host networks, heritage culture competence is associated with equally fundamental issues, such as bridging the gaps between past and present and fostering feelings of belonging that may contribute to psychological safety and that may be highly influential for their health trajectory in the long run [70]. Both processes are thus important in the trajectories of resettlement.

Aamir is a 17-year-old boy from Afghanistan. He arrived in Belgium three years ago after a hellish journey of two months. First, he stayed in an asylum center for more than a year. This was a horrible experience for him. Aamir's asylum procedure is difficult; he has already received two negative answers. For a couple of months, he's been living with Belgian foster parents who want to adopt him. Since Aamir has been living with them, he has been able to gain more mental distance from his family in Afghanistan. He says it is often too painful to think about his family, because they are still living in constant danger. He also says that it is difficult to keep in touch with his family, because the internet connection in the war zone his family is living in is very unstable.

Aamir feels a lot better with his foster parents, the only people in Belgium he trusts. Aamir considers them his family. In Aamir's current uncertain situation, it is very challenging for him to connect the different worlds he is living in. First of all, in terms of both his families. At this point, his Belgian 'family' is very present. They embody the image of the future and hope. It does not seem to be a conscious choice, but his Afghan family is somewhat in the background. This seems to be a way of surviving this extremely difficult situation. The foster parents' context is also ambiguous. They do not have children of their own. Aamir has come into their lives by chance and there was a connection right from the start. They are enjoying the affectionate bond that is developing, but they also try to navigate between his own family and his situation in Belgium. It is also hard for them to accept the idea that Aamir might be sent back to Afghanistan. Aamir has already integrated well into their family and circle of friends. These are positive changes for Aamir, but he finds it difficult to share them with his Afghan family.

Culturally, Aamir succeeds in uniting these worlds to a certain extent. He has a number of Afghan friends, and he has also applied himself to Afghan cooking. Being occupied with his cultural identity does not feel threatening to him; it is enriching.

Although Aamir has less contact with his Afghan family, it is still his dream to get his family here to offer them a future. If he can experience stability and finds out that he can stay in Belgium, there might be more room to connect both his lives.

High levels of unmet needs for mental health services and the disruptive effect of the asylum reception system can be offset, at least in part, by good quality family-based care [70]. However, only a minority of URMs experience foster care, with most lodged in shared housing – which can be very challenging [69]. Good quality family-based care is important; on the other hand, extra challenges are raised for the youngster in the complex negotiation between cultural adaptation and the relation with their background culture and family. Macro contexts of the receiving societies thus play a pivotal role in young refugees' adjustment processes and the care for refugees, given that, amongst other things, the type of residence permits URMs have (and the related procedures and policies), the organization of childcare services and the access to education all have an important impact on young refugees' trajectories in the host country [70].

Conclusion

Unaccompanied young refugees are a group of children and adolescents with highly diverse backgrounds, expectations, reasons to migrate, families and so forth. Although they are often seen and approached as a homogenous group (e.g., in legal status and in care and reception structures), their heterogeneity is much more important, in particular when looking at their care and support needs. A complex range of different, cumulative factors and experiences, both in the past and in the current living situation, impacts their wellbeing and needs to be considered when setting up specific care arrangements and psychosocial interventions. Specific attention here needs to be given to the element commonly shared by all of them: the fact that they are without parents and living in a 'strange' country. This not only means that they often lack the day-to-day presence of parental support, but also that they need to negotiate between on one hand asking for and receiving familial support (although from a distance) and on the other hand giving support themselves to their familial context and/or responding to familial expectations. To what extent they are able to find this balance is a complex process, affected by individual factors in the young refugee (such as their mental health, resilience and independence), familial factors in the past and the present (e.g., ways of expressing support and advice, openness to talking about expectations, types of expectations and the possibilities of adapting these to the child's capacities and current living circumstances) and the broader macro context of the receiving societies (e.g., educational opportunities for newcomers, daily stressors created by current reception services). Future research and in-depth exploration is needed to unravel this complexity further and to gain more insight into how these different factors interrelate and also impact URMs' wellbeing in the short term and the longer term.

The complexity and the dynamic nature of these family relationships and dynamics require the continuous reflection of all professionals involved (e.g., social workers, guardians, teachers, psychologists), in particular given the strong evidence that the wellbeing and integration processes of young newcomers strongly benefit from finding a balance between maintaining their own cultural heritage (links with the past context) and creating bonds with the new society, including new social networks. Yet broader migration policies, including the way care and reception structures for URMs are designed, also need to reflect on how parental and familial relationships can be maintained in a beneficial way for all parties involved without having a detrimental impact on the legal and juridical situation and the related residence documents of the young refugees involved.

References

1. UNHCR, *UNHCR Global Trends Forced Migration in 2017* (Geneva: United Nations High Commissioner for the Refugees, 2017).

2. I. Derluyn and M. Vervliet, The wellbeing of unaccompanied refugee minors. In D. Ingleby, A. Krasnik, V. Lorant and O. Razum, eds., *Health Inequalities and Risk Factors among Migrants and Ethnic Minorities* (COST Series on Health and Diversity, Vol. 1) (Antwerp/Apeldoorn: Garant, 2012), pp. 95–109.

3. I. Derluyn and E. Broekaert, Unaccompanied refugee children and adolescents: The glaring contrast between a legal and a psychological perspective. *International Journal of Law and Psychiatry*, 31(4) (2008), 319–330.

4. I. Derluyn and E. Broekaert, On the way to a better future: Belgium as transit country for trafficking and smuggling of unaccompanied minors. *International Migration*, 43(4) (2005), 31–56.

5. I. Derluyn, V. Lippens, T. Verachtert, W. Bruggeman and E. Broekaert, Minors travelling alone: A risk group for human trafficking? *International Migration*, 28(4) (2009), 164–185.

6. I. Derluyn, E. Broekaert and G. Schuyten, Emotional and behavioural problems in migrant adolescents in Belgium. *European Child & Adolescent Psychiatry*, 17(1) (2008), 54–62.

7. A. Hjern, H. Ascher, V. Vervliet and I. Derluyn, Age assessment of young asylum seekers – science or deterrence? In J. Bhabha, J. Kanics and D. Senovilla Hernández, eds., *Research Handbook on Migration and Childhood* (Cheltenham: Edward Elgar Publishing, 2018). pp. 281–293.

8. European Migration Network, *Policies on Reception, Return and Integration Arrangements for, and Numbers of, Unaccompanied Minors: An EU Comparative Study* (Brussels: European Migration Network, 2010.) http://ec .europa.eu/dgs/home-affairs/what-we-do/n etworks/european_migration_network/ reports/docs/emn-studies/unaccompanied- minors/0._emn_synthesis_report_unaccom panied_minors_publication_sept10_en.pdf

9. H. Crawley, *When Is a Child Not a Child? Asylum, Age Disputes and the Process of Age Assessment* (London: Immigration Law Practitioners' Association, 2007).

10. A. Hjern, M. Brendler-Lindqvist and M. Norredam, Age assessment of young asylum seekers. *Acta Paediatrica*, 101(1) (2012), 4–7.

11. K. De Graeve, M. Vervliet and I. Derluyn, Between immigration control and child protection: Unaccompanied minors in Belgium. *Social Work & Society*, 15(1) (2017).

12. M. Vervliet, E. Broekaert and I. Derluyn, The aspirations of Afghan unaccompanied refugee minors before departure and at arrival in the host country. *Childhood:*

A Global Journal of Child Research, 22(3) (2015), 330–345.

13. C. Clark-Kazak, Challenging some assumptions about 'refugee youth'. *Forced Migration Review*, 40 (2012), 13–40.

14. R. Kohli and R. Mather, Promoting psychosocial well-being in unaccompanied asylum seeking young people in the United Kingdom. *Child & Family Social Work*, 8(3) (2003), 201–212.

15. European Migration Network, Policies, practices and data on unaccompanied minors in the EU Member States and Norway. European Migration Network Synthesis Report for the EMN Focussed Study 2014 (Brussels: European Migration Network, 2015).

16. Fundamental Rights Agency, Separated asylum seeking children in European Union Member States: Comparative report (Vienna: European Union Agency for Fundamental Rights, 2010).

17. M. Vervliet, J. Lammertyn, E. Broekaert and I. Derluyn, Longitudinal follow-up of the mental health of unaccompanied refugee minors. *European Journal of Child and Adolescent Psychiatry*, 23(5) (2014), 337–346.

18. M. Fazel, R. V. Reed, C. Panter-Brick and A. Stein, Mental health of displaced and refugee children resettled in high-income countries: Risk and protective factors. *The Lancet*, 379(9812) (2012), 266–282.

19. T. Bean, I. Derluyn, E. Eurelings-Bontekoe, E. Broekaert and P. Spinhoven, Comparing psychological distress, traumatic stress reactions and experiences of unaccompanied refugee minors with experiences of adolescents accompanied by parents. *Journal of Nervous & Mental Disease*, 195(4) (2007), 288–297.

20. I. Derluyn, C. Mels and E. Broekaert. Mental health problems in separated refugee adolescents. *Journal of Adolescent Health*, 44(3) (2009), 291–297.

21. S. L. Lustig, M. Kia-Keating, W. G. Knight, P. Geltman, H. Ellis, J. D. Kinzie et al., Review of child and adolescent refugee mental health. *Journal of the American Academy of Child & Adolescent Psychiatry*, 43(1) (2004) 24–36.

22. M. Vervliet, M. Jakobson, M. Meijer, T. Heir, E. Broekaert and I. Derluyn, The mental health of unaccompanied refugee minors at their arrival in the host country. *Scandinavian Journal of Psychology*, 55(1) (2014), 33–37.

23. I. Correa-Velez, S. M. Gifford and A. G. Barnett, Longing to belong: Social inclusion and wellbeing among youth with refugee backgrounds in the first three years in Melbourne, Australia. *Social Science & Medicine*, 71(8) (2010) 1399–1408.

24. T. S. Betancourt and W. T. Williams, Building an evidence base on mental health interventions for children affected by armed conflict. *Intervention*, 6 (2008), 39–56.

25. A. Verelst, M. De Schryver, E. Broekaert and I. Derluyn, Mental health of victims of sexual violence in eastern Congo: Associations with daily stressors, stigma, and labeling. *BMC Women's Health*, 14(1) (2014), 106.

26. K. Bolland, *Children on the Move: A Report on Children of Afghan Origin Moving to Western Countries* (New York: Unicef, 2010).

27. Human Rights Watch, *Unwelcome Guests: Greek Police Abuses of Migrants in Athens* (Geneva: Human Rights Watch, 2013). www.hrw.org/report/2013/06/12/unwelcome-guests/greek-police-abuses-migrants-athens

28. A. Isakjee, S. Dhesi and T. Davis, *An Environmental Health Assessment of the New Migrant Camp in Calais* (Birmingham, UK: University of Birmingham, 2015).

29. I. Keygnaert, A. Dialmy, A. Manço, J. Keygnaert, N. Vettenburg, K. Roelens et al., Sexual violence and sub-Saharan migrants in Morocco: A participatory assessment using respondent driven sampling. *Globalization & Health*, 10 (2014), 32.

30. I. Derluyn, E. Broekaert, G. Schuyten and E. De Temmerman, Post-traumatic stress in former Ugandan child soldiers. *The Lancet*, 363(9412) (2004), 861–863.

31. M. Hodes, D. Jagdev, N. Chandra and A. Cunniff, Risk and resilience for

psychological distress amongst unaccompanied asylum seeking adolescents. *Journal of Child Psychology & Psychiatry*, 49(7) (2008), 723–732.

32. J. Huemer, N. Karnik, S. Voelkl-Kernstock, E. Granditsch, K. Dervic, M. Friedrich et al., Mental health issues in unaccompanied refugee minors. *Child & Adolescent Psychiatry & Mental Health*, 3 (2009), 13.

33. J. Herman, *Trauma and Recovery* (New York: Basic Books, 1992).

34. K. E. Miller and A. Rasmussen, War exposure, daily stressors, and mental health in conflict and post-conflict settings: Bridging the divide between trauma-focussed and psychosocial frameworks. *Social Science & Medicine*, 70 (1) (2010), 7–16.

35. M. Wessells and C. Monteiro, Psychosocial assistance for youth: Toward reconstruction for peace in Angola. *Journal of Social Issues*, 62(1) (2006), 121–139.

36. E. Montgomery and A. Foldspang, Discrimination, mental problems and social adaptation in young refugees. *European Journal of Public Health*, 18(2) (2008), 156–161.

37. C. Watters, *Refugee Children. Towards the Next Horizon* (London: Routledge, 2008).

38. E. Montgomery, Trauma and resilience in young refugees: A 9-year follow-up study. *Development & Psychopathology*, 22(2) (2010), 477–489.

39. I. Keygnaert, N. Vettenburg and M. Temmerman, Hidden violence is silent rape: Sexual and gender-based violence in refugees, asylum seekers and undocumented migrants in Belgium and the Netherlands. *Culture, Health & Sexuality*, 14(5) (2012), 505–520.

40. M. Vervliet, J. De Mol, E. Broekaert and I. Derluyn, 'That I live, that's because of her': Intersectionality as framework for unaccompanied refugee mothers' experiences. *British Journal of Social Work*, 44(7) (2014), 2023–2041.

41. S. A. O. Thommessen, P. Corcoran and B. K. Todd, Experiences of arriving to Sweden as an unaccompanied asylum-seeking minor from Afghanistan: An interpretative phenomenological analysis. *Psychology of Violence*, 5(4) (2015), 374–383.

42. A. M. M. Wallin and G. I. Ahlström, Unaccompanied young adult refugees in Sweden, experiences of their life situations and well-being: A qualitative follow-up study. *Ethnicity & Health*, 10(2) (2005), 129–144.

43. I. Derluyn, S. Vindevogel and L. De Haene, Toward a relational understanding of rehabilitation and reintegration processes of former child soldiers. *Journal of Aggression, Maltreatment, and Trauma*, 22 (8) (2013), 869–886.

44. L. De Haene and I. Derluyn, Vluchtelingenkinderen: Naar een relationeel perspectief op pedagogische praktijk in de context van gedwongen migratie. In P. Smeyers, S. Ramaekers, R. van Goor and B. Vanobbergen, eds., *Inleiding in de Pedagogiek, deel I. Theorieën en basisbegrippen* (Amsterdam: Boom, 2016), pp. 235–249.

45. C. Mels, I. Derluyn and E. Broekaert, Social support in unaccompanied asylum-seeking boys: A case study. *Child Care Health Development*, 34(6) (2008), 757–762.

46. R. M. Milardo, Families and social networks: An overview of theory and methodology. In R. M. Milardo, ed., *Family and Social Networks* (Newbury Park, CA: Sage, 1988), pp. 7–25.

47. T. A. Wills, Social support and interpersonal relationships. In M. S. Clark, ed., *Prosocial Behavior* (Newbury Park, CA: Sage, 1991), pp. 265–289.

48. C. Suárez-Orozco and M. G. Hernández, Immigrant family separations: The experience of separated, unaccompanied, and reunited youth and families. In C. G. Garcia-Coll, ed., *The Impact of Immigration on Children's Development* (Basel: Karger, 2012), pp. 122–148.

49. J. Brannen, K. Dodd, A. Oakley and P. Storey, *Young People, Health and Family Life* (Buckingham, UK: Open University Press, 1994).

50. R. Blieszner and R. R. Hamon, Filial responsibility: Attitudes, motivators, and behaviors. In J. Dwyer, ed., *Gender, Families, and Elder Care* (Thousand Oaks, CA: Sage, 1992), pp. 105–119.

51. K. Atkin, W. I. U. Ahmad and L. Jones, Young Asian deaf people and their families: Negotiating relationships and identities. *Sociology of Health and Illness*, 24(1) (2002), 21–45.

52. C. Suárez-Orozco, I. Todorova and J. Louie, 'Making up for lost time': The experience of separation and reunification among immigrant families. *Family Process*, 41(4) (2002), 625–643.

53. L. De Haene, N. T. Dalgaard, E. Montgomery, G. Grietens and K. Verschueren, Attachment narratives in refugee children: Interrater reliability and qualitative analysis in pilot findings from a two-site study. *Journal of Traumatic Stress*, 26(3) (2013), 413–417.

54. B. Oppedal and T. Idsoe, The role of social support in the acculturation and mental health of unaccompanied minor asylum seekers. *Scandinavian Journal of Psychology*, 56(2) (2015), 1–9.

55. R. Dekker and G. Engbersen, How social media transform migrant networks and facilitate migration. *Global Networks*, 14 (4) (2014), 401–418.

56. L. Komito, Social media and migration: Virtual community 2.0. *Journal of the American Society for Information Science and Technology*, 62(6) (2011), 1075–1086.

57. M. Brekke, Young refugees in a network society. In J. O. Bærenholdt and B. Granas, eds., *Mobility and Place: Enacting Northern European Peripheries* (Ashgate: Aldershot, 2008), pp. 103–114.

58. N. Elias and D. Lemish, Spinning the web of identity: The roles of the internet in the lives of immigrant adolescents. *New Media & Society*, 11(4) (2009), 533–551.

59. J. Dreby, Honor and virtue: Mexican parenting in the transnational context. *Gender and Society*, 20(1) (2009), 32–59.

60. T. Luster, D. Qin, L. Bates, D. J. Johnson and M. Rana, The Lost Boys of Sudan: Ambiguous loss, search for family, and re-establishing relationships with families. *Family Relations*, 57(4) (2008), 444–456.

61. C. L. Costigan and D. P. Dokis, Relations between parent-child acculturation and adjustment with immigrant families. *Child Development*, 77(5) (2006), 1252–1267.

62. C. Chroummanivong, G. E. Poole and A. Cooper, Refugee family reunification and mental health in resettlement. *Kōtuitui: New Zealand Journal of Social Sciences Online*, 9(2) (2014), 89–100.

63. C. Nakeyar, V. Esses and G. J. Reid, The psychosocial needs of refugee children and youth and best practices for filling these needs: A systematic review. *Clinical Child Psychology & Psychiatry*, 23(2) (2017), 186–208.

64. C. Rousseau, M. Rufagari, D. Bagilishya and T. Measham, Remaking family life: Strategies for re-establishing continuity among Congolese refugees during the family reunification process. *Social Science & Medicine*, 59(5) (2004), 1095–1108.

65. O. Suárez-Orozco, H. J. Bang and H. Y. Kim, I felt like my heart was staying behind: Psychological implications of family separations & reunifications for immigrant youth? *Journal of Adolescent Research*, 26(2) (2011), 222–257.

66. R. Kohli, What unaccompanied asylum-seeking children say and do not say. *British Journal of Social Work*, 36(5) (2006), 707–721.

67. J. Goodnow and J. A. Lawrence, Children and cultural contexts. In M. Bornstein and T. Leventhal, eds., *Handbook of Child Psychology and Developmental Science* (Hoboken, NJ: Wiley, 2015), pp. 746–788.

68. J. Wade, A. Sirriyeh, R. Kohli and J. Simmonds, Preparation and transition planning for unaccompanied asylum-seeking and refugee young people: A review of evidence in England. *Children*

and Youth Services Review, 13(12) (2012), 2424–2430.

69. S. Keles, O. Friborg, T. Idsoe, S. Siri and B. Oppedal, Resilience and acculturation among unaccompanied refugee minors.

International Journal of Behavioral Development, 42(1) (2018), 52–63.

70. M. Stein, *Young People Leaving Care: Supporting Pathways to Adulthood* (London: Jessica Kingsley, 2012).

Mobilizing Resources in Multifamily Groups

Trudy Mooren and Julia Bala

Introduction

Refugees and asylum seekers exposed to cumulative stress due to organized violence, forced migration and then lengthy asylum procedures have a significant risk of suffering from a number of serious complaints [1–3]. Post-traumatic stress disorder (PTSD), and comorbid anxiety and affective symptoms in particular, are most commonly observed consequences of the interaction of accumulated trauma and ongoing stressors, internal vulnerabilities, lack of resources, dysfunctional family coping strategies and poor adaptation. Many families find it difficult to deal with the losses and adjust to new social surroundings in the country of arrival while lacking the support of family relationships. Having family members nearby can be refugees' strongest motivation to build a new life in the host country. They want to take care of each other and invest in the future. Families can be viewed as dynamic systems that constantly seek a balance between stressors or challenges and coping resources and strengths [4]. Most family systems do their best to foster the personal development of all members. If families find themselves in a context where stressors outweigh their coping capacity, the interactions between individual family members can become harmful.

Understanding the impact of cumulative stress on refugee families can help efforts to enhance positive adaptation and strengthen family resilience. The way in which a family copes with the sequelae of political violence followed by forced migration and how it adapts to a new situation is affected by family members' perceptions of stressful events, the available resources and the presence or absence of effective coping strategies. Moreover, the aftermath of traumatic experiences for families needs to be understood in the context of risk and protective processes that hinder or promote the development of children and families in the pre- and post-migration period and in the sociopolitical and cultural contexts of the countries of origin and arrival [5]. This multifocal contextual prism opens up possibilities for integrating individual, family, multifamily and community interventions [6].

In this chapter, we describe a systemic approach to prevention and psychosocial interventions for traumatized refugee families that has been developed in our institute. Foundation Centrum '45 is a national expertise center in the Netherlands for the diagnosis and treatment of groups that suffer from complex psychotrauma, including members of the first, second and third generations of World War II survivors, veterans, police officers and refugees. Although the importance of the family as a unit in the aftermath of trauma has been stressed, there is little evidence for the efficacy of family-oriented interventions in the field of psychotrauma, for refugees in particular [7]. Our work with multifamily groups has its roots in the literature on family or systemic work and has been inspired by developments

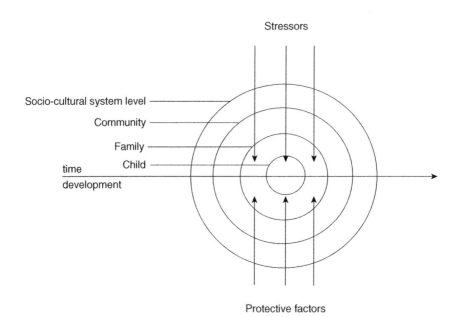

7.1 A family perspective on coping with traumatic events
Adapted from E. A. Carter and M. McGoldric, *The Changing Family Life Cycle: A Framework for Family Therapy* (Boston, MA: Allyn and Bacon, 1989).

in the field of psychotrauma and resilience [8]. The aim of this chapter is to provide a scientific and clinical rationale for prevention and intervention using multifamily groups in refugee populations. This chapter focuses on families adjusting in difficult times. Both the strains families face and the competences they develop are addressed. First, we briefly describe the accumulation of experiences with which refugee families are confronted. The second part describes the family-group interventions we have implemented, including case examples.

The Impact of Accumulative Stress on Families

Refugees may have experienced severe stress and loss at different points in their histories. As well as experiencing threats and violence in their countries of origin, refugees face loss or separation from family members due to death, imprisonment, combat, kidnapping or flight. The violence often does not stop when they leave their homes. Refugees face constant dangers, such as human trafficking, dependence on others and a long, risky journey. Moreover, families leave their social networks and close relatives as well as their possessions, often without giving information about their whereabouts because of the perceived danger. Worry about family members who have disappeared or who were left behind and grief for significant others they have lost are often intertwined with anxieties and uncertainty due to the unpredictable outcomes of asylum procedures.

For many refugees, the legal process of applying for asylum in a Western country is lengthy, and during it they are often faced with uncertainty, social exclusion and discrimination. Those who are granted refugee status are faced with the challenge of rebuilding their life in new surroundings. This process will be a source of hope and some optimism, yet at the same time difficulties at school or with finding a job as well as worries about family members and friends may cause depressive feelings or nostalgia and hamper families' adaptation. Family members need to learn a new language, get accustomed to local rules and cope with the uncertainties of their new life. Children usually adapt faster to their new surroundings than their parents, and may take over parental tasks, sometimes causing the adults in a family to feel dependent. It can lead to role reversal and when it continues for a long time there is a risk of the parentification of the children. Most refugee families miss the social and emotional support of their extended family at this particularly difficult time. Some refugees live for years in harsh circumstances, enduring, for instance, poverty and difficulty obtaining jobs or continuing their education.

Post-traumatic Family Adaptation

Traumatic experiences affect individual members, the family as a whole and different family subsystems [9]. Several family members may experience or witness the same or various traumatic experiences, but even if only one family member is directly traumatized, the family as a whole is affected. Traumatized refugee families are confronted with several challenging tasks: finding a way of coping with the painful past, redistributing roles and tasks that used to belong to the extended family, redefining relationships within the changed family structure, adjusting to a new environment and reorienting towards the future. After a traumatic event, members of the family try to make sense of disruptive experiences by searching for causal explanations and evaluating how the experience will affect their present life and future and their capacity to cope with the consequences. How family members define and frame a problematic situation will have an influence on their way of dealing with it [10]. Parents, especially, often struggle with many questions: how to make sense of their experience, whether or not to talk about painful issues from the past, what to tell their children and how to explain what has happened.

Refugee parents and children are searching for different ways to deal with their own intrusive memories, intense emotions and the changed behavior of other family members suffering from trauma- or stress-related reactions. The sequelae of trauma and the ways in which family members cope depend on developmental age, gender and the family's cultural beliefs (see Figure 7.1). Family members' reaction to each other's changed behavior can aggravate or minimize traumatic stress symptoms and facilitate or hinder the recovery of traumatized family members. Children may be frightened by their parents' unexpected impulsive or irritated reactions or the reenactment of traumatic experiences and nightmares; they may also be confused by parental withdrawal or dissociating behavior. Parents, in response, can become worried about withdrawal, regressive behavior and separation anxiety in their children or feel overwhelmed by their children's sudden outbursts of anger. Family members may become distant or over-involved and be unable to support each other or to contain or help regulate the emotions of other family members. The daily lives of refugee families can be dominated by prolonged grief due to loss, increased hostility and/or a permanent state of anxiety.

Even though many refugee parents chose to flee with the motivation of protecting their children, many traumatized parents exposed to chronic, cumulative stress realize that they do not always manage to adequately take care of their children in the way they would like to. Parents emphasize that when they are overwhelmed with intrusive memories, depressed, anxious or worrying about a stressful situation they are unable to give as much attention to their children as they would wish, they are not as emotionally available as they used to be and they sometimes react to their children with irritation. A mother of a young boy from West Africa explained:

> When I am stressed and feel bad, Ramon comes and talks to me, but when my head is full I want to be alone … I become irritated and push him away. He then becomes upset and starts crying. When I am stressed I become angry easily and will start screaming at him. Later I feel guilty. I would like to take good care of him.

There is growing evidence that cumulative and chronic or enduring (traumatic) stress, trauma-related symptoms and psychiatric comorbidity can seriously undermine parental functioning and parent-child interactions [11–14]. Refugee parents with more symptoms of post-traumatic stress are less sensitive and structured and more hostile to their children [12] in comparison to norm-groups of parent-child dyads. Parents' post-traumatic symptoms have been found to be directly related to insecure or disorganized attachment and developmental problems in their children [15] and to psychological distress and increased vulnerability to PTSD in their children [16]. Clinical practice has demonstrated that the cumulative stress experienced by refugee families negatively affects parent-child relations and family functioning, but research findings also suggest that family processes are pivotal to adaptive post-traumatic adjustment [17, 18].

Fostering Resilience

Resilience is being defined as a dynamic, interactive and process-oriented concept, implying continuous interactions within and between multiple systems [19–22]. Family resilience involves, according to McCubbin and McCubbin [23], a process of continuous adjustment, crisis management and adaptation over time. Families that manage to adapt well in the aftermath of adversity tend to share the characteristics of cohesion, flexibility, effective communication, problem-solving and the capacity to utilize external resources and cultural traditions [24–26]. Positive adaptation is also dependent on the broader context, for instance, the extent to which a family is subjected to discrimination or other forms of social exclusion.

The adaptation capacity of traumatized refugee families may have been diminished by long-term, cumulative stress that has reduced individual and family resources and by the loss of social support. Many parents feel powerless and helpless at times, weakened by post-traumatic or long-lasting stress reactions. When referred to treatment and asked what they find helpful in difficult times, many traumatized refugee parents emphasize that their resources are depleted and their efforts to cope with disruptive life events are no longer sufficient. Exploring and mobilizing hidden or dormant resources is a challenge for refugee families and their therapists. Reactivating resilience processes and enhancing positive adaptation is more likely to be successful if the therapist believes that even when not all problems can be solved, resilience can be forged [27]. Even if one cannot change a situation, one can choose how to react to it [28]. Helping families to use their strength and build up their protective capacities also means increasing their flexibility, managing the balance between togetherness and separateness, and promoting mutual support, problem-solving and conflict resolution [29]. When confronted with stressors, family members may try to cope by changing the situation, regulating their emotions, adjusting their perceptions of the problems or searching for external resources [30]. If the family is caught up in a lengthy asylum procedure with an uncertain outcome, therapeutic options include attempting to change perceptions, working on emotional regulation and activating social support. Much like individuals who have to cope with (traumatic) stress, families may need, first, to be able to regulate their emotions, then, second, to come to terms with what has happened and to cease to feel overwhelmed by memories of the (recent) past and, finally, to be empowered to solve problems in daily life in their new surroundings and gain confidence.

Multifamily Groups in Practice

Aims of Intervention

In Centrum '45, multifamily therapy for traumatized refugee parents and children focuses on the consequences of traumatic experiences, forced migration and current stressors that hinder or facilitate the adjustment of family members. Building on both stress-coping paradigms and systemic perspectives, the aim is to enhance the positive adaptation and resilience of traumatized refugee families, improve functional parenting and enhance parent-child relations. Interventions are directed at reducing trauma- and stress-related reactions and improving parenting competencies. This entails working with interactions and relationships, working in the here and now and taking social context into account, as well as increasing empowerment – which we define as a sense of self-efficacy embodied in the phrase "Yes, you can" – despite internal and external problems. The aim is improvement of family relationships and fostering communication within and among families and others. Multifamily group therapy may be combined with individual trauma-focused therapies, such as cognitive behavioral therapy, narrative exposure therapy (NET) or eye-movement desensitization reprocessing (EMDR). Multifamily groups are organized in various settings. Within Centrum '45 there are multifamily therapy groups for refugee families with one or more traumatized family members, families with children aged 0–5 years, refugee families at high risk of being expelled from the country, victims of human trafficking and their newborns and other target groups, such as veterans. In addition, early-intervention and short-term programs are run based on family groups in collective reception centers and in the community.

A multifamily group for traumatized parents of infants and toddlers with weekly meetings over six months aims to reduce unwanted trauma-related intergenerational effects on parent-child relations, enhance sensitive parenting and secure attachment. The short-term mentalization-based multifamily groups, implemented in asylum centers for families with limited chances of getting a permit to stay, are enhancing families' ability to cope with long-lasting uncertainty and ongoing stress. These groups focus on strengthening positive parenting and parent-child relations despite extremely stressful conditions, and they foster resilience, including intra- and interfamilial support. The aim is to reinforce and strengthen social networks among families living in comparable circumstances. The difference from multifamily *therapy* groups is the lack of individualized family goals and treatment plans in these outreaching groups.

What is Multifamily Therapy?

Multifamily therapy, a combination of family- and group-oriented interventions, entails the participation of six to eight families in regular sessions focused on coping with family consequences of traumatic experiences and cumulative stress. As a general rule, a 'family' includes all persons living together, and all family members are welcome in the meetings. The number of sessions may be fixed or open-ended, depending on the problems. The families working together have in common a certain difficulty or problem related to trauma, long-lasting stress and uncertainty, live in a collective center or have just arrived in a new community, and have a family member with PTSD, anxiety or depression or problems of attachment with a child born as a result of sexual violence. These experiences and related responses or symptoms have caused relational difficulties within the family, and it is these that are the focus of the intervention. The therapists organize activities, such as exercises, games or assignments, in order to elicit and enhance interactions between family members. Improving family interactions is the starting point for supporting families to help each other and a means of promoting adjustment. Multifamily group sessions typically have a clear structure; they start with an ice-breaker, continue with activities that are focused on core issues and end with a reflection task [31–33].

Why Family Groups?

Family groups with (traumatized) refugees offer many possibilities for empowering, broadening coping strategies and strengthening protective processes within and between families. Mutual support is one of the most powerful ways to facilitate refugee families' adaptation and change in the face of adversity [34]. Multifamily groups help to overcome isolation and stigmatization, open up multiple perspectives, foster the transition from helplessness to being helpful to others and in control, promote mutual support and allow families to discover and practise new competencies in a safe place as well as giving them hope [32]. Systemic mentalization-based and behavioral interventions are planned on multiple system levels. Opportunities for pathways for the reduction of intergenerational effects of trauma on parenting and parent-child relationships are created including mentalization, emotional regulation, coping with stress and activating resources, thus enhancing child development.

How to Run Family Groups: Creating a Context for Support and Change

Creating a "context for change" is a principle of multifamily therapy (MFT [32]). First of all, this means evoking an atmosphere that resembles a naturalistic environment, so facilitating interactions as they occur in daily life [32]. Group members can then experiment with behavioral alternatives, supporting each other and asking for support when needed. During this process of experimentation, other families in the group can help by providing feedback, both compliments and suggestions. The families in the group form a supportive buffer that gives group members the space to change. Usually a network of families starts to emerge. This refers to the second dimension of the significance of a naturalistic setting. Bringing families together in group work may mirror bonds within and support provided by extended family and communal life. As an example, a Dutch community group of families from Eritrea created a frequently used WhatsApp group.

One member of the family group for Eritrean refugees used WhatsApp to contact group members for advice regarding her husband's toothache. It was the weekend, and she and her husband wanted to know where to go for medical assistance. They received an immediate response telling them that emergency medical and dental services are always available, even at weekends.

In the spring of 2016, a family group for Syrian refugees was organized in a medium-large Dutch town with community support. A cohesive social network was soon established. During summer a year after, a community organization invited the Syrian families on a boat trip at a nearby lake. Many families accepted, and they brought other families with them. They enjoyed the trip very much. One mother recounted how having a pleasant experience on the boat, in a safe group, helped her to overcome her painful memories of the hazardous journey across the Mediterranean Sea.

To create a context for change, the following structural principles are: structured sessions; an informal, safe atmosphere with jointly defined group rules; work within subgroups; and the therapist as stage manager, remaining distant and enabling families to work with each other.

Structured Sessions

Multifamily group sessions develop according to a clearly defined structure. There is an introductory ice-breaking activity, which is intended to be energizing, pleasant and interactive. This is followed by a core activity, usually centered on a theme that is significant to the group. Lastly, the session concludes with a reflection and exchange, during which the therapist supports what the group members have learned from their experiences in the session.

Safety

In the initial phase of multifamily group therapy sharing, negotiation and clear mutual expectations are crucial. It is helpful to offer an introductory meeting at which the program and the therapists or facilitators are introduced to potential participants; this is also an opportunity to give information about rationales and goals, procedures, schedules and location. Some information about families can be acquired, such as children's ages, school schedules and language. The interpreters may also be introduced; multicultural multifamily groups usually include several interpreters.

As in any therapeutic group setting, a number of rules need to be agreed so that members feel safe enough to contribute; this is particularly important in groups for people who have experienced trauma and who tend to be reluctant to trust others. The rules are defined by the group members themselves. Common rules include: everyone will be respected for what they say; people will be listened to and given a chance to speak; matters discussed during the group sessions will not be shared outside the group.

Efforts are made to enhance participants' sense of safety by creating an informal atmosphere, for example, having breaks during which food and drinks are available and working with nice, child-friendly materials and playful exercises. The aim is nevertheless to create a working context that makes it easier for family members to open up and share their strengths and difficulties.

Working with Subgroups

The perception of safety can also be enhanced by giving meetings a clear structure. Groups can be split into subgroups (e.g., children of similar age, mothers, fathers, parents or families), but the group is always together at the start and the end of a session and during breaks. Where parenting has been undermined by post-traumatic or long-lasting stress, the choice is made to work with parents on increasing their awareness of the effect that their trauma- and stress-related reactions have on their relationships with their children. Building up their skills for coping with stress and increasing their self-esteem to become "good enough" parents despite internal and external difficulties turns powerlessness into challenge. Particularly sensitive issues can be discussed apart from the rest of the group.

The Therapist as Stage Manager

The multifamily therapists refrain from acting as experts, although they are in charge of setting up group sessions. In family group work, the therapist prepares and organizes the activities and exercises. The therapist plays a facilitative role, encouraging interactions between families, highlighting problematic interactions, enhancing experimentation and inviting reflection. When necessary, the therapist intervenes and orchestrates the interactions, providing support, feedback and help. A multifamily group therapist observes the exercises and steps in when there is an opportunity for new behavior or change. If the therapist maintains a background position, family members will be more active, while a positive belief in families' own resources is being expressed.

Cultural Diversity

Sometimes, multifamily groups are composed of families sharing a national background and sometimes of families from different home countries. Multifamily therapy with families from different parts of the world creates room for multiple perspectives. Sharing problems and experiences increases families' sense of being acknowledged and strengthens perceptions of safety and trust. The juxtaposition of different opinions, thoughts and ideas generates multiple perspectives and, within a safe context, new ideas. The presence of participants with different cultural backgrounds, living circumstances, ages and genders helps to challenge fixed ideas, prejudices and assumptions. These assumptions may have been rooted in cultural beliefs. Exchanging perspectives and perceptions facilitates a shift in ideas.

Working with Diverse Languages

A multicultural group in which the family members do not share the same language requires the inclusion of more interpreters. Up to three or four interpreters can help the group to function smoothly. When one interpreter translates a family member's comment to the group (in Dutch), the other interpreters translate it for other families in their own language. This double translating can slow down the group process, but experienced interpreters manage to coordinate and attune with each other, as in an "orchestra," starting and ending at the same time. Family members are asked to talk in short segments to avoid prolonged translating moments. It is preferable that the same interpreters remain with each family during the group.

A short meeting with the interpreters before the group starts allows for creating a working alliance, for providing a short explanation about the functioning of the group and its aims [33], and for discussing possible difficulties. The presence of several interpreters in a large group can create some discomfort during the first meeting. Starting the group with a playful ice-breaker and learning each other's names will facilitate the inclusion of the interpreters. Interpreters are involved during discussion and reflection, but withdraw themselves from participation in exercises or activities. Prolonged, spontaneous exchanges between interpreters and parents, for example, can become "barriers" between families [32] or family members and interfere with the multifamily activities. Some settings or techniques in MFT (interviewing each other, fathers and mothers apart) can be more difficult to apply when none of the parents speaks a little of the shared language like Dutch or English, and this requires creativity and flexibility from the therapist and the interpreters.

Outcomes

Multifamily groups are generally well accepted by the participants and increase knowledge of the problems at stake, improve collaboration with mental health professionals and community workers and decrease stigmatization [18]. Results that have been reported from multifamily groups are members showing more understanding towards each other, improvements in family dynamics, the development of supportive relationships between families, the reduction of stigma in relation to various issues and lower levels of stress among group members [18, 32]. A recent Delphi study [34] summarized the positive outcomes of MFT for traumatized refugee and veteran families: increased understanding within families, deescalation of family conflicts and improved parenting. Practitioners in the study listed the following reasons for applying MFT to families confronted with trauma: people with similar problems find it easier to understand what someone is going through, generation of hope and multiple perspectives, sharing and connecting with other people, increased mentalization and families becoming experts in their own processes.

Mechanisms of Change

How do multifamily groups contribute to improved interactions and relationships in the aftermath of traumatic experiences and in the context of ongoing post-migration stress? Five mechanisms of change can be distinguished: (1) motivation and commitment, (2) emotional regulation, (3) mentalization, (4) coping with stress and (5) activation of resources and social support.

Motivation and Commitment

It is helpful to start with psychoeducation, as it increases awareness of the consequences that individual responses to trauma and loss have on other family members and on relationships. Realizing that their sorrow, intrusive memories, anxieties and increased irritability have a direct impact on their children motivates parents to change. Because participants have often been under stress for a long time, they sometimes perceive their burden of stressors as overwhelming; group members recognize that they share similar difficulties and this creates a sense of being 'in the same boat.' Problems may be categorized according to the extent to which they can be solved. Acknowledging the fact that some problems are not possible to solve or are beyond the control of participants, listing them helps the participants to start devoting more attention to solvable problems. These could subsequently be highlighted and the ideas and solutions provided by group members explored.

Pleasurable experiences are an indispensable source of stress relief for group members. Joint playful activities allow family members to explore ways of understanding and supporting each other in a safe setting; they can discover how to reexperience moments of pleasure and joy together, discuss how to solve problems and deal with the consequences of past and ongoing stress. Hope also fosters intimacy and growth at both individual and relational levels. The strategy is to empower family members by counteracting the sense of helplessness and powerlessness that they frequently experience. Noticing minimal positive changes in other families strengthens group members' motivation and hope that, despite their difficulties, they will find better ways of coping with multiple stressors and their consequences. If participants attribute their small successes to their own actions, this should increase their sense of agency.

Emotional Regulation

Parents' capacity to tolerate and regulate their own internal, affective experiences helps them to tolerate and regulate the experiences of their children [35]. States of hyper- and hypoarousal can undermine reflexive parental capacities. These states can trigger parental hostility or lead to withdrawal and emotional unavailability; both responses have a severe negative impact on parental sensitivity. Parental sensitivity is one of the crucial conditions for secure attachment quality and child development [36]. Warmth, emotional connectedness and the ability to read and respond to one's child's cues are precisely the capacities that can be blunted by the stress caused by daily hazards. Fostering harmony and balance of stressors and resources is an important starting point for intervention. Looking at one another with genuine interest and curiosity is a welcome experience for both adults and children. Gaining more control over intense emotions, including anxiety and irritability caused by actual stress, depressive or dissociative withdrawal, overwhelming anger or anxiety, can gradually help parents to stay within the 'window of tolerance' and become more emotionally available to their children and prioritize their children's needs. Parents suffering from lack of sleep, PTSD or depression may be irritable and hostile towards their children.

> During the "Rewind the clock" anger management exercise, parents recollect a situation when they lost control, including their thoughts and feelings at the time. Then they are asked to rewind the clock 10, 15 or 30 minutes and describe how they felt and what they thought. In groups, they exchange ideas about what might have helped them to calm down when they first became aware of thoughts or feelings of anger. The exercise can also be done as role-play. It allows parents to identify moments that lead to dissociation or depressive withdrawal and build up skills to handle overwhelming emotions. Parents can practise new behavior in a group in various settings, supported by other parents.

Mentalization

The multifamily therapy developed in London [31, 32] underlines the importance of mentalization. Mentalization can be defined as the ability to recognize that one's perspective is different and separate from those of others. Mentalization involves being aware of the thoughts, intentions and needs of another person and acting accordingly ("having one's mind in mind"), as well as the capacity to include the awareness of one's own affect and cognitions. Only when one understands that their own thoughts and feelings are different from those of another person is one able to empathize more. The literature stresses the development of mentalizing capacities in relational attunement, mirroring and containment [37, 38]. It requires practising exploring and therefore knowing oneself and, based on that, being able to understand the needs of another. To increase mentalizing capacity and parental emotional availability, the group will be encouraged to offer feedback and can thereby be used for 'mirroring' purposes.

> In one multifamily group session in an inpatient facility, two mothers were asked to swap children for a period of play. The mother of a two-year-old son playing with a girl aged seven exclaimed: "This is so easy, so nice; I can actually enjoy interacting with this child." Reflecting on what made it easy, she became more aware of the fact that her son was still learning how to express himself verbally, that this requires patience from her and that she needed to find different ways to enjoy interacting with him, knowing that in time they will have more opportunities to enjoy doing things together.
>
> A mother from Armenia who was living in a collective center for asylum seekers participated in a family group activity with her youngest daughter. In one exercise, the participants were asked to fill out a mind map of each other's thoughts, and the mother indicated that her daughter had been in a car accident, but because she had been afraid to overwhelm her mother emotionally she had been reluctant to tell her mother about the accident, which had made her mother feel very concerned and sad.

The role of the coordinating therapist is to facilitate the interactions between participants; to stimulate reflection so that, based on their own feelings, thoughts and experiences, participants come to a better understanding of the intentions of the other person. This increases parental sensitivity to children's needs and a sense of connection and intimacy, the vehicle for attuned interpersonal interaction.

Coping with Stress and Activation of Resources

Coping with stress involves an internal perception of adversity, the weighing of impact and risk and a search for resources. Psychoeducation about stress and the extent to which stressors can be reduced or coping resources enhanced will be helpful. Relaxation techniques and physical exercises designed to reduce physical tension can improve coping. Encouraging family members to share experiences they found helpful will help to enrich the coping options available to group members. Various stress management activities can be introduced, for example, distraction exercises, questioning other group members about successful coping strategies and useful resources, making a family poster of strengths and filling a family treasure box.

> During one of the community-based family group sessions, parents were asked to pick a postcard depicting an effective way of coping with stress. Then, in turn, they were invited to show the group their card and explain their choice. One of the mothers, a refugee from Syria, presented a card depicting a mountainous landscape with snowy peaks, blue lakes and green forests. She shared precious memories of hiking through the mountains, camping and picnicking. She explained that thinking of these moments and of the mountains helped her to cope with daily stresses, although at times she also felt sorrow.

In family groups that we have run as part of an outreach preventive program in collective refugee centers, we have used the metaphor of a bucket and a treasure box.

The bucket represents the numerous difficulties and hazards that are experienced by asylum seekers. The treasure box represents a wealth of resources for coping with these difficulties. Only when difficulties (filling the bucket) have been addressed properly will there be room to start sharing coping resources. The starting point is to recognize the problems in the bucket and categorize them into those that one can tackle oneself, those that one cannot currently do anything about and those that one cannot influence directly. Families are invited to consider what they can change to strengthen family relations and family resources despite their difficult circumstances and ongoing stress. This metaphor resembles the stress-coping paradigm: Optimal adaptation requires a balance between stressors and resources [39].

Family group exercises create opportunities for family members to discover new ways to communicate with each other, become more cohesive, solve problems together and support each other in the here and now. In the 'frozen statue' exercise [32], family members work as a group to present themselves as a sculpture.

> The parents of 12-year-old Zara and 15-year-old Karel, from the Caucasus, are positioning themselves in the middle of the group, distant from each other. The mother's eyes are fixed on the ground. Karel is a long way from the rest of the family, facing away from them. His father is motionless but looking desperately from one family member to another. The loneliness and disconnection of all family members was immediately apparent, leading to the painful realization that during the lengthy period of adversity they had experienced all the family members had become distant from each other. When asked how they would like it to be different, the parents and children moved closer and embraced each other.

Exploring how to bring family members closer together is a step towards strengthening family cohesion. Even traumatized parents who repeatedly emphasize that nothing can help them to cope with painful pasts, troublesome presents and insecure futures often manage, with the help of the group, to start exploring their hidden resources or acquiring new ones.

> During one exercise, family members are asked to think of things that help them in difficult situations and depict them on two or three cards, using pictures from magazines. These cards are then shared with the group. When there are 20–30 cards on the table as a visible representation of coping resources it is difficult to step back to the position that nothing can help.

Social Support

Many refugee families arrive from countries where tasks and responsibilities around upbringing are divided among members of their extended family. Separation and loss of social ties and of a supportive network, forced by migration, evokes grieving for loved ones and often missing their emotional and social support. Frequently, refugee families, often single parents, remain isolated for a long time due to diminished trust, language barriers and withdrawal from social contact because of nostalgic feelings, sorrow or depression. Sharing the same problems, difficulties and worries creates the feeling of "being in the same boat," bringing families closer together. Working in various settings (two families together, fathers or mothers, children and parents together and apart as a parental group or sub-group) also mimics the changing forms of interactions within the extended family. This naturalistic setting enhances small steps in establishing new contacts, in experiencing a feeling of belonging and in reducing social isolation. When evaluating the group, family members highly value the presence of other families, and they learn from them by observation, feedback and advice. Many parents and children experience MFT as a large temporary supportive family, and some of them remain connected with each other after the group ends.

Moreover, mutual support and feedback and the discovery and building of competencies strengthen parents' self-esteem and give them hope that, internal and external problems notwithstanding, they can learn to protect and support their children. Changed interactions will continue to impact family daily life. Gained experiences tend to generalize to situations outside of the group meetings. An increase of trust and self-esteem ("Yes, I can") functions as a booster for coping with daily or new stressors. Closing sessions with a 'party or reception' exercise [32] that involves the participants circulating and complimenting each other can help to increase family members' self-esteem.

Conclusion

This chapter has described the use of multifamily therapy and prevention groups to enhance family adjustment in the aftermath of trauma and loss. Refugee families have gone through multiple traumatic and stressful experiences and face the challenge of adjusting to new surroundings. Despite all these difficulties, many families manage to reestablish their disrupted lives. Others are, as a consequence of the accumulation of stressful events, at high risk for dysfunctional family relations and poor parenting. The effects of these dysfunctions on the children will continue to disturb both individual *and* family functioning and hamper treatment and recovery. The aim of the multifamily group intervention is to support positive post-traumatic and post-migration family adaptation.

Multifamily therapy and preventative groups focus on the relational effects of trauma, long-lasting stress and adversity. Multifamily groups are both a technique and a context for change. Groups can be created according to the needs and capabilities of the target refugee population in a culturally sensitive way. Multifamily groups are a powerful way of supporting intra- and interfamilial relationships and reestablishing optimal parenting. There is a need for further systematic evaluation and research, including in non-Western regions. Strengthening familial and parenting competencies will benefit the development of children who have a vulnerable outlook on the future.

References

1. M. Fazel, J. Wheeler and J. Danesh, Prevalence of serious mental disorder in 7000 refugees resettled in western countries: A systematic review. *The Lancet*, 365(9467) (2005), 1309–1314.

2. M. Fazel, R. V. Reed, C. Panter-Brick and A. Stein, Mental health of displaced and refugee children resettled in high-income countries: Risk and protective factors. *The Lancet*, 379(9812) (2012), 266–282.

3. R. V. Reed, M. Fazel, L. Jones, C. Panter-Brick and A. Stein, Mental health of displaced and refugee children resettled in low-income and middle-income countries: Risk and protective factors. *The Lancet*, 379 (9812) (2012), 250–265.

4. M. A. McCubbin and J. M. Patterson, The family stress process: The double ABCX model of family adjustment and adaptation. *Marriage and Family Review*, 6(1–2) (1983), 7–37.

5. J. Bala and S. Kramer, Intercultural dimensions in the treatment of traumatized refugee families. *Traumatology*, 16(4) (2010), 153–159. DOI:http://10.1177/1534765610369262

6. T. Measham, J. Guzder, C. Rousseau, L. Pacione, M. Blais-McPherson and L.

Nadeau, Refugee children and their families: Supporting psychological well-being and positive adaptation following migration. *Current Problematic Pediatric Adolescent Healthcare*, 44(7) (2014), 208–215. DOI:http://10.1016/j.cppeds.2014.03.005

7. O. Slobodin and J. T. de Jong, Family interventions in traumatized immigrants and refugees: A systematic review. *Transcultural Psychiatry*, 52(6) (2015), 723–742. DOI:http://10.1177/1363461515588855

8. T. Mooren and M. Stöfsel, *Diagnosing and Treating Complex Trauma* (London: Routledge, 2016).

9. L. J. Kiser and M. M. Black, Family processes in the midst of urban poverty: What does the trauma literature tell us? *Aggression and Violent Behavior*, 10(6) (2005), 715–750.

10. F. Walsh, *Strengthening Family Resilience* (New York: Guilford Press, 2006).

11. K. Appleyard and J. D. Ostrovsky, Parenting after trauma: Supporting parents and caregivers in the treatment of children impacted by violence. *Infant Mental Health Journal*, 24(2) (2003), 111–125.

12. E. van Ee, R. J. Kleber and T. Mooren, War trauma lingers on: Associations between maternal PTSD, parent-child interaction and child development. *Infant Mental Health Journal*, 33(5) (2012), 459–468.

13. L. De Haene, H. Grietens and K. Verschueren, Adult attachment in the context of refugee traumatization: The impact of organized violence and forced separation on parental states of mind regarding attachment. *Atttachment and Human Development*, 12(3) (2010), 249–264. DOI:http://10.1080/14616731003759732

14. S. J. Price, C. A. Price and P. C. McKenry, eds., *Families and Change: Coping with Stressful Events and Transitions* (Thousand Oaks, CA: Sage, 2010).

15. E. van Ee, M. Sleijpen, R. J. Kleber and M. J. Jongmans, Father-involvement in a refugee sample: Relations between posttraumatic stress and caregiving. *Family Process*, 52 (4) (2013), 723–735.

16. J. Lambert, J. Holtzer and A. Hasbun, Association between parents' PTSD severity and children's psychological processes. *Journal of Traumatic Stress*, 27 (5) (2014), 9–17.

17. A. Nickerson, R. A. Bryant, D. Silove and Z. Steel, A critical review of psychological treatments of posttraumatic stress disorder in refugees. *Clinical Psychology Review*, 31(3) (2011), 399–417.

18. S. Weine, N. Muzorovic, Y. Kulauzovic, S. Besic, A. Lezic, A. Mujagic et al., Family consequences of refugee trauma. *Family Process*, 43(2) (2004), 147–160.

19. D. Cicchetti, Resilience under conditions of extreme stress: A multilevel perspective. *World Psychiatry*, 9(3) (2010), 145–154.

20. M. Rutter, Resilience as a dynamic concept. *Development and Psychopathology*, 24(2) (2012), 335–344.

21. M. Sleijpen, J. Haagen, T. Mooren and R. J. Kleber, Growing from experience: An exploratory study of posttraumatic growth in adolescent refugees. *European Journal of Psychotraumatology*, 7(1) (2016), ArtID: 28698. DOI:http://dx.doi.org/10.3402/ejpt.v7.28698

22. F. Walsh, ed., *Normal Family Processes*, 4th ed. (New York: Guilford Press, 2015).

23. L. D. McCubbin and H. McCubbin, Resilience in ethnic family systems: A relational theory of research practice. In D. S. Becvar, ed., *Handbook of Family Resilience* (New York: Springer, 2013), pp. 174–196.

24. D. H. Olson, Multisystem assessment of stress and health (MACH) model. In D. R. Catherall, ed., *Handbook of Stress, Trauma, and the Family* (New York: Brunner-Routledge, 2004), pp. 325–347.

25. A. S. Masten, Global perspectives on resilience in children and Youth. *Child Development*, 85(1) (2014), 6–20.

26. M. Ungar, *Working with Children and Youth with Complex Needs: 20 Skills to Build Resilience* (New York: Routledge, 2015).

27. F. Walsh, Family resilience: A framework for clinical practice. *Family Process*, 42(1) (2003), 1–18.

28. V. Frankl, *Man's Search for Meaning* (Boston, MA: Beacon Press, 1992).

29. D. R. Hawley, The ramifications for clinical practices. In D. S. Becvar, ed., *Handbook of Family Resilience* (New York: Springer, 2013), pp. 30–50.

30. M. A. McCubbin and H. I. McCubbin, Theoretical orientations to family stress and coping. In C. R. Figley, ed., *Treating Stress in Families* (New York: Brunner-Mazel, 1989), pp. 3–45.

31. E. Asen, Multiple family therapy: An overview. *Journal of Family Therapy*, 24(1) (2002), 3–16.

32. E. Asen and M. Scholz, *Multi-family Therapy: Concepts and Techniques* (London: Routledge, 2010).

33. C. Rousseau, T. Measham and M. R. Moro, Working with interpreters in child mental health. *Child and Adolescent Mental Health*, 16(1) (2011), 55–59.

34. E. van Ee, Multi-family therapy for veteran and refugee families in the Netherlands: Understanding complex interactions. *BMC: Military Medical Research*, 5(1) (2018), 25. DOI:https://doi.org/10.1186/s4 0779-018-0170-9

35. A. Slade, Parental reflexive functioning: An introduction. *Attachment & Human Development*, 7(3) (2005), 269–281.

36. M. A. J. Zeegers, C. Colonnesi, G. J. J. M. Stams and E. Meins, Mind matters: A meta-analysis on parental mentalization and sensitivity as predictors of infant-parent attachment. *Psychological Bulletin*, 143(12) (2017), 1245–1272.

37. P. Fonagy and A. W. Bateman, Mechanisms of change in mentalization-based treatment of BPD. *Journal of Clinical Psychiatry*, 62(4) (2006), 411–430.

38. A. N. Schore, *Affect Dysregulation and the Repair of the Self* (New York: W. W. Norton & Company, 2003).

39. T. Mooren and J. Bala, *Goed ouderschap in moeilijke tijden [Good parenting in difficult times]* (Utrecht: Pharos, 2016).

Working through Trauma and Restoring Security in Refugee Parent-Child Relationships

Mayssa' El Husseini and Elisabetta Dozio, Malika Mansouri, Marion Feldman, and Marie Rose Moro

Situations of mass violence are the origin of large population movements. People fleeing danger, repression and persecution seek refuge in neighbouring countries or in areas free from conflict within their national territory. People migrate from their countries to seek protection, a safe place where they hope to rebuild their lives.

This process is impeded by different challenges. Refugees must deal with their own traumatic experiences, which are intimate and personal but which also relate to collective trauma that can destroy a sense of belonging to a community and weaken shared values based on communal cultural determinants. Moreover, we have to take into consideration the traumatic experiences inherent in the migration trajectory itself, where refugees most often experience cumulative traumatic events during their journey.

Finally, once refugees arrive in a foreign country, they have to re-adapt to a new life and are more often confronted by hostilities.

In this chapter, we explore the process of refugee parent-child psychotherapy in working with the sequelae of collective violence and exile from a twofold perspective: the consequences of the disruption of cultural meaning systems and cultural belonging that is invoked by collective violence, and the loss invoked by migration itself. Both these perspectives on the psychosocial impact of forced dislocation have been thoroughly articulated within ethnopsychoanalytic literature [1–11].

This chapter introduces these ethnopsychiatric notions as a frame of reference for developing transcultural psychotherapy and addresses how these sequelae of collective violence play out in transcultural parent-child psychotherapy with refugees. Hereto, we describe how these structural changes in the holding environment defined by the culture and the community, along with the parents' traumatic journey through migration, expose the children to various vulnerability factors: disruptions in parental responsiveness and sensitivity as well as strains in the possibilities of identification with a solid parental figure. We then explore the process of evaluating and addressing this vulnerability in transcultural psychotherapy with refugees, providing a safe space to work with the silent suffering in parent-child relationships [12].

Collective Trauma

Refugees leave their native countries when they are persecuted and/or when their lives or the lives of their families are threatened. In most cases, these circumstances are a result of conflict or other violent and extreme situations that often impact the entire population. Such events, which cause utter suffering to an entire community or country, are considered collective trauma [13].

In war trauma, violence manifests in a brutal and sudden way, striking the community deeply in its fundamental cultural and social tissue. Through these disruptions, violence simultaneously brutalizes each individual in their personal self and in their sense of belonging to the community [14]. The individual is annihilated. They can no longer identify with a valuable self because violence was directed at them with the intentional objective of destroying them as a subject in order to destroy an entire community. As a result, the individual can become suspicious of the other because they can no longer recognize themselves or recognize the other in a shared identity system. Consequently, community ties become severed or completely damaged. In war, it is not only belonging to one's own community, region and country that is questioned but, more generally, being human.

Collective violence, extermination and genocide transgress human existence, infringing, questioning and going beyond the bounds of established moral principles and the social order. They undermine the certainty of what was once understood to be 'human'; the prohibition of murder as a necessary condition of human life collapses [15]. There is a disruption at the individual and collective level in the ontological connotation of belonging to humanity. Individuals and communities feel defenceless in the face of the threat of death [16].

Systematic violence against individuals communicates to the victims how they are valued or devalued as human beings by defining their place in society and by compromising their sense of social identity and sense of belonging to society. Collective violence, through the massification of violence and the fragmentation of individuals, attacks the body and the psyche but also the whole socio-cultural order. The victims come out of this process annihilated and isolated, without any fixed points of reference or possibility of repair. The culture that bound individuals to one another, which allowed people to attribute meaning to norms and to the rules and ties between families and communities, is deeply weakened and perhaps even destroyed.

Large-scale violence targets social ties and cultural practices as much as it targets individual bodies and psyches. It is often carefully thought out with the aim of destroying the functions and attributes of culturally constituted meanings [17].

During episodes of mass violence, fathers and mothers, who are often forced to witness aggression against their children, are damaged in the most fundamental cultural parental function – that of protecting their own children. Men are humiliated and assaulted before their families; mothers are victims of sexual violence and can no longer recognize in themselves their symbolic function as protector and provider. Children forced to perpetuate violent acts against their parents are condemned to individual annihilation and to rejection by the family or community. Suddenly dominated by hatred, neighbours who once lived in peace and solidarity become able to commit horrible acts of violence against one another, making future social cohesion unthinkable and condemning all to reciprocal mistrust.

These disrupt the role of culture and community in its ability to alleviate violence, to nurture and facilitate the grieving process and to protect ethnic and cultural identities targeted by acts of violence. Here, cultural identities are shaped and re-shaped by the experience of trauma. The personal, historical and cultural memory influenced by collective violence then becomes a primary vehicle in intergenerational transmission that perpetuates trauma within the cultural fabric and meaning systems. For instance, it can emerge in the collective escalation of gender-based violence or domestic violence.

Trauma of Migration: An Ethnopsychiatric Perspective

In addition to multiple traumas experienced in their country, refugees face the trauma of migration itself and the experience of dramatic and traumatic events that occur during migration. For many, their journeys to host societies are marked by events such as the loss of loved ones or prolonged periods of uncertainty about the future or about their own survival and that of their families. Additionally, many migrants experience detention, torture, enslavement and sexual violence during their trajectory.

Nathan [3] argued how every migration process, whether voluntary or forced, constitutes a traumatic experience marked by a rupture with the country of origin, by the modification of relational links and by difficulties in cultural identification. Migration alone is not pathogenic; it is the multiple ruptures and abandonments that make migration traumatic.

Moreover, refugees and/or migrants do not necessarily react to the experience of migration with the same expression of suffering. The potentially traumatic events endured in the migration process will impact each person differently. Reactions depend not only on personal history, particularly the individual's pre-migratory history and sense of personal resources, but also of their capacity to be resilient – where resilience enables an individual to respond to the traumatic situation and to rebound by learning to adapt and to live despite the traumatic rupture [18].

The trauma of migration, combined with the violence that led to the critical decision to leave or escape one's native country, may create a feeling of loss and lack of self-confidence and has a severe impact on the cultural identity of refugees. The cultural framework of reference, which gives meaning to representations of existence, has been weakened by migration and by the systematic mass violence that took place at the country of origin and/or during the migratory journey. This rupture of the cultural framework may lead to a failure in the internalized cultural structure of individuals who are no longer able to decode external reality and associate it with a recognized cultural and identity system.

The breakdown of the cultural system of reference, and consequently of internal representations, makes the migration process traumatic. The individual is upset, disordered by a feeling of instability, confusion or anxiety [19]. The rupture in the thinking capacity takes place in the refugee's inner world, caused by the disconnection between external and internal representations. These processes lead refugees to be affected by the specific attribute of the migration trauma or 'the appearance of a remarkable internal psychic cleavage and its consequences on the feeling of identity' [20].

In addition to the breakdown of internal and external representations, migration is characterized by fractures on two axes: the axis of space and the axis of time. Consequently, the resulting trauma of migration is structured on these two same axes [21].

In relation to 'time', the trauma is revealed in a conception of time that goes beyond the traumatic experience of migration itself. A traumatic event takes on a meaning for an individual in its aftermath that represents a later historical and subjective context in which the individual can give the traumatic event new meaning. The event is re-shaped and revisited during a latency period whose length can vary. It can be very long, and the trauma can manifest itself long after the migration itself, or even in the space of the following generations through intergenerational transmission. In its aftermath, it is possible to assess the presence of migration trauma and the effects on the conflict between internal psychic space and its external reality, as well as the impact on a refugee's capacity to adapt to a different cultural context. This latency period continues into the post-migration phase, where refugees realize how accommodations and adaptations will lead them to the introjection of new values and new rules of living together, often at the expense of their own cultural identity. This process of accommodation subjects refugees to a radical upheaval that disconnects them from their intimate being. In the effort to adapt to the new conditions of life and value systems, the refugee can undergo a distortion of their own identity to the point of borrowing an imaginary identity, which allows them to maintain an intimate connection with their culture of origin in part of their own psychic life while adapting to a new cultural reality [20].

In the first phase of migration, this adaptive 'strategy' makes it possible to reconcile the external threat of annihilation and the intimate need to protect cultural identity. In the second phase, the adoption of a new identity is a short-term solution that can allow refugees to harmonize their external and their internal world after having gone through a process of grieving and elaborating on personal losses. After this initial period, if the refugee fails to reconcile their inner and external worlds, they can reinforce their defences against the external world and find themselves in a situation of marginality and exclusion, without any references or landmarks. In this case, they cannot adapt to the new space.

Beyond 'time', the dimension of 'space' can also influence the ability of a refugee to adapt to their new situation as an individual or, on the contrary, exacerbate their reactions, which can result in a total refusal of the host culture (marginalization) or in an over-investment in the host culture at the expense of the preservation of their cultural identity of origin. These two opposing and extreme attitudes prevent cultural interweaving of the refugee and their new reality. The 'space dimension' should also be considered as a broader concept that goes beyond geographical, cultural or linguistic space [21], including the 'psychic space'. In the foreign space in the host country, refugees can have access to their psychic space, represented by the extended family or cultural group, with its rites, its history and its heritage. This inner 'family' dimension allows for integration into a new socio-cultural world made up of collective ideas that are specific to the host community. Interiorized family and cultural group core objects constitute a solid attachment ground for a safe identity construct, hence allowing malleable identity adaptive transformations. Collective violence experienced by refugees can destroy this internal space and destroy the sphere of the family and the rites that once provided the references and landmarks for acting in a collective sense of community. In this case, the possibility of becoming part of a new external reality in adapting the internal identity is highly threatened as the internal world is demolished. Weakened by this internal destruction, the refugee will face difficulties in implementing a functional strategy of adapting to a new life system.

Trauma and Migration in Refugee Mothers during the Perinatal Period

Female refugees are particularly vulnerable, as they may be in charge of young children and infants or pregnant in the migration and resettlement phase. The physical and psychological vulnerability of the perinatal period refers to the special condition of a woman, around the birth of the baby, theorized by Bydloswki as 'psychic transparency' [22]. From the first moments of pregnancy, the psychic apparatus of a future mother has privileged access to old internal conflicts, to the more archaic of cultural norms, and to the deeper desires that can easily rise to the surface through a new, heightened awareness brought on by pregnancy. The migration process potentiates this 'psychic transparency', creating psychological upheaval in the pregnant woman and then in the exiled young mother [23].

Pregnancy and birth are initiatory periods of life. These moments fall within shared cultural norms. Migration and the migration journey may make it impossible to uphold cultural norms, rituals and traditional protection mechanisms for mother and baby. Migration can limit access to groups and to support, as family and community members are separated, scattered or have disappeared altogether.

Women may find themselves alone during this vulnerable period, where traditionally their mother or family group would have supported them. The welcoming of the baby cannot always be done in respect of tradition and the norms that provide the baby with protection but which also welcome it into a cultural community that shares the same system of values. Refugee women and mothers are not only affected by trauma experienced in their country of origin or during the perilous journey to foreign lands, but also by a sense of loneliness and anxiety exacerbated by the intra-psychic experience of pregnancy and motherhood.

In general, the occurrence of depression and anxiety in women can increase during pregnancy [24]. Migration, trauma and exposure to violence as well as limited social support increase the risks of vulnerability. Female refugees may be confronted with the loss of a child due to the violence in their country of origin or due to the loss of a child that did not survive the perils of the migratory journey. The grief for these children can be extremely long and painful. Moreover, a new pregnancy can re-activate these painful memories.

For all these reasons, the mother-child relationship might be severely compromised. Refugee mothers will not have access to the psychological resources that help them provide care for their children. Clinical studies [12, 25] show that the family's adaptation to a foreign environment, often perceived as hostile, can be expressed through a child's fragility. It also highlights the specific exposure of the first child born in the host society [12]. Moro's study documents how an immigrant woman's first pregnancy in France may end in the child's death, either in utero, at birth or in the first days of life. Hence, the risk of death is not imaginary or fantasized. It can occur in reality and it weighs on some children of refugees. It may therefore constitute one element of the child's vulnerability.

In this context, the protective effect of cultural practices is strained or non-existent. Every culture has its own specific mothering techniques. Transformed progressively by each generation, every mothering technique introduces multiple variables into the caregiving system that have different consequences for the child's psychic development [26, 27]. These mothering techniques are inherent to the cultural framework that supplies them and keeps them operational. They are part of the cultural patterns, the transmitted cultural structures [2]. Cut off from this human environment, they sometimes lose their meaning, become rigid and are no longer effective. They are intimately linked to the cultural group as a whole, to the women's and mothers' groups. This is the basis for our clinical premise that the mother's insecurity is linked to the loss of support from her own cultural framework. Adding to the fragility of the cultural holding of the refugee mother, in host communities, notably in France, such culturally coded mothering techniques are also subject to disqualifying critics.

Children Affected by Trauma and Migration?

Collective violence and migration have as many adverse effects on children as they do on adults. Children are profoundly impacted when they are victims of violence and aggression or when they suffer the loss of loved ones or sudden separation from other members of the family. Indirectly, they are also seriously impacted by the destruction of their social system and community-based value-sharing spaces such as schools, all of which leads to the loss of landmarks in a world that (for children) becomes meaningless [28].

With parents in survival mode, refugee children are left alone with their inner emotional state, without the possibility of expressing their suffering or asking questions to gain a better understanding of what has happened to them and their families. Fleeing to a new life in a foreign country is difficult for adults, but the suffering experienced by children is often underestimated.

A child's ability to play is a sign that always reassures adults, who project this behaviour as a child's ability to deal more easily with an external context or to ignore external conditions altogether. In this manner, children are perceived as not experiencing the same level of suffering as adults. Unfortunately, the way that refugee children play often involves repetitive gestures, dynamics or drawings that are actually symptomatic expressions of traumatic repetition [12]. In this re-enacting play, they reproduce the traumatic events they experienced or the violence they witnessed.

Refugee parents, impacted by events, affected in their individual and collective identities and weakened in their ability to protect their children, may become in themselves a source of trauma for their children. Children who are not contained by a family nucleus or a cultural group feel isolated, excluded from the larger community of humans, and lose confidence in everything that gave meaning to their world that was once the foundation of their construction of identity. The external reality, nonsense and exclusion [29] breaks into the inner reality of the child, who cannot distinguish between external and inner reality.

Even infants are involved in this process of traumatization. Indeed, the trauma of parents can be transmitted not only to their children, but to future generations of children. There have been many studies on the subject of intergenerational transmission of collective trauma in historical contexts such as the Holocaust and its impact on its survivors, the Vietnam War and its impact on its veterans, the 1948 Nakba and the expulsion of Palestinians from their homeland [30–36]. In more recent years, studies have focused on the intergenerational transmission of trauma in countries affected by massive events of violence, including ethnic cleansing and genocide, such as Burundi, Rwanda, Cambodia and Sierra Leone. All of these studies underline the need to understand the mechanisms of transmission in order to limit its potential negative impact on an entire community or country for generations [37–40].

The ongoing research into intergenerational transmission of collective trauma has highlighted different theoretical models that may help explain the pathways of trauma transmission, including the inextricable link between the impact of exposure to traumatic events on parenting and child development. Based on the assumption that an infant or child is completely dependent on parental care and that an infant or child will express themselves in different ways depending on their environment, parental representations, behaviours and patterns of communication with a child or an infant may operate as factors in the process of trauma transmission. A trauma experienced by parents may directly impact their children through parent-infant interaction, in which parents may reflect their traumatic experience on their children. An infant or child, in turn, may respond with fear and internalize their parents' traumatic reaction as their own emotional state. This mechanism of transmission was confirmed in a recent study that suggests the strong impact of maternal trauma on the mother-child attachment relationship and consequently on child development [41].

The Polarity of the Migrant Condition

In further understanding these dynamics of transgenerational trauma transmission, it is relevant to point to the potential interplay between vulnerability and adaptation. The immigrant child is confronted with a two-fold fragility: the child's own vulnerability, linked to the cleavage in cultural belonging and the loss invoked by migration, and parental vulnerability invoked by migration. Yet this instability provokes movement and can therefore have positive consequences: everything is precarious, but everything is still possible. Here, the migrant condition, because of its instability, enables adaptation. Migrant children are thus faced with a polarity between fragility and adaptive trajectories in resettlement. Examining the plight of the children of immigrants, the French sociologist Schnapper, studying immigrant children's social interaction, concluded that 'those who surmount it derive an added profit in the rationale of self-affirmation and in the search of distinction, but the risk of failure is statistically high for those who do not possess the same individual and social advantages' (Schnapper, 1991, p. 198 [42]).

In subsequent studies, Moro studied samples of immigrant children's school trajectories in France, documenting prototypes of children doing either well or fairly well in schools, or 'sacrificed' children who underperform [9, 43]. For children with good or fairly good school performance in these studies, three key factors are related to school success: (1) the child lives in a sufficiently secure milieu, rich in stimulation; (2) the child finds adults within their own environment who help them to adapt to the new world; and (3) the child is endowed with singular personal capacities and a good deal of self-esteem. For the first two factors, the initial situation of imbalance finds contextual elements to re-establish a new order and thereby encourages the development of creative potentialities. Moreover, in these study's samples, some migrant children perform better than their native peers on the same social plane. On the other hand, within some immigrant families one child performs brilliantly well at school while the others, who nonetheless live in the same conditions, develop scholastic failure. A number of factors explain this differential achievement, including child personality, degree of child vulnerability, child position in the family and parental investment. Here, one specific factor has been consistently identified: immigrant children with successful school trajectories have someone in their entourage who plays the role of 'initiator'. It may be a teacher, an older sister or a kind neighbour. These persons from the 'exterior world' enable the child early on to develop meaningful stable relationships between events in the outside environment. These enable the child to interiorize rationales of the exterior world and hence to integrate knowledge about this outside world more easily. If this world is not recognized at least in part as a world to which you belong, how can you relate within yourself to the rationale proper to this universe?

Next to these well-performing children, Moro's studies also indicated a group of immigrant children who appear to be 'sacrificed'. These sacrificed children sometimes have good intellectual capacities that they are unable to express. They don't necessarily have manifest psychopathological disturbances, but they don't allow themselves to succeed. They don't succeed in becoming children who are perfectly integrated into the French scholastic world.

In another study, Moro documented the onset of adolescence as a developmental transitional phase that may pose a risk for the occurrence of vulnerability during this phase when the child is beset by internal conflicts [44]. Puberty throws the child of immigrants harshly into insoluble problems of filiation. They wonder what their place is. Are they like their father? Their grandfather? Are they foreign to their own filiation? For the adolescent child of immigrants – 'as for any child who, for one reason or another, cannot occupy a well-defined place in his own filiation – adolescence is a particularly difficult moment' (Moro and Nathan, 1989, p. 715 [10]). Here, adolescents' acting-out behaviours, suicidal risks and drug addiction are vehicles of youngsters' attempts to avoid this cleavage, but result in repeating the trauma of migration.

In sum, living in exile and a transcultural condition, like any condition of liminality, in a way potentiates differences between oneself and the other. Rather than linearly impacting children's psychic and cognitive structuring, this liminality invokes two potential outcomes: submitting to the risk or mastering the risk under certain external and internal conditions, given or acquired. In conceptualizing this polarity, Moro [12, 43] proposed the image of the exposed child as a concept to depict the specific condition of vulnerability which the immigrant child develops.

The Exposed Child

Philosophers have taught us that knowledge in a particular discipline can advance by integrating concepts and images from other sciences. In light of this, we would like to propose a heuristic model to conceptualize the child of immigrants in a dynamic way, a model Moro refers to as the 'the exposed child'. The child of immigrants is exposed to a specific risk – the transcultural risk. Mythology gives us several examples of children exposed to a danger – most often confined to the waters in a chest. Exposed to a life-or-death risk, the child, if he surmounts it, becomes a hero. This notion of exposure is found in the legends of Dionysus, Karna, Moses, Paris, Perseus, Sargon, Telephesus and, of course, Oedipus [45]. Exposure is a kind of abrupt acculturation.

We found this image with the immigrant parents and their child, and we experimented with its operability in specific psychotherapies. It is as if the parents thought – consciously or not – 'we've brought a child into a foreign and possibly hostile world'. Later, the child will think – consciously or not – 'I've managed to grow up in this different world from my parents, so I've made myself by myself, without help; I've made myself, maybe even created myself'. Others will think, 'I can't grow up in this world that is so different from my parents''. This concept is a source of anxiety, inhibition, self-destructive acts and the reiteration of traumas.

The image of the exposed child aims to account for a double polarity: there is a transcultural risk, which, if the child and its family surmount it well, reverses itself and becomes a dynamic and creative process. Poorly surmounted, the risk will lead to illness or to the child hiding their potential symptoms. In our understanding, it is in this case that the child bears the traumatic family experience of migration.

On the psychological level, emigration is a borderline situation; it has tangible consequences but also 'dormant' effects that are neutralized by other factors like social parameters. On the epistemological level, when we describe the emigration of the parents as a vulnerability factor in the child, we are not talking about linear and absolute causality. The 'emigration' factor is not an independent variable but a specific external and internal element. Growing up in a transcultural situation is a risk factor for psychic structuring. Therefore, on the methodological level, an immigrant parent and their child can only be observed and can only be treated by integrating these additional elements of the parents' original culture and their immigration. On the clinical level, the migratory phenomenon's double polarity enables us to anticipate the possibilities of a reversal of this process of vulnerability and, consequently, the therapeutic strategies for transforming this vulnerability into a strength.

Transcultural Psychotherapy for Exposed Refugee Children and their Parents: Working with the Destruction of Cultural Belonging and the Trauma of Migration

The Technical Setting

In our transcultural consultations at Cochin Hospital in Paris and Avicenne Hospital in Bobigny, we work especially with babies, children, adolescents and families. We invite the entire family to the session: the mother, the father, the child, the other children, other family members and the team that referred the family to us. They settle into a group formed by the principal therapist and the co-therapists of varying nationalities and ethnic groups, speaking a wide range of languages. Sometimes, especially for families from Africa where a myriad of languages and dialects can come into play, an outside interpreter proves necessary. The patient is always given a chance to speak in their own language when that is desired.

This multi-professional and polyglot group (with psychiatrists and psychologists) fulfils three essential functions for the family and child [46, 47].

First, It is made up of many diverse representations of otherness, of women and men, of white people and black people, of mixed-race people, of close relatives, of close relatives of relatives and so on to distant relatives. These parcels of otherness embodied by group members and represented in space enable the family to experiment with another form of otherness that is neither threatening or destructive but on the contrary is an otherness that is representable and creative.

Second, The group provides a second function regardless of the planned clinical situation: that of holding. Once the family is sufficiently held by the group, it can in turn hold the child. The same logical process is recognizable: A is to B what B is to C. With the child acknowledged in their otherness and effectively held, an exchange relationship can then be established.

Third, The group provides the materialization of the passage from one universe to the other. This is a very important function for the child, who often identifies with the interpreter and leans on them to do this difficult work of linking (outside/inside).

The cultural representations surrounding the baby can be divided into three levels of complexity. First, there are representations concerning the nature of the infant (ontological level). What is a baby? What do they need? What is a mother? What is the father's role/ place? Second, there are etiologic theories concerning the nature of the infant's disorder – retarded development, sleeping problems, mother-infant difficulties – and such theories may reflect belief systems involving jinxing, witchcraft, attack by a jinn and so forth. Third, there are cultural representations of care. Depending on the ontological and etiological level, the parents' expectations do not necessarily correspond to what is proposed: protection, humanization, divination, breastfeeding or bottle-feeding, massaging or not, going to a healer or a doctor.

Furthermore, as mentioned before, certain migrations are traumatic and the arrival of an infant forces the parents to face this trauma in order to construct their parental position harmoniously. All postpartum pathologies and the different forms that they can take depending on the cultural origins of the mother prove this: inhibitions are related to witchcraft theories and, on the contrary, excitement is linked to the representation of possession. Finally, the therapist should elaborate their position concerning the difference in culture not to apply ethnocentric judgements either to the parents or to the child. The elaboration of this cultural counter-transference is indispensable in order to establish an efficient framework to permit parents to talk about their suffering with their own choice of words and images.

In this set-up, the two worlds that structure the child can be used, and bridges between these worlds can be built. The parents' world with its specific cultural representations of the child, its disease, the causes and the way to treat it, and the outside world with its own rationales. The therapeutic process consists of allowing the child to rebuild a filiation (insertion in the generations) and affiliations (insertion in groups). Affiliation requires a necessary and transitory passage through the parents' cultural representations. Rebuilding a filiation without reference to affiliations is not enough for the children of immigrants. Relying on cultural representation opens the way for conceiving these affiliations to help the child to build their own road, which for the child of immigrants will be of mixed colour.

We illustrate our previous theoretical elaboration with a clinical vignette, that of Elavie, a war baby of a young mother who fled from conflicts in Kinshasa, the Democratic Republic of Congo, to find herself in a maternity service in Paris, fearing the risk of deportation.

Clinical Vignette: Elavie

A Parisian maternity hospital made an emergency call to us concerning a situation about which they were worried and which clearly upset them. The care team was anxiously waiting for us and immediately presented a young woman who had arrived the previous night from Roissy airport with no identification papers, confused, dazed, speaking very little French, and also pregnant. She was weeping and complaining of pains. She was urgently transported to the maternity hospital and gave birth three hours later.

The therapist approached her bedside and found a slight young woman with very light skin, obviously scared and completely immobile. The therapist introduced herself and asked the woman if she spoke French. She seemed to understand but preferred to talk Lingala, her mother tongue. The therapist was accompanied by an interpreter accustomed to working together, and the rest of this first encounter was conducted in Lingala.

A War Baby

The young mother is named Alfonsine and is barely 18. She weeps a lot during the interview, and more than anything she is afraid of being put on a flight back to Congo. She says that if they send her back there she will be killed. She does not know exactly how she has got to where she is: a member of her family put her on a flight with a single ticket, without identification papers and without telling her where she was going. The therapist is struck by the fact that Alfonsine is not looking at her baby (a little girl) and asks no questions about her, even though she has just been born. She is clearly concerned that the mother says that the baby has no name yet and adds: 'This baby is a stranger.' Alfonsine goes on, 'If you want, you can give the baby a name; you can even give her your name; it will protect the baby.' Alfonsine's interpretation of therapist concern for the baby girl as a mode of protection simultaneously shows her distress, her projected concern for the child and her ability to lean on others for support, in particular on the therapist. Where has this baby come from? Alfonsine replies that this is a 'war baby', with no real father, and she bursts into tears, hiding her face. The origin of the baby appears clear: the baby reminds her of a traumatic event, probably rape. All three adults fall silent, and the baby stops crying. On therapist instructions, the interpreter draws closer to her and suggests that the interview be terminated for today. Alfonsine then says that she wants the team to stay nearby but to stop talking. She then asks the team to carry the baby a little because her own arms are tired. The interpreter and the therapist carry the baby around in turn. She is a small baby, very physically active and alert, who holds her head well and is seeking to suckle. The mother, who has dried her tears, watches the team members carrying the baby. For the first time there is a direct visual interaction between the mother and her baby. At this moment the therapist recalls Serge Lebovici often saying that the challenge is to convert the 'capabilities' of the child into performance [25]. Clearly this baby without a name is extremely capable, and shows it, but the mother cannot really see this. Perhaps she wants a nurse to give the baby some milk? She agrees: for the time being she wants the team to give this baby some milk in a bottle, 'as they do in France', she remarks. In the last part of the encounter, when the baby is with the nurse, Alfonsine, terrified, tells the team of her fear of the night and darkness, that she is afraid of being touched, and that she has difficulty eating and often vomits. It all started about nine months ago. She is from Kinshasa and fled the fighting with her mother and brothers. Her father stayed in Kinshasa. On the road one night they met some 'militiamen' (the term she uses). The men raped her in front of her brothers and her mother, and then raped her mother. Her own rape was terrible, but it was even more terrible to see her mother raped; that is the experience that returns to her at night. The images of this event haunt her and return as soon as she closes her eyes. Her family continued on their way despite this. She was afraid that she or her mother might have contracted AIDS.

Life resumed; her body hurt, but life resumed. 'It was possible,' she says, astonished and frightened. It seems to us that in this 'it was possible' there is a touch of wonder. Her mother told her that the main thing was that they were together and alive. Then, much later, they all headed back towards Kinshasa. How much later? She does not remember. They all made their way back except her mother, who died first, of old age, exhaustion or something else. One night, when they were very close to Kinshasa, they met armed men along the road. One of them, she remembers, had a voice she knew, maybe a neighbour from home or someone she went to school with. She would rather not know. It was this man who raped her in front of her brothers. This time it was even harder. She screamed and asked them to kill her. After the rape, she begged her brothers to leave her there and go on. She wanted to die; she wanted to be left alone. She wanted to join her mother.

She has talked too much for today, she says. She does not want the team to go; she is afraid of being alone; she wants us to stay and remain silent. She looks at the interpreter and says: 'You have a way of looking at me that is like my mother.' This note, which is at once poetic and transferential, moved the therapist as much as the interpreter, taken aback by this sudden comparison. It moved the therapist because it showed that this young mother had not lost her ability to dream and to connect to representations of safety in caregiver-child relationships. The therapist begins to imagine her before the trauma: 'Tell us about your mother.' 'My mother,' she says, 'married very young, a young man that she had chosen without her father's agreement. I was born from that.'

The nurse brings the baby back, calm and satisfied, and she is put back in the cot near her mother. The therapist and the interpreter suggest returning the next day to continue putting words to things. Clearly Alfonsine shows post-traumatic suffering that expresses itself in her body, her sleep, her death wishes, her reminiscences. The repeated rapes, the rape of her mother, the loss of her mother and perhaps other events have left major sequelae. These sequelae affect her individual identity, her sexual identity and her ability to become involved with a baby born from these circumstances.

Following this meeting, the therapist initiates therapeutic consultations, long sessions of about two hours where they do not always talk; sometimes all four are quiet together. The baby punctuates the sessions. These consultations enable Alfonsine, first of all, to elaborate these extreme traumas that have left deep marks. Clearly some will affect her future destiny, but some can heal if they can find an acceptable inscription in her life narrative and will be transmissible without feelings of shame to her daughter.

For Alfonsine, the first stages are cathartic. She relates her traumatic memories with numerous details that are sometimes violent for the listener, too, because it is the mark of trauma that it is traumatic to those hearing the narrative – of course, to a lesser degree. The experience is not comparable, but the mark of the trauma exists for the other person in the encounter and even signals that an encounter has taken place. After the catharsis phase, the symptoms gradually alleviate but do not disappear completely. Then, in a second phase, she starts to ask what she is going to do with the child: keep it while it is the living incarnation of her rape? Give it up? Doing so, she says, will increase her shame even further.

This phase is followed by painstaking work on the tree of life of this baby. Alfonsine remembers her mother and summons her in her dreams. In the following interview, she tells the therapist and the interpreter that her mother 'came to see her in the night' and that she wants her to keep the child with her.

A Very 'Capable' Baby

This baby looks well; the therapist tells the baby so as she looks at her. The therapist imagines that the baby is smiling. The therapist observes furtive visual interaction between the mother and the baby and, above all, interactions involving touching and carrying: for the first time, Alfonsine has put the baby on her back, for a moment only; she did it because the baby was crying, and that soothed the child. The therapist tells her what she sees, and Alfonsine smiles, hesitating to admit that she is breastfeeding. 'Maybe that's why she looks so well,' she says, almost jokingly. She began breastfeeding with a feeling of transgression mixed with guilt. She says later that she was afraid we would find her odd, breastfeeding a baby born from rape. This is the time when the relationship is forming, and early interactions are occurring that should not be missed because they contribute to the construction of parenthood.

Here we can see a basic mechanism at work in the early formation of the child's self, which Lebovici propounded as early as 1961: the reciprocal investment between the child and the mother means that if the mother invests in her child, that investment has an effect on the mother, which in turn alters the child's experience, and the same is true in reverse, for the child. This explains the primary importance of reciprocal investment and the fact that these constructions are necessary. There is an investment by the care team and by the authors' team in this little girl, and this investment draws out investment from the mother, leading her to re-invest in successive stages.

She is to give this little girl her mother's name and her own milk. Her mother herself bore her maternal grandmother's name, which means 'beginning'. Throughout the therapeutic interaction, the little girl was made human by milk and by her ancestors. The little girl will in return make her mother human, this mother who felt sullied by rape but consoled (her word) by the beauty of the child, by its capabilities, which she now perceives as performances, and by the child's very existence. She will now invest in this child as a positive sign of destiny, after hesitating as to her meaning and the ties between them. She is asking more and more questions about the child's development. The therapist asks a colleague – a psychologist – to give her a development scale, the Brazelton scale for assessing abilities in infants. When the scale is administered in the presence of the therapist, it is a fine moment for Alfonsine, who is proud to see everything that this little girl is capable of. At times she has tears in her eyes. Later she tells the therapist that the tears came when she thought of her mother. She is thinking that this little girl, born from horror, has come to console her after the death of her own mother. This is a first stage in the construction of the tree of life that gives the little girl a difficult, complex, ambivalent but authentic place. From her existence, the roots can grow out. The child has played an active part, imposing herself by her vivacious energy and her ability to initiate interactions with her mother and the world.

In the interview that precedes her departure for a mother-and-infant home, Alfonsine tells the therapist that she sometimes feels full of sad thoughts when she sees the baby, but that she feels she is a mother even so. And there is no doubt that this nascent maternal identity, hinged on the primary maternal concerns that are within her and filling her with a new feeling, will help her to restructure in another mode, deeply altered by the traumas but not annihilated, full of a painful otherness but able to invest in the future incarnated in this unwanted, unexpected, rejected baby that has come to be recognized as a part of herself and her history, however painful. She sometimes has feelings of anger when the baby cries at night, but she also remarks that they are the cries of life. The cries recall others, her own, but now she is able to differentiate meanings.

Alfonsine still lives in France. She has been able to find a cousin, with whom she now lives with her daughter. Her daughter now has two first names: the first, the grandmother's name, is 'Lingala', opening to a reconnection to cultural belonging. The second was added when she arrived at her cousin's. It was a name composed by all the women living around this child. The name they have given contains the notion of life and vitality (*élan*, *vie*) – 'Elavie'.

Conclusion: Moving from Vulnerability to Creativity in the Therapeutic Space

From what has been said, we can conclude that the child of immigrants has to face several vulnerability factors triggered by two core dimensions within the parents' life experience:

the impact of collective violence on the disruption of cultural meaning systems and cultural belonging and the loss invoked by migration itself.

For the children of immigrants, any therapeutic technique that does not take their cultural singularity into account only contributes to reinforcing the cleavage that exists between their two referential worlds. We thereby contribute to their de facto exclusion from the receiving society and to their marginalization. Taking their cultural background into account leads, on the contrary, to favouring personalized, case-based strategies, the learning process and participation in the receiving society. Coming from abroad, these children are called upon to live in a different world from that of their parents, thus to be linked to multicultural worlds. Our role as therapists is to help immigrant children to bridge the gap between their referential worlds and not to set these worlds against each other. In this way we can think in terms of mastering the transcultural risk. Our role as clinicians is to conceptualize a set-up that contains their otherness and transforms it into creativity.

References

1. G. Devereux, *Essais d'ethnopsychiatrie générale* (Paris: Gallimard, 2007).

2. G. Devereux, *Ethnopsychanalyse complémentariste* (Paris: Flammarion, 1972).

3. T. Nathan, *La folie des autres: Traité d'ethnopsychiatrie clinique* (Paris: Dunod, 1986).

4. T. Nathan, La fonction psychique du trauma. *Nouvelle revue d'ethnopsychiatrie*, 8 (1987), 7–9.

5. T. Nathan, Migration et rupture de la filiation. In A. Yahyaoui, ed., *Troubles du langage et de la filiation chez le maghrébin de la deuxième génération* (Grenoble: La pensée sauvage, 1988).

6. M. R. Moro, *L'enfant exposé* (Grenoble: La pensée sauvage, 1989).

7. M. R. Moro, *Parents en exil: Psychopathologie et migrations* (Paris: PUF, 1994).

8. M. R. Moro, *Psychothérapie transculturelle des enfants de migrants* (Malakoff: Dunod, 1998).

9. M. R. Moro, *Enfants d'ici venus d'ailleurs: Naître et grandir en France* (Paris: La Découverte, 2002).

10. M. R. Moro and T. Nathan, Le bébé migrateur: Spécificités et psychopathologie des interactions précoces en situation migratoire. In S. Lebovici and F. Weil-Halpern, eds., *Psychopathologie du bébé* (Paris: PUF, 1989), pp. 683–722.

11. M. R. Moro and T. Nathan, Ethnopsychiatrie de l'enfant. In S. Lebovici, R. Diatkine and M. Soulé, eds., *Nouveau traité de psychiatrie de l'enfant et de l'adolescent* (Paris: PUF, 1995), pp. 423–46.

12. M. R. Moro, *Aimer ses enfants ici et ailleurs: Histoires transculturelles* (Paris: Odile Jacob, 2007).

13. C. Lachal, Le comportement de privation hostile. *L'Autre*, 1(1) (2000), 77. https://doi.org/10.3917/lautr.001.0077

14. M. De Clercq, Les répercussions psychiatriques et psycho-sociales des catastrophes et trauma graves. *Médecine de Catastrophe: Urgences Collectives*, 2(3–4) (1999), 73–8. https://doi.org/10.1016/S1279-8479(00)80006-3

15. N. Zaltzman, ed., *La résistance de l'humain*, 1st ed. (Paris: PUF, 1999).

16. D. Benhaim, Meurtre, héritage traumatique, transmission. *Variations. Revue internationale de théorie critique*, 12 (2008). DOI:http://10.4000/variations.244

17. M. M. Suarez-Orozco and A. C. Robben, Interdisciplinary perspectives on violence and trauma. In A. C. Robben and M. Su'arez-Orozco, eds., *Cultures under Siege: Collective Violence and Trauma* (Cambridge, UK: Cambridge University Press, 2000), pp. 1–42.

18. B. Cyrulnik, *Un merveilleux malheur* (Paris: Odile Jacob, 2007).

19. T. Baubet and M. R. Moro, L'approche ethnopsychiatrique. *Enfances & Psy*, 4(12) (2000), 111–17.

20. A. Eiguer, Migration et faux-self: Perspectives récentes. *L'information psychiatrique*, 83(9) (2007), 737–43.

21. F. Duparc. Traumatismes et migrations. *Dialogue*, 3(185) (2009), 15–28.

22. M. Bydlowski. La transparence psychique de la grossesse. *Études freudiennes*, 32(29) (1991), 66–213.

23. M. R. Moro, D. Neuman and I. Réal, *Maternités en exil: Mettre des bébés au monde et les faire grandir en situation transculturelle* (Paris: La pensée sauvage, 2008).

24. World Heath Organization, ed., *Mental Health: New Understanding, New Hope*, repr. (Geneva: World Health Organization, 2002).

25. S. Lebovici and M. Lamour, Les interactions du nourrisson avec ses partenaires. *Encyclopédie Médico-Chirurgicale, Psychiatrie*, 37(190) (1989), B60.

26. H. Stork, *Enfances Indiennes: étude de psychologie transculturelle et comparée du jeune enfant* (Paris: Paidos/Le Centurion, 1986).

27. H. Stork, *Introduction à la psychologie anthropologique* (Paris: Paidos/Le Centurion, 1999).

28. S. Tomkiewicz, P. D. Eunson and L. Kreisler, L'enfant et la guerre: enfance majuscule. In M.-P. Pollpot, ed., *La résilience: le réalisme de l'espérence* (Paris: Fondation pour l'Enfance, 1997), pp. 3–34.

29. M. Feldman, *Les enfants exposés aux violences collectives* (Toulouse: Erès, 2016).

30. M. R. Ancharoff, J. F. Munroe and L. M. Fisher, The legacy of combat trauma. In Y. Danieli, *International Handbook of Multigenerational Legacies of Trauma* (New York: Springer, 1998), pp. 257–76.

31. D. Bar-On, J. Eland, R. J. Kleber, R. Krell, Y. Moore, A. Sagi et al., Multigenerational perspectives on coping with the Holocaust experience: An attachment perspective for understanding the developmental sequelae of trauma across generations. *International Journal of Behavioral Development*, 22(2) (1998), 315–38.

32. S. Coates, J. Rosenthal and D. Schechter, *September 11: Trauma and Human Bonds* (New York: Routledge, 2013).

33. C. C. Swenson and A. Klingman, Children and war. In C. F. Saylor, ed., *Children and Disasters* (New York: Springer, 1993), pp. 137–63.

34. J. Chaib, Transgenerational transmission of trauma in the Palestinian camp of Shatila, research paper (Paris 13 University, 2010).

35. M. El Husseini, Y. Ghosn, G. Assaf, L. Issa and D. Yammine, Prevalence of psychological disorders in children and adolescents in the Palestinian refugee camp of Al-Buss, Lebanon, research paper (Handicap International in Lebanon, 2010).

36. S. Jabr, *Derrière les fronts: chroniques d'une psychiatre psychothérapeute palestinienne sous occupation* (Paris: Premiers Matins De Novembre, 2018).

37. T. S. Betancourt, R. K. McBain, E. A. Newnham and R. T. Brennan, The intergenerational impact of war: Longitudinal relationships between caregiver and child mental health in postconflict Sierra Leone. *Journal of Child Psychology and Psychiatry*, 56(10) (2015), 1101–7. https://doi.org/10.1111/jcpp.12389

38. N. P. Field, S. Muong and V. Sochanvimean, Parental styles in the intergenerational transmission of trauma stemming from the Khmer Rouge regime in Cambodia. *American Journal of Orthopsychiatry*, 83(4) (2013), 483–94. https://doi.org/10.1111/ajop.12057

39. M. Roth, F. Neuner and T. Elbert, Transgenerational consequences of PTSD: Risk factors for the mental health of children whose mothers have been exposed to the Rwandan genocide.

International Journal of Mental Health Systems, 8(1) (2014), 1.

40. S. J. Song, W. Tol and J. de Jong, Indero: Intergenerational trauma and resilience between Burundian former child soldiers and their children. *Family Process*, 53(2) (2014), 239–51. https://doi.org/10.1111/fa mp.12071

41. M. Bosquet, B. Egeland, E. Carlson, E. Blood and R. J. Wright, Mother–infant attachment and the intergenerational transmission of posttraumatic stress disorder. *Development and Psychopathology*, 26(1) (2014), 41–65. http s://doi.org/10.1017/S0954579413000515

42. D. Schnapper, *La France de l'intégration* (Paris: Gallimard, 1991), pp. 10–11.

43. M. R. Moro, *Nos enfants demain: Pour une société multiculturelle* (Paris: Odile Jacob, 2010).

44. M. R. Moro, Éloge de l'altérité. *L'Autre*, 1 (1) (2000), 5–9.

45. O. Rank, *Le mythe de la naissance du héros*, Vol. 117 (Paris: Payot, 1983).

46. M. R Moro, Q. De La Noë and Y. Mouchenik, *Manuel de psychiatrie transculturelle: Travail clinique, travail social* (Grenoble: La pensée sauvage, 2006).

47. M. R. Moro, R. Riand and V. Plard, *Manuel de psychopathologie du bébé et de sa famille* (Grenoble: La pensée sauvage, 2010).

9 Trauma Narration in Family Therapy with Refugees

Working between Silence and Story in Supporting a Meaningful Engagement with Family Trauma History

Lucia De Haene, Peter Adriaenssens, Nele Deruddere, and Peter Rober

Merdan and Dilnaz are both refugees. Father Merdan is a Turkish Kurd; mother Dilnaz is Syrian-Kurdish. Both parents were engaged in the military struggle for Kurdish rights and an independent Kurdish territory. Merdan is the son of an influential Kurdish leader and intellectual who lived through long-term imprisonment and torture during Merdan's adolescence. After his father's release from prison, Merdan joined the paramilitary forces and became an important leader of the partisans. Thirteen years ago, he escaped to Belgium. His asylum claim is still pending, with the message from the Belgian authorities that his request will not be responded to in order not to compromise relationships with the Turkish government. Dilnaz became a member of the Kurdish partisans as a young woman and met Merdan during military mobilization, when he was taking care of two injured militants. They became lovers and continued to wait for each other after Merdan fled to Belgium. When Dilnaz later escaped from Syria to Europe, she was granted recognition as a refugee. Upon arrival in Belgium, she reunited with Merdan.

During an initial individual therapeutic trajectory with Merdan, our therapeutic team met the family's children for the first time when the father inadvertently brought them to our consultation. Elin and Jine, two girls of seven and six years old, were born in Belgium. Merdan explicitly encouraged his daughters to talk with us while positioning his chair a bit further away from us and his children, as if to materially create a space for them to talk. Elin, the oldest daughter, spoke hesitantly about her trajectory in school, where she had refused to speak out loud for a long time but where she has now started to have friends and loves to learn. She expressed her experience of disconnection from her peers sometimes, especially when she felt her friends did not seem to understand how painful war can be, 'like the war in Syria.' When we asked her whether she was following the Syrian war, she responded:

'In school, I looked for Kurdistan in the world map, but I couldn't find it.'

'Do you know what it is, Kurdistan?'

'No,' she responded.

Merdan had been observing the unfolding conversation closely, and he expressed how they had never spoken about these themes at home. He added:

'I cannot speak to them about the difficult things. They know I was part of the guerila, but I can't tell them more.'

We invited the family members to collaborate further on Elin's work in trying to understand, an idea Elin seemed to like a lot. She eagerly asked when they would come back.

Shaping the transmission of trauma histories within family relationships often occupies center stage in refugee family members' engagement with their family history in diaspora. It confronts family members with intricate questions on how to talk and not to talk about past and present traumatic predicaments in family relationships, how to shape the transmission of transgenerational family histories in parent-child relationships, and how to construct ways of remembering and witnessing atrocity and injustice while at the same time allowing for the reconstruction of future perspectives on family members' lives in exile. In this chapter, we explore how therapeutic practice with refugee families may support family members in shaping processes of trauma narration that provide ways of restoring stability, meaning, and continuity.

The first section presents an overview of theoretical and clinical research on trauma narration and its intersection with empirical findings on trauma communication in refugee families, evolving into an understanding of refugee families' dynamics of trauma narration as relational regulation of simultaneously approaching trauma and maintaining a safe distance from it within family relationships. A second section shifts the focus to therapeutic practice and aims at exploring how this relational understanding of trauma narration may inform therapeutic work with refugee families. This section articulates a phased approach to supporting modes of trauma narration within family relationships, delineating consecutive modes of therapeutic dialogue that enable the reconstruction of meaning and continuity in engaging with family trauma history. A third paragraph further explores this approach through a clinical case analysis[1] in the further therapeutic trajectory with Merdan's family.

In developing this approach, we draw from our ongoing therapeutic practice with refugee families at the Faculty Clinical Center PraxisP, Faculty of Psychology and Educational Sciences, University of Leuven (Belgium), in collaboration with the Centre for Marital and Family Therapy and the Unit Child Psychiatry at the University Psychiatry Hospital. Our team provides transcultural trauma care for refugee families, aiming to support refugee families in coping with and giving meaning to traumatic suffering. Drawing from clinical approaches within the fields of family therapy, transcultural psychiatry, and trauma care, and in close interconnection with our ongoing research on refugee family relationships, we emphasize the role of family relationships as a primary vehicle of coping with traumatic suffering and shaping cultural adaptation in exile. In our therapeutic work, family therapeutic sessions can be complemented with individual child, parent, couple, or community sessions. We collaborate intensively with family or community doctors, psychiatrists, social welfare organizations, asylum centers, schools, and cultural brokers. This focus on intersectoral cooperation is inspired by recent collaborative approaches to mental health care in marginalized communities [1].

---

[1] In the case analysis, a narrative account of subsequent sessions is based on detailed written notes by the first author (therapist) and third author (co-therapist), made during and immediately after sessions, with this narrative account resulting from a comparison and integration of both independently developed notes, reviewed by the second author (co-trainer). All identifying details have been omitted.

Trauma Narration within Refugee Family Relationships: The Relational Regulation of Moving between Narration and Silence

Within the broad clinical literature on refugee trauma care, the reconstruction of continuity and meaning is often primarily tied to the therapeutic process of trauma narration. The reconstruction of traumatic memories throughout the narration of a coherent, meaningful life story in the clinical space is emphasized as a central reparative mechanism [2]. Clinical literature predominantly locates this process of trauma narration within individual treatment modalities. Within the context of therapeutic practice with refugee families, however, the question on how to work with families on the narration of traumatic life experiences arises. How can we work with families on the process of trauma narration from within a primary engagement with family relationships as spaces of restoration?

In recent family therapeutic literature, scholars increasingly emphasize a systemic understanding of trauma narration that moves beyond a focus on narrating trauma as a process of individual biography. Scholars have articulated the intersecting of personal, relational, collective voices in the narration of disruptive life events [3, 4]. This emphasis invites an understanding of trauma narratives as not merely accounting for the individual's lived experience, but simultaneously reflecting the voices of family and community members in understanding suffering. In refugees' stories of collective violence and exile, this relational construction of trauma narratives also entails the expression of cultural or political interests, referring to cultural notions of self or to political narratives of resistance, loyalty, and hope [5]. Through this intertwining of personal, familial, and collective voices, trauma narration develops as a process of coauthoring stories of disruptive life events rather than reflecting an individual narrator's biographical account [6]. Furthermore, studies address how family relationships in the aftermath of trauma are imbued with an ongoing dialectic of both approaching and distancing traumatic memories [7, 8]. Reflecting Herman's seminal interest in understanding human response to traumatization from within the tension of a dual imperative of both remembrance and forgetfulness of trauma [9], these authors emphasize how family relationships are characterized by their members' continuous engagement with both witnessing and avoiding traumatic life experiences. They address how family interaction operates within a continuous tension between silencing and disclosing traumatic life experiences [10, 11]. At the level of relational interaction, this tension invokes a process of relational attunement or the joint regulation of coping with painful memories through a continuous search for the right distance from these painful memories: close enough, but not too close so as to avoid emotional flooding [12]. An analogous process of interactive dynamics of relational attunement has been observed in refugee families coping with traumatic memories, in which the family members sensitively monitor what is safe and bearable for each other in approaching traumatic memories, hereby invoking a careful balancing between both narration and silence around trauma [13].

Recent findings on trauma communication in refugee families resonate this emerging understanding of relational attunement in approaching and avoiding traumatic memories within family communication and document the multilayered meaning systems underpinning patterns of communicating on traumatic life histories within family relationships. Exploring patterns of shared silence around traumatic life events in refugee families [14, 15], studies have indicated the role of cultural notions of active forgetfulness as well as family members' orientation towards protecting each other from reliving harm. Further, silence on traumatic family histories may be lived as a vehicle of mobilizing meaningful future perspectives. Here, refugee parents share a pattern of silence as a way to transmit their hopes for creating prosperous future perspectives in the host society, their emphasis on transgenerational cultural continuity, or their profound wish to resist the reiteration of collective violence in their children's later lives (see also chapters in this volume: Chapter 3 by Cissé, De Haene, Keatley, & Rasmussen; Chapter 4 by Kevers & Rober). Studies have equally documented the process of modulated disclosure in refugee families, a communicative pattern pertaining to a partial transmission of trauma narratives [16, 17]. This modulated transmission of trauma narratives may relate to a parental strategy of adapting to children's developmental abilities, with a recent study showing how this pattern of child-focused trauma communication was associated with refugee children's attachment security [18]. Equally, modulated disclosure may involve the transmission of collective narratives of violence and displacement inflicted upon the families' (ethnic/cultural) community while concealing the personal involvement or injury, or it may take the form of tacit memory practices shared within the family, in which family members share in a silent attunement around material, symbolic markers of remembering [19].

To summarize, this body of findings on intrafamilial trauma communication indicates how refugee families construct unique strategies of narration or silence around their family trauma history. Equally, these studies indicate the relational regulation of traumatic experience within family relationships, invoking an understanding of refugee families' practices of trauma narration as relational manifestations of simultaneously approaching trauma and maintaining a safe distance from it. In this relational process, family members are engaged in navigating and negotiating the dual imperative to forget and to remember, telling and performing coauthored stories that emerge from their interaction and joint, potentially nonverbal, meaning-making.

Trauma Narration in the Therapeutic Relationship with Refugee Families: A Phased Approach to Working between Narration and Silence

The perspective of a relational understanding of trauma narration as a complex process involving multilayered meaning systems and interactive dynamics of navigating between narration and silence between family members invites a therapeutic position that respectfully joins with the family's continual balancing between addressing and avoiding the sharing of traumatic life histories in family interaction. This joining with the dynamics of disclosure and silencing of trauma histories in family relationships and exploring their meaning invites different foci of intervention in therapeutic dialogue. Below, we develop a phased approach to supporting trauma narration within family interaction. This phased approach delineates four consecutive modes of therapeutic dialogue that enable the reconstruction of meaning and continuity in shaping trauma narration within family relationships. While the use of these interventions may be circular throughout the therapeutic trajectory, the phased approach reflects a gradual exploration of trauma narration within family relationships and assumes that the preceding intervention is necessary to ensure conversational safety that allows clients to move into the next mode of the phased approach.

Exploring and Joining Family Narration

First, joining with the particular ways of approaching or avoiding the sharing of traumatic history aims at validating the unique pattern of narration that the family system engages in and performs in dealing with traumatic predicaments. Rather than assuming predefined strategies of reconstruction, such a therapeutic position acknowledges the potentially reparative role of both disclosure and silence [19, 20] and primarily aims at developing a careful exploration of the specific intrafamily modes of approaching traumatic family history.

Validating Protection and Care

Second, this exploration of intrafamily patterns of trauma narration supports the therapeutic dialogue to shift to acknowledging and voicing the protection and care that underpin family members' strategies of narrating and silencing trauma [11]. Here, the therapeutic dialogue connects to ways of narrating or avoiding traumatic predicaments in family interactions, and it invites family members to jointly explore how these strategies are imbued with their orientation towards restoring a sense of safety and sense of future in coping with atrocity [10].

Inscribing Relational Meaning within Family Trauma History

Third, through this exploration of valid reasons shaping family patterns of trauma narration, through giving words to the care, protection, and hope underlying patterns of trauma narration, the therapeutic dialogue may create a dialogical space to voice the multilayered meanings within ongoing relational processes that evoke and represent family trauma history within family relationships. Here, family members are supported in exploring how particular relational processes may be imbued with meanings that allow for a meaningful engagement with trauma history within family interaction: performing transnational family interaction, sharing transgenerational communal histories, mobilizing cultural meaning systems and orientations towards preserving cultural legacies in exile, or coping with current social predicaments in diaspora may form an integral part of intrafamily strategies of approaching and avoiding trauma in family relationships. For example, therapeutic dialogue may explore how trauma histories resonate in family members' engagement with religious or collective identity affirmation, in familial interaction around symbolic markers of a silenced traumatic past, or in children's active interest in turning their parents' and their communities' collective predicament into futures in which a restoration of hope and justice can emerge. This exploration of relational meaning-making around families' traumatic pasts does not necessarily consist of supporting refugee families' open disclosure on traumatic predicaments in past and present. Rather, this joint exploration focuses on a shared 'working around trauma' [20]: investing traumatic experience with dynamic layers of meaning and giving voice to those relational meanings that are shaped and performed within family members' approaching and avoiding of traumatic family histories [21].

Voicing the Untold in Traumatic Experience

Finally, this inscribing of relational meanings within trauma history may support a therapeutic dialogue in which refugee family members and therapists move towards acknowledging and giving words to spaces of the untold in family interaction. Here, the therapeutic position balances between respectfully acknowledging family members' hesitations to speak and at the same time voicing the therapists' inner resonances that may allow family members to finds words for unspoken layers of emotion and experience and that can support novel ways of understanding the role of traumatic experience in shaping their ongoing constructions of their selves in relationships [22–24].

In developing this phased approach, therapeutic intervention does not focus on exploring the content of family trauma history. Rather, these four modes of therapeutic intervention often focus on ongoing interactive patterns within family relationships through exploring how traumatic experience is coped with and given meaning within relational dynamics in spousal, parent-child, or transnational family relationships. This interest in shaping a shared engagement with trauma narration through exploring the imprint of trauma history in ongoing family relationships is often supported through the use of enactment [24, 25], in which the therapist mobilizes the emotional intensity of interactions in the here-and-now of the session to explore family members' coping with traumatic experience in individual and relational functioning. Throughout these four consecutive interventive modes, carefully exploring the enactment of family coping and meaning-making of trauma histories in the here-and-now of the session may create spaces for shaping forms of trauma narration in family communication that restore members' sense of meaning and safety. In the next paragraph, we further explore this phased approach and its four consecutive modes of working with trauma narration through a case analysis of the therapeutic work with Merdan's family.

Working between Narration and Silence as Relational Spaces of Restoration: A Case Analysis

Case Analysis (a): Words for Fear without Words

In the weeks following the first meeting with the children, their mother's home region in Syria was marked by an upsurge of violence. In a meeting with Merdan and Dilnaz, Dilnaz tells the therapist (1st author) and co-therapist (3rd author) that she has stopped working and that her days are now filled by following media channels, agonizing about her family members and the ongoing threat to their lives.

Throughout the unfolding dialogue, we aimed at an exploration of how family members developed relational modes of engaging with the ongoing violence in Dilnaz's home region, invoking pervasive threat within the transnational family bond. In exploring these relational strategies, the therapist (1st author) did not primarily focus on inviting Dilnaz's story about the threatening predicament in Syria, but primarily focused on developing an understanding of how this story and her pain was shared and not shared within ongoing partner communication. Through this exploration, the therapeutic dialogue highlighted the relational attunement at stake in Merdan and Dilnaz's engagement with the traumatic predicament that simultaneously represented ongoing threat and echoed the long-term history of their communities' oppression:

> Dilnaz recounted how she couldn't bear to be present at work anymore and to observe other people continue living their lives: 'Everything just goes on here, while over there …'. Unable to continue, Dilnaz started to cry loudly and had difficulty breathing.

Merdan came in immediately, started to detail the current political situation and broadened this story by explaining the geopolitical stakes of different countries involved.

The therapist (1st author) asked: 'Merdan, may I ask you on what just occurred here between you and Dilnaz, is this how it happens in between you at home? Is this how it occurs, that her words stop and that she gasps for breath, and that you start words where her words stop, and that you start explaining, detailing? That you search for words?'

Merdan responded: There are so many questions I cannot answer. I know I can't answer. And then I just try to explain. He then shifted into continuing his clarification of the political situation, extending his arguments to the ongoing predicament of the Kurdish diaspora in Europa.

'May I understand that if Dilnaz starts to cry, if her words stop, if there are no more words, that you, Merdan, start to talk on the political situation?' asked the therapist, and both parents nod.

Through this intervention of *exploring and joining family narration*, the therapeutic dialogue shifted to exploring the partners' relational attunement in speaking about traumatic suffering in spousal interaction. In observing how Merdan's political speech seemed to regulate Dilnaz's suffering in approaching the ongoing traumatic predicament of her family members, the therapist focused on the enactment of a shared communicative pattern that unfolded in the session. This allowed for the conversation to further explore the shifting positions of sharing and avoidance of overwhelming fear on the faith of family members within the spousal relationship: a process of relational attunement in which Merdan moved into a vocabulary of addressing the political predicament at those moments where Dilnaz's expressions of suffering approached a fear she was hardly able to voice, a fear without words for the death of a family member in her home country. Giving voice to the attunement between both vocabularies representing either cognitive or affective response to trauma prevented splitting and rather supported the integration of both modes of coping.

The therapist turned to Dilnaz and asked: 'How do you experience this, that Merdan starts to talk when your words stop?'

She responded: 'It helps me not to disappear in this pain,' and the therapist added: 'Merdan's words are helpful; they are comforting.'

Here, Merdan bent his body forward, quickly and repetitively moving his hands.

The therapist came in: 'Merdan, it feels as if your body is telling us that all of your words, all of your attempts to comfort, are not always comforting? As if you feel you cannot comfort Dilnaz, or as if underneath your words you are feeling a lot of pain too?'

With a loud voice, he responded: 'Of course.' And then, quietly, he uttered: 'I am so afraid too, for what could happen. Maybe even more afraid than she is.'

Dilnaz said: 'I know you understand, but it is not the same for us. It is my mother, it is my brother.'

Merdan responded: 'Now it is your family, but one day it will be mine. Then the violence against us will shift over there.'

'It doesn't matter anymore now who will have the victory over the land', said Dilnaz. 'The only thing that matters now is the people who try to escape, to survive, or who are killed.' She continues to voice her fear for her mother in her home region, where militia are violently attacking Kurdish residents, violating women and killing children.' She cried, shivered, and talked in a loud voice: 'If I think the militias are knocking on her door, demanding coffee from her, if I think they are in her house. I can see on my phone how everything is shaking because of the bombs; I don't know whether the bombs fell on her house when the mobile connection falls away suddenly; I don't know …' Dilnaz's words stopped; she cried, heavily breathing.

For a few seconds, we remained silent, until the therapist said: 'It feels as if this fear, that you also feel right now sitting here, is without words, this fear for everything that could happen in this ongoing injustice in Syria, fear without words.'

Dilnaz cried silently, and when the co-therapist asked both of them how they deal with these phone calls that overwhelm Dilnaz with fear, Merdan recounted how he tried to soothe Dilnaz. The therapist added: 'You try to find words; you try to find words that can make this fear without words less fearful.' Then Merdan quietly whispered: 'But I know that one day, someone will die.'

Dilnaz and Merdan remained silent. Then the therapist reflected: 'Merdan, if you say here that one day someone will die, that seems as if you are doing something different than trying to give words that soothe and that try to fill the silence of the fear without words. Saying that you feel someone will die one day, are those words that express what is not said in Dilnaz's fear?'

Dilnaz responded: 'Merdan understood what I feel. But he never told me this before. This is the first time he does.'

The therapist said: 'Now Merdan gives words to the fear without words. The fear that someone will die.'

Dilnaz nodded, and the therapist continued: 'It seems as if Merdan tries to find words in different ways: Words that explain and that try to soothe your fear, and words that try to express what you fear and what you can't say in words.'

In this sequence, the therapeutic intervention of *validating protection and care* aims at exploring the shared relational strategy of avoidance as a story of restoring safety in partner communication, hereby validating Merdan's care expressed by his strategy of shifting into political language when confronted with Dilnaz's overwhelming pain. The therapeutic dialogue further unfolded into a conversational space in which Merdan could connect to those voices of fear without words within his inner experience, his shared fear of future traumatic loss and his silenced fear of his spouse's gradual disconnection from the will to live in witnessing the destruction of her family and community in her home country.

The therapist continued: 'Merdan, there is something that I would like to understand, something you said a few moments ago here. Can you help me understand your expression that maybe you are more afraid than Dilnaz?'

He nodded and quietly said: 'I am so afraid about her. I see how much she suffers. I am so afraid for the day that someone will die; I am so afraid she will maybe not be able to breathe anymore.'

'As if she would in a way stop breathing if a family member would die in Syria?' the therapist asked. When Merdan nodded and bent his body towards his lap, the therapist asked Dilnaz how it feels to hear Merdan say this.

Her head bent down, Dilnaz quietly responded: 'It's true. He understood. Then I will not want to breathe anymore, if Mom dies there.'

Then she continued: 'But I know that there are parts in me that want to continue living. I want to be there for the children.' She added: 'It is so difficult to live right now. I could have protected them because of my fighting skills. I know how to do it. My mother and brother don't know how to do it; they were never involved in the resistance.'

'Listening to you, I wonder how the safety of your life here is also a source of guilt?' asked the therapist.

Both Dilnaz and Merdan confirmed explicitly and expressed their guilt at not being involved in the resistance against the militia.

The co-therapist (3rd author) asked: 'May I think that your experience of being unable to protect your family members deprives you of a sense of meaning, that it brings you close to hoping you would be over there, even if there is destruction?' They both nodded and we remained silent for a little while.

In developing a space of containment for Dilnaz's embodied closeness with death in her continuous perspective on the potential death of her family, she voiced her balancing between the wish to live and not to live, the imperative to live as a mother for her children and not to live as the daughter of her mother if she were to lose her life. Here, the therapist explored this lived experience by inviting an understanding of this double imperative as balancing on a lived experience of guilt. This *inscribing relational meaning within family trauma history* explored how ongoing traumatic suffering was profoundly related to the lived experience of guilt within transnational family and community relationships, developing into a shared expression by both parents of their deep sense of guilt in living in the safety of exile while facing the threat of the slaughter of family members they are unable to protect. In containing their strong expressions of guilt, the therapeutic dialogue may have enabled the sharing of their silent experience of the senselessness of their exile, as their exile was the space itself where they felt disarmed from the strength that would have enabled them to protect family members. In this sequence, the interventions of *inscribing relational meaning within family trauma history* were closely tied to the unfolding of a therapeutic dialogue that enabled the *voicing of the untold in traumatic experience*. Here, in holding their embodied experience of survivor guilt [26], the therapeutic dialogue may have provided a holding space for Dilnaz's fragile sense of life purpose as embedded within a profound encounter with meaninglessness in the face of atrocity and its disintegration of social worlds [27]. Words for unspoken fear unfolded, in which the therapist engaged her inner experience to voice potential layers of meaning for the untold, the fear of traumatic loss, and how this imbued their own lives with an embodied loss of connection to life in exile. In this sharing of words for fear without words, the therapeutic dialogue aimed at supporting the spousal relationship as a space for fragments of restoring safety, for relational stories of sensitivity and the holding of suffering.

Case Analysis (b): Moving Anger to Future in a Communal Space of Holding

The week after the session with Merdan and Dilnaz, we contacted them to invite the family to participate in a reflecting team session [28] with a group of 18 psychotherapists in the context of a postgraduate specialization course in psychotraumatherapy. As part of this postgraduate training, the therapist (1st author) was preparing a training day on refugee trauma care together with her colleague and child psychiatrist affiliated to the University Hospital (2nd author). The idea of inviting the family to a reflecting team session with the postgraduate training group developed from our shared idea that pursuing the work on trauma communication with the family in a group of psychotherapists would operate as a relational context of witnessing [29] that could provide containment and acknowledgment of pain.

Both parents agreed, and we organized a meeting with them to prepare for the reflecting team session. They both agreed that all parts of their story could be shared with the group, expressing how they wished to account for the predicament of their communities in Syria and refugees' suffering in exile to a group of psychotherapists who might encounter other refugee families in their future work. Merdan also emphasized that he felt it was important for Dilnaz to find a space to speak about her suffering, but he wanted to protect his children from witnessing this. Here, he proposed to organize the reflecting team session in two parts: a first part with Merdan and Dilnaz aiming to provide a space of holding for Dilnaz, and a second part with the whole family; Merdan, Dilnaz, Elin, and Jine.

In starting the session, Dilnaz and Merdan were invited to sit down in the chairs that stood in a circle in the middle of the wider circle of trainees and the co-trainer (2nd author). In the middle of the circle, Dilnaz and Merdan sat together with the therapist (1st author), co-therapist (3rd author), and the interpreter.

At the start of the reflecting team session, both Dilnaz and Merdan explicitly engaged with the reflecting team as a circle of witnesses through initiating the therapeutic dialogue and voicing their past and present predicaments:

> Dilnaz expressed the ongoing suffering in their home because of the destructive violence inflicted upon her family and community in her home country, Syria. She addressed the injustices that are part of daily life in her home region: the violation of women, the killing of university students, the murder of young children whom she refers to as 'our children.' Merdan continued and testified of the historical violence against Kurds throughout centuries, emphasizing how the oppression of Kurdish communities was met with neglect and silence across Europe for many decades and only now received some attention because of the current economic and security interests of western countries.
>
> Dilnaz added: 'It is different between us. It is my land now where the destruction is. It's my land; they are the places where I played as a child. It's the land where my father is buried that is now a place of war.' She started to cry when she says: 'Sometimes I think my father is angry now and wonders why my mother and brother are not visiting his grave anymore.'
>
> The therapist (1st author) asked: 'Would it be right to say that this violence is not only about the destruction of your memories, of your belonging, but also feels like disconnecting you from your father, who is buried in that land?'
>
> Dilnaz nodded. 'And this is not the same for Merdan, because it is my land.'
>
> Merdan responded: 'It was my land 25 years ago. This is part of a long history of violence against the Kurdish people. What happens now on your land with our children is what I experienced as a child in my country. This violence is repeated across generations.'
>
> Listening to the different perspectives on narrating the ongoing violence in Dilnaz's home country and how Merdan seemed to connect Dilnaz's suffering to a shared collective predicament of a community to which they both belong, the therapist reflected: 'It seems I hear two languages spoken here: the language of pain and unspeakable fear, and the language of the partisans, of political resistance against the historical injustice inflicted upon the Kurdish.'
>
> 'Yes,' said Dilnaz, 'that's how it feels.'
>
> 'Can you help me understand those two languages?', the therapist asked. 'How do these languages live in your home?'
>
> 'It feels like the language of a father and a mother,' reflected Merdan. He continued: 'Those languages are in constant tension inside of me.'
>
> 'It's the language of being a mother and daughter,' added Dilnaz. She started to cry and told us how she is trying to live, but how parts of her seemed unable to continue living because of what is happening to life in Syria, where life is threatened. 'Even the children where I work remind me of our children there, who are not protected. It is maybe strange to say this here, but I can only wonder: Why are these children protected and why not ours?'

In this sequence, the therapist (1st author) aimed at *exploring and joining family narration* and invited an understanding of how they seemed to engage in this witnessing of their suffering in different vocabularies, the language of partisans and political resistance and the language of suffering and the intimate, embodied pain of family bonds threatened by violence. In Merdan's language of partisans, he accounted for their shared history of oppression, voicing the collective predicament of the Kurdish community across generations and country borders. This language of partisans may reflect how, in the aftermath of collective violence, survivors may evoke personal trauma histories through narrative modes that emphasize collective suffering [4], echoing cultural notions of a relational self as deeply embedded within communal bonds [30]. In the therapist's inner dialogue, Merdan's language of partisans equally resonated the interweaving of past and present in a process of trauma narration at times when violence and injustice reawakens in exiled refugees' home regions [13], evoking how ongoing violence may reactivate stories of past violence and burden the present lived experience with the reliving of personal persecution. In her turn, Dilnaz's language of suffering explicitly disconnected from the political and armed struggle she was representing before her exile. In her refusal to experience the land of the current violence as a land of aggression against the Kurdish, a land shared with father, in emphasizing how this land was now the land of her family's suffering, she disconnected from the political purposes of the resistance struggle. Here, Dilnaz located her suffering in the intimate bonds as a daughter and a sister within transnational family bonds, stripping the suffering from a larger web of political meanings. Within the therapist's experience, her expressions of profound suffering provoked by the pervasive threat of loss transmitted a shared experience of humanity beyond cultural or political identities [31], the experience of the shattering of family ties in the face of atrocity. At the same time, this language of suffering that she explicitly disconnected from political or cultural struggles seems to have operated as a reconnecting to political agency within the developing interaction with the reflecting team. Dilnaz's account implied a transmission of suffering to all conversational partners, positioning the reflecting team members as representatives of her host society in which the ongoing atrocity in her home region received scant public attention. This dimension of counteracting the silencing of the Kurdish predicament in their country of exile was equally resonating in Merdan's language of partisans, where his account was explicitly addressing the long-term neglect of the oppression of the Kurdish community in Europe as well as the selective interest recently in response to growing security interests. Locating the exploration of relational processes of trauma narration in a reflecting team may have supported these fragments of political agency in both parents, supporting their engagement with a transmission of their suffering to a host community of listeners.

> The co-therapist (3rd author) asked: 'Dilnaz, you express how deep your pain is as daughter of your mother, and how the pain of being her daughter living here while she is threatened is what fills your home continuously. Could it be that Elin and Jine feel the pain of you as your daughters, like you feel as your mother's daughter?'
> Dilnaz cried, and both parents spoke about their continuous attempts to keep their children at a distance from their suffering but that the children know about the violence. The co-therapist wondered: 'Would you agree if I say that you try to protect them by not talking about what is happening in Syria, but that the walls of protection you have built with so much care seem to be destroyed by the images of violence that break through the walls of your home?'

Merdan agreed and added: 'I want to protect them from the pain; I want them to lead a safe and good life. But I also hope they may know about this pain.'

'It is important for you to be protected from this suffering, but at the same time you want to transmit the story of suffering to your children,' reflected the co-therapist.

Dilnaz nodded: 'I think they understand, because they come close to me very often; they come to sit on my lap or hug me when I am afraid or sad.'

The therapist reflected: 'As if they understand a lot of painful things are happening.' When Dilnaz nodded, the therapist added: 'And as if they want to pull you to life?' 'Maybe,' responded Dilnaz.

In this fragment, the co-therapist (3rd author) shifted the conversation to reflect on ongoing parent-child interactions. Through interventions aiming at *exploring and joining family narration* within the parent-child dyad and *validating protection and care* across generations, the co-therapist invited Dilnaz to reflect on how her profound embodied connection with her mother could support an understanding of the children's felt experience of Dilnaz's pain. This opened a space to reflect on their children's experience of their mother's suffering in exile and how ongoing mother-child interactions indicated their silent care for their mother's gradual disconnection from a sense of purpose. Through acknowledging the mutual orientation towards protecting each other in both parents and children, the therapeutic dialogue evolved into an initial *inscribing relational meaning within family trauma history*, in which the parents explored how they wished to inscribe their children's lives within family trauma history. Here, Dilnaz and Merdan expressed their ambivalence in shaping the role of their trauma history in their children's future trajectories. They accounted for their hope that their children would be protected from traumatic suffering, holding a representation of their flight as ensuring safety in their children's future, while simultaneously expressing their wish that their children would not forget, evoking their hope that their children would become actors of remembering the plight of their parents and their community. In this initial exploration, the parents voiced how their children's current and future engagement with the family's trauma history was imbued with their hopes for shaping a meaningful inscription of traumatic experience in parental life histories.

The therapist turned to the co-trainer (2nd author), who was sitting in the wider circle of reflecting team psychotherapists. The therapist asked him: 'We are speaking together about how to find a way to speak to children about the war and the suffering it brings into their home. I hear two languages that speak of the pain of Dilnaz and Merdan, the language of partisans and the language of fear and guilt. I wonder, can we bring in the group as witnesses? How can we represent a community of witnesses?'

For a while, the co-trainer remained silent, until he said: 'What I feel is anger. A word that has not been said here.' He spoke slowly, came into the small circle, sat down on his knees next to Dilnaz, and uttered again: 'I feel so much anger.' Dilnaz started to cry; Merdan bent his head close to his lap.

The co-trainer asked the group in the wider circle: 'Who among you felt anger while listening here?' Silently, all raised their hands.

In this intervention of *voicing the untold in traumatic experience*, the co-trainer (2nd author) opened a space for an unspoken experience in both parents' expressions of traumatic suffering. His reflection on his inner resonating of anger throughout Dilnaz and Merdan's stories provided an acknowledgment of the not-yet-spoken lived experience [32]. Through kneeling down with them, he embodied the weight of their plight, humbly expressed his solidarity, and was present in a profound validation of their silent indignation. Both parents' response to his voicing and holding of the unspoken anger indicates how the co-trainer connected to a profound experience in the relational processes of witnessing past and present trauma. This holding and validation of the unspoken was further amplified by the co-trainer's mobilization of the reflecting team: their silent raising of hands in the wider circle of witnesses may have resonated cultural coping strategies of addressing pain within communal spaces [33]. Here, in its providing of a strong context of holding evoked by clients' mobilization of empathy towards an audience representing their host community, the circle of witnesses resonated the encounter between home and host societies, allowing for a lived experience of trauma narration not as mere process of autobiography but as relational story emerging from the interaction between the speaker and a community of listeners [34].

> The co-trainer continues to explore anger as a space of the untold between parents: 'Anger leads to distance between people. Anger makes you, Father, sit with your back turned away from you, Mother. Anger needs a language, otherwise it makes people sick. Why can't the anger be spoken?'
>
> He moves to sit down on the ground in front of them: 'If I would be seven years old and I would be sitting here, then I would feel how much I would like to sit here, in between you, and how the anger is creating distance between you. It makes you turn away from each other,' and he brings their arms together, crossing the space between their chairs. 'There is so much anger that seeks to get out.
>
> 'Anger seeks a dream, it seeks a goal. And your children need an image of their future. What are your dreams for your children's future? What do you dream for them?'

Throughout this unfolding of therapeutic dialogue, the co-trainer further shifted the therapeutic dialogue to an orientation towards the children's position in the ongoing dynamics of approaching and avoiding trauma within family interaction. His bodily movement between a position close to the parents, voicing their disconnection in coping with their anger, and sitting down on the ground, symbolizing the children's position, further mobilized the parents' sensitive engagement with the impact of their shared silence on the children's lived experience of safety. Here, while the co-trainer's words invited the parents to explore their hesitation to speak about lived experiences of anger, he simultaneously mobilized them to reshape their anger into a meaningful future perspective, a dream that could voice the legitimacy of their indignation while being stripped of its distancing or aggressive power. Through inserting the perspective of their children's position and development, the therapeutic dialogue supported Dilnaz and Merdan in *inscribing relational meaning within family trauma history* and reshaping their silent anger into meaningful future perspectives, in mobilizing their anger as a source of meaningful dreams for their children while allowing for a space to restore a sense of agency in counteracting the felt experience of meaninglessness into fragments of hope. In the further conversation, both parents initiated their reflection on envisioning their children's future and how the dream for their future was interwoven with transgenerational trauma histories:

> Merdan responded: 'I want to avoid they make the choice for the military struggle; I don't want them to make the choice I've made. I want them to learn what is right; I want them to be sensitive to injustice and to fight against injustice, but without repeating my life story.'
>
> 'What about you?' asked the co-trainer of Dilnaz.
>
> 'I would like them to become persons with a good heart, persons who help others.' Here, Dilnaz started to bring in fragments of their history of oppression and collective violence as

part of the Kurdish community in Turkey and Syria. She recounted the burden of the responsibility she felt as a young girl when becoming a member of the military struggle, separated from her family in Syria, and told the group about Merdan's father, an important intellectual, community leader, and politician, who was imprisoned for many years during Merdan's childhood. His father had wished that Merdan would not enter the military struggle but continue to fight for Kurdish rights in writing and intellectual debate, with 'the pen as our weapon,' but after Merdan's father was released, Merdan distanced himself from his father's wish and became part of the armed forces.

Dilnaz continued: 'We want the girls to know about the injustice, but we want to protect them against this pain.'

Through reflecting on their dreams for a future involved in justice, Dilnaz and Merdan may have given words to their unspoken anger: an anger that not only reflected indignation about atrocity and the shattering of humanity in past and present oppression, but a refraining from expressing anger in a life history where anger was so closely tied to aggression and a profound orientation towards not reiterating violence in their children's future lives [13]. Further, the developing conversation about their dreams for their children seems to have created a space in which they could bridge vocabularies of collective and intimate suffering in spousal interaction, as Dilnaz turned to fragments of collective violence shaping the shared predicament of the Kurdish community and voiced Merdan's profound suffering on the sequelae of this communal plight within the intimate relationship with his father. Here, Dilnaz expressed her emerging understanding of how sharing future dreams with their children would imply addressing complex moral questions on the legitimacy of violence in resisting injustice, and how similar questions had been negotiated in parent-child relationships in the previous generation, at times when both parents, during their transition into young adulthood, had witnessed the oppression and atrocities inflicted on their own parents and had given shape to their responses of both loyalty and autonomy. Her account indicates the process of *inscribing relational meaning within family trauma history* in therapeutic dialogue, acknowledging how the investment of parent-child relationships with meaningful future perspectives would involve fragments of transmitting stories of trauma in its intersection of collective and personal meanings. In the therapeutic space, Dilnaz and Merdan joined in a holding of how their children's engagement with the collective predicament of Kurdish oppression would be intricately intertwined with their daughters' responses to their parents' personal trauma histories, bridging languages of partisans and suffering.

Case Analysis (c): A Family Story Book

We invited the children, who had been playing and drawing outside, to come in. When welcoming the children, the co-trainer (2nd author) asked Elin and Jine whether they thought they knew what we had been talking about. Both girls remained silent for a while, and the co-trainer added: 'If you remain silent like this, then I feel we don't have to explain anymore, then I know for sure that you know what we have been talking about.'

The therapist (1st author) said: 'We asked Mom and Dad to come here today and work together about the worries of being a refugee. Do you know what that is, a refugee?'

Jine, the youngest daughter, responded: 'People who go from one country to another.' 'But they go because of war.' Elin added.

The co-trainer said: 'You understood it well: but they go because of war. Can you explain that a little more?'

Elin uttered: 'That stupid people start a war, and then people have to leave from the war.'

'And what about us here today; what do you think we have been talking about?' asked the co-trainer.

'I don't know,' Elin said quietly. The co-trainer came to sit behind her chair.

'About refugees,' Elin added.

Both girls moved from their chairs, Elin onto her mother's lap and Jine onto her father's lap.

The co-trainer sat down close to the family, with each parent holding a child close to them. 'I can see it is safe to sit there,' he said. 'Is this how you would sit at home?'

'Maybe yes,' Dilnaz said. Elin added: 'Sometimes we come down to give a hug, or to say something, and then we go back upstairs.'

'Yes,' confirmed Jine, 'because then we are shy, so we go back upstairs.' The girls went back to their chairs. The co-trainer wondered: 'What do you know about your mom and dad? Do you dare to ask them: Where were you born?' He went to sit down next to Elin.

Jine responded: 'Mom was born in Syria.' Elin said: 'Dad was born in Turkey.' Dilnaz and Merdan listened carefully. Jine added: 'Mom is from Afrin.'

'So is there a war over there?' asked the co-trainer.

'I don't know,' whispered Elin.

'Would you dare to ask?' added the co-trainer.

'No,' Elin quietly responded.

The therapist (1st author) expressed: 'I think Elin listens a lot and hears a lot; I think there is a lot inside of her, but it feels as if she is concerned to talk about it because it could be hurtful for Mom and Dad.'

The co-trainer touched Elin's head with his hand and said: 'There is a lot going on in here, in this little head. But it keeps silent, just like Mom and Dad keep silent.'

The co-trainer stood up and addressed Dilnaz and Merdan: 'Your children need a story. They need your story.'

It is silent for a while, and the co-trainer added: 'There is a history to feel proud of, and your children need your story.'

After a short silence, he continued: 'Elin and Jine, maybe in the next weeks you can talk with Mom and Dad, and then come back here and tell us about what you've learned.'

The therapist (1st author) suggested: 'Could it be an idea that Elin and Jine would work on a book, like journalists, a book of their family's story?'

'But we don't have paper!' responded Elin. The therapist reflected: 'Maybe Elin says she is not sure Mom and Dad like the idea of making a book as journalists?'

Both Dilnaz and Merdan confirmed to their girls 'We will make the book.'

Elin said: 'I also would like to have parts of the newspaper in our book, about the war in Afrin.'

Jine added: 'But we don't have glue!'

Dilnaz responded: 'We will go and buy glue!'

The therapist reflected: 'It seems that today, every one of you expressed their hesitation about sharing the family story, and at the same time I never heard Mom and Dad say this strongly that they want to work on the family book with you, Elin and Jine. And I wonder: could it be an idea that everyone in the wider circle here writes down a reflection for you to add to your book, for you to know that your book is held by many people?'

When the group agreed, we concluded: 'There will be mail to add to your family book!'

In this fragment, therapeutic interventions further the *exploring and joining family narration* and *validating protection and care* with a particular focus on parent-child relationships, shaped through a careful engagement with the shared avoidance of traumatic predicaments in family relationships and giving words to the protective orientations imbuing the children's joining in their parents' silence. In his positioning on the floor, next to the children or behind their chairs, the co-trainer embodied his resonating with the children's lived experience of the family's silence on past and present trauma. As he was sitting next to their chairs and speaking to their parents about his inner understanding of the children's silencing, the co-trainer's words attempted to give words to the meaning of the children's silence, both as a shared relational strategy transmitted from parents to children and as the children's active position of attempting to care for their parents, protecting them from their silent fear of what could be part of past and present stories of trauma [13].

This invitation to amplify sensitivity and responsiveness to the unspoken in parent-child relationships developed through a balancing movement of the therapeutic position between validating the care underlying the relational process of avoidance in family relationships and actively inviting family members to open ways of trauma narration that could provide children with a meaningful story of past, present, and future. Hereby, the therapeutic dialogue shifted into interventions that invited an *inscribing relational meaning within family trauma history*: the co-trainer (2nd author) engaged in mobilization of the parent-child relationship as a space of shaping meaningful relational stories of trauma within family relationships and of projecting indignation invoked by injustice into meaningful future perspectives. Through giving voice to his understanding of the children's developmental and relational position with parent-child relationships imbued with avoidance, the co-trainer brought another language for shaping the transmission of trauma stories into therapeutic dialogue: he invited parents to tell stories about their roots in family, communal, and cultural bonds to their children. His reference to the children's need for a story did not aim to push for the disclosure of traumatic suffering but aimed at jointly shaping a language that could allow for a safe distance from traumatic experience while at the same time enabling the children to feel connected to family roots and future. In the conversation that unfolded, the therapeutic dialogue invited a symbolic engagement with this transmission through jointly working on a family book. Here, the figure of the book brought in a creative and playful language from which to develop fragments of trauma narration. This shift into creative language may have supported the shift to the mode of action in coping with traumatic suffering in family relationships, reversing the powerlessness into agency and authorship. This invitation to coauthor their family story aimed at inviting them to shape their unique vocabularies of trauma narration that could operate as vehicles of transmission while equally ensuring their agency in deciding upon what would become part of the family book and what wouldn't. Both parents strongly supported the perspective on jointly working on the family book in responding to their daughters' subsequent voices of hesitation that were reflected in their expressions of having no paper or glue, indicating the children's active participation in the family's relational regulation of wishes to approach and avoid trauma in a process of mutual protection. Here, the therapeutic dialogue may have supported parents in their active expression of their sensitive responsiveness to their children's silent concerns and fears of their parents' suffering, to their need of a family story to feel part of. The oldest daughter's explicit reference to including parts of newspapers on the violence in Syria indicates how she broadened the children's need of a story to the complex intersection between past and present trauma stories within the family.

In closing the reflecting team session, the invitation to the members of the wider circle aimed at amplifying the role of containment and acknowledgment of suffering in the family's wider social fabric, expressing how their story should not be silenced in social spaces of their country of exile and developing a symbolic social holding through adding letters from host society members to their family book.

Case Analysis (d): Transmitting History in Relational Stories of Restoration

In the next family session with the therapist (1st author) and co-therapist (3rd author), a naming and validating of the continuing hesitation to share in a family story of past and present traumatic predicaments evolved into a gradual transmission of fragments of the family history and present:

Jine explained how she had been collecting pictures, and how she had brought together pictures of Mom and Dad in military uniform. The therapist reflected: 'So it is not only a journalist, but also a photographer working on your family book?' Both girls giggled and nodded.

'But I didn't speak about it with Mom and Dad,' Jine said.

'You were just working silently as a photographer, searching for pictures?' Jine nodded.

'How about your work as a journalist?', the therapist asked Elin.

She explained how she had been keeping newspaper articles on the violence in Afrin. Elin quietly added that she did not show the articles to her mom and dad yet. 'The book is still empty, because I first prepared questions. But they are not ready yet, so I didn't write them down; they are just in my head. They need to be right first.' Both parents listened very carefully.

'I wonder if what you tell us, Elin and Jine, is that the photographer and journalist feel a bit unsure about their work. As if they are afraid to ask questions that are not right?' asked the therapist. Both girls nodded. The therapist continued: 'Can you help me understand why you are concerned about asking wrong questions?'

The girls responded with silence.

The therapist reflected: 'Maybe you are afraid they could make Mom and Dad sad?'

'Yes,' said Elin, and both girls approached Dilnaz's chair almost simultaneously, where Dilnaz had started to cry silently.

Dilnaz addressed both therapists: 'I don't want them to know this pain.' She cried and continued: 'And, you know, the pain is not just history. It's not over. It is now! And I don't want them to know this pain.'

Elin and Jine stood behind Mom, each holding one of Dilnaz's shoulders.

The therapist responded: 'When I listen to you, I hear you say how difficult it is to work on the family book if so much of this pain is not just part of your history as a family, but is also part of your present as a family. And you want to protect them from this pain. And Dilnaz, when you are telling us this, I see two girls who listen attentively, who come close to you almost immediately when you feel pain, and who come to protect you. They feel the pain you want to protect them from.'

Jine expressed: 'We see it, even when the tear is not even rolling from her eye, but when the tear is waiting in the corner of her eye.'

The therapist turned to Dilnaz: 'They feel your pain, but they don't know words for your pain. They don't know what your tears are telling. And maybe they try to find words for your tears inside of themselves, because they are trying to understand what your tears are about.'

And maybe what they are thinking is frightening too. Maybe their thoughts are difficult to bear, when they are searching for what your tears may be saying.'

Elin and Jine nodded. 'Yes,' Jine said.

The therapist reflected: 'I am wondering whether the work on the family book could be a bit too difficult for the journalist and photographer. Maybe it is burdensome for their work if they feel that some parts of the book are too painful for Mom and Dad, and if they are afraid to ask questions that are painful for Mom and Dad.'

Elin and Jine nodded.

The therapist asked: 'Maybe we can agree on parts of the book that are not too difficult, parts that are nice to work on, and ask the journalist and photographer to work on those parts, and we can then continue to think, together with Mom and Dad, about how to address the parts that are more difficult and what could be words or parts of stories that feel safe for Mom and Dad to share in your book, and that could help Elin and Jine give some meaning to the pain they feel in Mom and Dad?'

Throughout this initial exploration, the girls recounted how the invitation to create a family book had supported them to shift into a position of approaching traumatic predicaments in their family history. With the youngest daughter engaging with her parents' background in military struggle and the oldest daughter documenting newspaper items on the ongoing violence in her mother's home country, they had together engaged in orienting the family book on both past and present trauma. Here, the therapeutic dialogue explored how the photographer and journalist had not shared their work with their parents but returned to the family's shared avoidance. Giving words to their fear of their parents' suffering that imbued their hesitation to pursue their work on the family book in parent-child interaction opened a space for the mother to express her profound orientation towards not instilling her suffering into her children in a family story that was this strongly affected by present atrocities. In her emphasis on the present violence in her home country, she accounted for the inhibition of her ability to engage in the sharing of a transgenerational family story that could not provide narrative closure in the face of the traumatic present.

In the therapist's inner dialogue, the hesitations expressed by the girls and Dilnaz resonated as hesitation on the extent to which the family book may have been too threatening for Merdan and Dilnaz, transgressing their authorship in shaping a relational story of trauma. Experiencing the potential violence of the family book if it was experienced as a mere push towards disclosure without ensuring a parental sense of safety and agency in monitoring transmission, the therapist's response aimed at holding Dilnaz's hesitation as a valid expression of protection while simultaneously inserting the children's position into therapeutic dialogue. She explicitly voiced the children's ongoing alertness to their mother's suffering and how the absence of meaning for her tears may evoke their silent fear, a reiteration of their mother's fear without words. These interventions of *validating protection and care* aimed to address dyadic transactions between Dilnaz's and the children's lived experiences, in which the shared avoidance of creating a family story was understood as a vehicle of shared protection. Giving words to the mutual protection underpinning avoidance created a safe conversational space to shift into *inscribing relational meaning within family trauma history*, where the therapist invited family members to create safe modes of partial disclosure of traumatic suffering within the parent-child relationship in order to shape spaces of meaning for these silenced predicaments that could allow family members secure and meaningful ways of inhabiting silence.

When all family members agreed, the co-therapist (3rd author) wondered whether it could be an idea to talk about the history of love between Mom and Dad. Elin decisively responded: 'Mom and Dad are not in love; we were just born here. They are friends.'

At this moment, Merdan and Dilnaz told their children about their story of falling in love with each other and how their love was forbidden by the system of the militia. They expressed how they could not write each other but decided to wait for each other for years, separated between Belgium and Kurdistan. While the girls listened and giggled with twinkling eyes, the mother and father told their children about how they found each other again in Belgium and then started their family.

'This is a very special story,' the therapist said to the girls. 'The first time you hear about this beautiful story of Mom and Dad being in love.'

Dilnaz reflected: 'It is just now that I realize I did not tell the girls about us, because love was not allowed by the system. I kept on thinking within the rules, even until now. When I think about it now, I understand the repression of the system continued until here; I was still thinking within the rules of the system and that's why I thought I couldn't tell them about it. We were not allowed to fall in love; we were not allowed to have children.'

The therapist reflected: 'Dilnaz, what you tell us now is also a part of the family book; this is part of your family history.'

'Yes,' she responded, smiling and with tears in her eyes, 'and this is so beautiful to talk about. When I think about it, I still can't believe I could become mother of these two girls.' Then, Dilnaz went on to talk about her past times in the militia, explaining to the girls how she felt responsible for fighting for justice for the Kurdish community when she was 17 years old, even while knowing the hardships that would be part of life in the resistance army. The girls listened carefully when their mother talks about her moral training in the militia and about her memories of strong expressions of solidarity in their group, the cohesion and care she felt when a fellow member who held even a tiny bit of sugar in her backpack shared it with the others, and the profound communal bonds this shaped across time and borders, even into exile.

Addressing the girls, who sat in front of their mother listening to her story, the therapist asked: 'When Mom is telling you their love was not allowed in the system they were part of, do you know what that is – a system?'

'No,' both girls responded. The therapist turned to Merdan and asked him to explain the meaning of a system to his children. After he told his girls about a system by referring to the rules of their classroom or a country, the therapist added: 'The story of Mom and Dad is a story of a love that was stronger than the system they were part of.'

Merdan started to cry, and the therapist asked him what his tears were telling. He expressed how fighting against injustice in systems was an important part of his life: 'I fought against the oppression of the Kurds and later, I resisted the rules in the system of our own military.' He remained silent for a while and then added: 'But if Elin and Jine would take distance from the system of our resistance movement, I am so afraid that they let go of our struggle. I hope they will not let go of Kurdistan.'

'You hope they will share in your dream of Kurdistan,' the therapist reflected.

'Yes,' said Merdan. 'But I also want them to know that always, always, you can find alternative ways to fight for justice.' Dilnaz cried listening to Merdan.

In concluding the session, the therapists offered the letters that were written to them by the reflecting team members to the family.

In this fragment, exploring the story of love between parents and inviting the father's reflection on the meaning of political systems in their parents' life histories aimed at a shared *inscribing relational meaning within family trauma history* within parent-child relationships and evolved into fragments of *voicing the untold in traumatic experience.*

Therapeutic interventions initiated a process of modulated disclosure, mobilizing modes of narrative reconstruction that supported the restoration of meaning while enabling a safe distance from traumatic life experiences. In the sharing of the love story between parents that was never told before, in Dilnaz's account of her time in the military, and in Merdan's expressions on the role of political systems, the parents engaged in a partial transmission of past predicaments of collective violence that supported their children's anchoring in their family history while at the same time projecting their dreams for their children's future coping with these parental stories of injustice. Dilnaz's reflection on the enduring silencing of the love story in exile as an expression of her continuing oppression by strict rulings in the military system enabled a moment *of voicing the untold in traumatic experience* that supported her transgression of these rulings in the here-and-now of the session, as a space of reconnecting with autonomy and the authorship of her life. This fragment of reconstruction developed as a relational story of restoring meaning, as her relationship to her daughters became the locus of her reclaiming of voice and freedom. In her unfolding story, she shifted to providing her daughters with a window into her experiences while being part of the militia. Her moving account of her life echoed hardship and violence but simultaneously enabled her children to connect to experiences of solidarity and communal ties in the face of injustice. In Merdan's reflection on the meaning of a 'system' in their life stories, he silently evoked his personal involvement in violence and simultaneously voiced the moral complexities of revolting against human rights abuses, addressing how the resistance against the injustice inflicted upon the Kurdish community may have evolved into injustice within the resistance itself. Through this *voicing of the untold in traumatic experience* in which Merdan shared burdensome moral questions imbuing his life story, he expressed his profound wish to safeguard threads of continuity in his daughters' lives, continuities of cultural and collective identities and of resistance against injustice. Here, implicitly reconnecting to their grandfather's position of developing resistance without violence, he invited his daughters to develop ways of continuing to imbue their future lives with an engagement with the Kurdish community but to shape this resistance without violence and aggression.

Throughout this unfolding dialogue, Dilnaz and Merdan developed a vocabulary of transmission and shaped a relational process of trauma narration that operated in a space beyond literal or detailed disclosure, a narrative spoken in the language of political agency and cultural continuity, of solidarity in the face of suffering, of cultural notions of self and community, and a joint emphasis on restoring justice. Here, both parents mobilized the parent-child relationship not only as a space of trauma narration, but as an intimate space of reclaiming political agency and a relational space restoring the possibility of meaning and humanity in life histories of atrocity and injustice.

Conclusion: A Therapeutic Relationship Moving between the Told and the Untold, Shaping Spaces to Inhabit the Untold

In this chapter, we described a phased intervention approach in working with trauma narration with refugee families, and reflected through a case analysis on working within this phased approach. Throughout the (often circular) use of four consecutive modes of intervention, therapeutic dialogue develops a gradual engagement with trauma narration within family relationships through the inscription of therapeutic dialogue in the unique relational patterns of narrating and silencing traumatic experience, the exploration of protection and care underpinning these patterns, inscribing relational meanings within trauma history, and creating a safe space for voicing the untold lived experience revolving around past and present traumatic experience. Throughout this phased approach, working on trauma narration does not primarily focus on the telling of family trauma stories in the there-and-then, but involves mobilizing here-and-now interactions in their present emotional intensity to support safe spaces of 'working around trauma' [20]. These conversations expand through time and require a careful movement between subsystems (e.g., couple relationship, parent-child dyad, extended family network) in jointly creating the family system's engagement with trauma narration.

Throughout these consecutive, circular modes of therapeutic intervention, the core instrument of this work is the therapeutic relationship itself. The therapeutic relationship becomes an integral part of relational transactions of both narration and silence, shifting between positions of approaching and avoiding trauma. This invokes the therapists' inner resonances that echo potential meanings of what is told and untold within family relationships and history. A central part of therapeutic positioning is the active reflection on how the therapeutic relationship becomes imbued with the families' balancing between narration and silencing of traumatic predicaments and how the therapists' inner voices resonate family members' constructions of the world, their constructions of understanding and coping with traumatic life stories in the context of transgenerational lineage and present exile. These resonances are brought into dialogue, where the therapist gives words to potential meanings and experiences imbuing family interaction, providing them with a space of welcome and recognition. Here, the therapeutic relationship mirrors the secure attachment relationship where a sensitive, responsive attachment figure mentalizes and provides words that are able to hold vulnerable experience, words that invest lived experience with meaning and enable regulation.

Throughout this therapeutic process of becoming part of the dynamics of approaching and avoiding traumatic experience and providing them with a mentalizing welcome, the therapeutic position moves towards a position of voicing the untold in traumatic experience. Through giving words to inner resonances, therapeutic intervention may provide a language to lived experience and emotions that are difficult to express, disconnected, or pushed to the margins in relational patterns of coping with trauma. This may develop through voicing resonances of guilt, despair, or indignation, or through explicitly bringing the child's perspective into therapeutic dialogue. In this latter insertion of the child's position, family members are invited to shift the process of trauma narration into a novel space of engagement with traumatic history: it supports parents in actively reflecting on how ongoing relational dynamics relate to children's developmental needs, acknowledges how these interactions are imbued with traumatic suffering, and invites parents to project this suffering into hope for their family's future. Here, refugee parents are invited to explore ways of transmitting representations of the family's past beyond a mere emphasis on its disruptive impact: they are supported in their ability to hold the ambiguities in which they live and to express a vision for their children's future within these ambiguities. Investing traumatic experience with hopeful future perspectives enables them to share in fragments of trauma transmission, parts of the untold that are expressed in imagining a future.

In gradually moving towards sharing these spaces of the untold, the therapeutic position often involves a certain transgression of the client system's trauma communication pattern. It is, however, not a transgression that pushes towards traumatic disclosure, nor a transgression of the untold that focuses on the content or events of traumatic life history: it is a transgression that aims to create a dialogical space for unspoken layers of meaning and experience that are related to living in the face of a traumatic past and present. Here, inscribing therapeutic dialogue in the dynamic tension between approaching and avoiding trauma evolves into therapeutic interventions that invite a meaningful engagement with the untold and that may enable restorative ways of inhabiting the untold. Importantly, this opening of spaces for the untold within the family's narration and silence of traumatic history is not understood as an objective description given to family members by the therapist as an external expert of what is at stake in the family. Rather, it operates as an invitation to dialogue: through carefully listening to and welcoming family members' responses, family members are primary partners in expressing whether the therapist's inner voices will come to operate as words for what was yet untold. Here, opening spaces for the untold does not imply a transgression that reiterates the position of powerlessness in the trauma victim but precisely aims at mobilizing agency and authorship.

Throughout this process, family members' authorship may also be supported by yet another dimension inherent to the therapeutic relationship, a relationship that holds the promise of not only resonating the intimate containment and regulation of a secure attachment dyad but also of mirroring a space of communal listening. Throughout the creating of a holding environment that mobilizes and voices the multilayered meanings revolving around traumatic experience, the therapeutic relationship always inherently carries the imprint of its broader social context, resonating the encounter between home and host societies and between cultural universes [35]. Here, authorship in family members may be mobilized through the way in which the therapeutic space represents the broader social nexus, providing a forum to speak out, to voice the suffering and hope evoked by atrocities, and to counteract the disruption of language that is so often evoked by collective violence imposing either silence or speech [36]. Here, the therapeutic space may hold the promise of yet another way of inhabiting the untold, the reclaiming of voice and language enabled by the presence of a circle of witnesses, a community of listeners [34].

References

1. L. Nadeau, B. Author and T. Measham, Addressing cultural diversity through collaborative care. In L. Kirmayer, C. Rousseau and J. Guzder, eds., *Cultural Consultation: Encountering the Other in Mental Health Care* (New York: Springer, 2014), pp. 203–221.

2. A. McFarlane and I. Kaplan, Evidence-based psychological interventions for adult survivors of torture and trauma: A 30-year review. *Transcultural Psychiatry*, 49(3–4) (2012), 539–567.

3. R. Kevers, P. Rober, I. Derluyn and L. De Haene, Remembering collective violence: Broadening the notion of traumatic memory in post-conflict rehabilitation. *Culture, Medicine and Psychiatry*, 40(4) (2016), 620–640.

4. M. Gemignani, The past if past: The use of memories and self-healing narratives in refugees from the former Yugoslavia. *Journal of Refugee Studies*, 24 (2011), 132–156.

5. M. Brough, R. Schweitzer, J. Shakespeare-Finch, L. Vromans and J. King, Unpacking the micro-macro nexus: Narratives of suffering and hope among refugees from Burma recently settled in Australia. *Journal of Refugee Studies*, 26(2) (2013), 207–225.

6. L. K. Kirmayer, Failures of imagination: The refugee's narrative in psychiatry. *Anthropology & Medicine*, 10(2) (2003), 167–185.

7. C. Rousseau, M. Morales and P. Foxen, Going home: Giving voice to memory strategies of young Mayan refugees who returned to Guatemala as a community.

Culture, Medicine and Psychiatry, 25(2) (2001), 135–168.

8. C. Sluzki, *The Presence of the Absent: Therapy with Families and Their Ghosts* (New York: Routledge, 2015).

9. J. L. Herman, *Trauma and Recovery* (New York: Basic Books, 1992).

10. L. De Haene, P. Rober, P. Adriaenssens and K. Verschueren, Voices of dialogue and directivity in family therapy with refugees: Evolving ideas about dialogical refugee care. *Family Process*, 51(3) (2012), 391–404.

11. P. Rober and P. Rosenblatt, Silence and memories of war: An autoethnographic exploration of family secrecy. *Family Process*, 56 (2017), 250–261.

12. A. Hooghe, P. Rosenblatt and P. Rober, 'We hardly ever talk about it': Emotional responsive attunement in couples after a child's death. *Family Process*, 57(1) (2018), 226–240. DOI:http://10.1111/famp.12274

13. R. Kevers, P. Rober, C. Rousseau and L. De Haene, Silencing or silent transmission? An exploratory study on trauma communication in Kurdish refugee families. *Transcultural Psychiatry*, (2019, under revision).

14. N. T. Dalgaard and E. Montgomery, Disclosure and silencing: A systematic review of the literature on patterns of trauma communication in refugee families. *Transcultural Psychiatry*, 52(5) (2015), 579–593.

15. E. Montgomery, Tortured families: A coordinated management of meaning analysis. *Family Process*, 43(3) (2004), 349–371.

16. T. Measham and C. Rousseau, Family disclosure of war trauma to children. *Traumatology*, 16(2) (2010), 85–96.

17. N. J. Lin, K. L. Suyemoto and P. N. Kiang, Education as catalyst for intergenerational refugee family communication about war and trauma. *Communication Disorders Quarterly*, 30 (4) (2009), 195–207.

18. N. Dalgaard, B. Todd, S. Daniel and E. Montgomery, The transmission of trauma in refugee families: Associations between intra-family trauma communication style, children's attachment security and psychosocial adjustment. *Attachment & Human Development*, 18(1) (2016), 69–89.

19. R. Kevers, P. Rober and L. De Haene, The role of collective identifications in family processes of posttrauma reconstruction: An exploratory study of Kurdish refugee families and their diasporic community. *Kurdish Studies*, 5 (2) (2017), 3–29.

20. C. Rousseau and T. J. Measham, Posttraumatic suffering as a source of transformation: A clinical perspective. In L. J. Kirmayer, R. Lemelson and M. Barad, eds., *Understanding Trauma: Integrating Biological, Clinical and Cultural Perspectives* (Cambridge, UK: Cambridge University Press, 2007), 275–294.

21. L. De Haene, C. Rousseau, R. Kevers, N. Deruddere and P. Rober, Stories of trauma in family therapy with refugees: Supporting safe relational spaces of narration and silence. *Clinical Child Psychology & Psychiatry*, 23(2) (2018), 258–278.

22. M. Elkaïm, *Si tu m'aimes, ne m'aime pas* (Paris: Points, 1989).

23. P. Rober, The therapist's self in dialogical family therapy: Some ideas about not-knowing and the therapist's inner conversation. *Family Process*, 44(4) (2005), 477–495.

24. P. Rober, *In Therapy Together: Family Therapy as a Dialogue* (London: Palgrave, 2017).

25. S. Minuchin and H. C. Fishman, *Family Therapy Techniques* (Cambridge, MA: Harvard University Press, 1981).

26. E. Bourgeois-Guérin and C. Rousseau, La survie comme don: Réflexions entourant les enjeux de la vie suite au genocide chez des hommes rwandais. *L'Autre*, 15(1) (2014), 55–63.

27. E. S. Uehara, M. Farris, P. T. Morelli and A. Ishisaka, 'Eloquent chaos' in the oral discourse of killing fields survivors: An exploration of atrocity and narrativization. *Culture, Medicine and Psychiatry*, 25(1) (2001), 29–61.

28. T. Andersen, The reflecting team: Dialogue and meta-dialogue. *Family Process*, 26(4) (1987), 415–428.

29. M. White, *Maps of Narrative Practice* (New York: W. W. Norton, 2007).

30. L. Kirmayer, C. Rousseau and J. Guzder, Introduction: The place of culture in mental health services. In L. Kirmayer, J. Guzder and C. Rousseau, eds., *Cultural Consultation: Encountering the Other in Mental Health Care* (New York: Springer, 2014), pp. 1–20.

31. P. Rober and L. De Haene, Intercultural therapy and the limitations of a cultural competency framework: About cultural differences, universalities and the unresolvable tensions between them. *Journal of Family Therapy*, 36(S1) (2014), 3–20.

32. P. Rober, Some hypotheses about hesitations and their nonverbal expression in family therapy practice.

33. D. Pely, Quasi-customary dispute resolution mechanisms in Israeli Darfuri refugees. *Conflict Resolution Quarterly*, 35 (1) (2017), 111–140. DOI:http://10.1002/crq.21198

34. L. K. Kirmayer, The refugee's predicament. *L'Évolution Psychiatrique*, 67(4) (2002), 724–742.

35. L. De Haene and P. Rober, Looking for a home: An exploration of Jacques Derrida's notion of hospitality in family therapy practice with refugees. In I. McCarthy and G. Simon, eds., *Systemic Therapy as Transformative Practice* (Farnhill: Everything is Connected Press, 2016), 94–110.

36. C. Rousseau, The place of the unexpressed: Ethics and methodology for research with refugee children. *Canada's Mental Health*, 41(Winter) (1993–1994), 12–16.

Journal of Family Therapy, 24(2) (2002), 187–204.

Exile and Belonging

Negotiating Identity, Acculturation and Trauma in Refugee Families

Jaswant Guzder

Introduction

In the course of our engagement with refugee and displaced families, family consultations and family therapy processes bear witness to child and adolescent identity vicissitudes. Though the reasons for referral may be related to mental health problems, including disorders, distress, legal or psychosocial variables or school-related issues, we are usually focused on strengthening coping, global functioning, the promotion of resilience and protection in our efforts to evaluate needs and give support during post-migration adaptation. While mental health problems in immigrants to high-income countries are often initially lower than in host culture populations, with child populations showing lower rates of disorders until later in their development, the subgroup of refugees or displaced migrants with significant pre-migratory trauma have higher rates of trauma-related disorders, chronic pain or somatic disorders [1] and are often referred to us from primary care or school settings. The issues of the child may be intertwined with peer groups, systemic or institutional issues, pre-migratory trauma, family dynamics, ethnicity or psychosocial stressors. This paper will use a case history approach to underline some of the challenges of working with identity shifts in the course of exile, adaptation and coping with resettlement. These case examples are based on families who had been referred to a teaching child psychiatry day hospital or cultural consultation service [2] and integrate cultural formulation and cultural axis, appreciating complex cultural variables as well as systemic and child psychiatric evaluation approaches [3].

Acculturation evolves across time, across life stages and across generations. Each family member, parent and child, deals with shifting agendas of identity, cultural hybridity and cultural frames of reference as part of the migration journey and process. It remains essential for therapists to be aware of cultural safety [4], entailing the clinician's sensitivity to 'any actions that diminish, demean or disempower the cultural identity and well-being of an individual'. From this perspective, therapists are oriented towards creating a working therapeutic alliance and acknowledging social and power gradients as reciprocal elements of therapist, institution and client relations, and they strive to empathize with each family member as the family re-structures itself and settles into the new predicaments of North American life.

Therapists or teams using a systemic approach engage family narratives with listening and empathic stances while monitoring their capacity for reflection, mentalization and transference responses. Refugees live with uncertainty and impart partial histories that usually involve complex narratives. Therefore, working with team reflection or co-therapy becomes advisable and supportive for competent therapeutic intervention, as well as facilitating support and balancing therapist perspectives on each member of the family system.

Frames of Reference in Transcultural Systemic Practice: Transgenerational Identity Shifts, Cultural Hybridity and Identity Influenced by Socio-political, Cultural and Resilience Variations

Despite North America's histories of immigration, it was not until 1974 that McGoldrick and others [5] prepared a volume of collected papers on identity and ethnicity relevant to the training of systemic therapists. McGoldrick also suggested the essential role of genograms in unraveling object relations and histories of ethnicities generationally [6]. Therapeutic encounters embrace explicit communication but also implicitly unknown agendas, whether silenced or denied in open dialogue, especially involving traumatic events, secrets, trust, cultural embedding and gendered hierarchies which may operate undetected [7]. Absent or distant family members, whether living or deceased, may also be significant to the understanding and problem-solving approaches of systems and can remain involved in influencing current family predicaments across time and distance. Ghosts or invisible significant others can exert significant influence on sharing in the discourse and decision-making [8].

Since the cultural embedding of personhood is shaped by collectivist or cultural frameworks of self [9], family narratives are helpful in unpacking issues of identities and family roles. The individualism characteristic of European–North American cultures mirrored in our therapeutic literature reflects an ethnocentric emphasis on an autonomous motif of personhood as a social experience of the self normative to western society. However, collectivism is more typical within many Asian, African and indigenous ethnicities and alters the family system narratives, structural and life cycle goals implicated in therapeutic approaches. In collectivist societies, interdependence and collective networking are more likely to be internalized as part of personhood and social identities from early development and in rituals of belonging. In exile, these divergent cultural patterns resonate with the acculturation of social patterns and aims of the life cycle, as validated and supported by a large body of research.

While there are many concepts of personhood that have been proposed and studied, Marcus [10], Roland [11] and Kitayama [12] have suggested that the *interdependent self* of Asian cultures (such as India and Japan) and the *independent self* typical of European–North American contexts pursue different life cycle aims, goals or aspirations. Individualism internalizes more self-directed or autonomy-driven priorities and emphasizes more personal evaluations of internal and social experience [9]. The emerging cultural psychiatry and family therapy literature is gradually becoming more conversant with ethnographies, southern global health concerns and interdisciplinary [13, 14] and intersectional [15] theoretical frameworks that depart from European–North American and colonial agendas.

The writings of Asian therapists, including Girindrasekhar Bose in the early 1900s, who established Indian psychoanalytic training [16, 17], and Sudhir Kakar [13], whose work *The Inner World: A Psychoanalytic Study of Childhood and Society in India* was the first work on Hindu childhood paradigms to outline an alternate cultural, clinical and social experience, challenged the Euro-North American ethnocentrism. Takeo Doi [18] in Japan offered alternate formulations more culturally specific to Japanese intimacy, dependence and relationships with authority. Doi introduced the concept of 'amae' [18] as a Japanese variation of attachment and dependence, powerfully evident in the therapeutic alliance as an experience of positive accompaniment with a parental figure, even in silence. These ethnopsychologies shared their specific Asian clinical experience relevant to our therapeutic frameworks and explored variations of therapist and client relationships.

A more recent research study in 2016 by Vignoles et al. [19] drew from samples in 33 countries and across 55 cultural groups and validated divergences between individualism versus collective social motifs. They reported that these divergences were mirrored by the dimensions of dependence and interdependence as domains of self-definition and person-hood across their sample. These domains of personhood are summarized in seven categories: self-definition (the self as unique versus similar to others); self-experience (self-contained versus connected to the group); decision-making (degree of others impinging on choices or decisions); autonomous care (self-reliance or dependence in taking care of oneself); variability or consistency across contexts (self-expression or harmony with others); communication with others (self-expression or harmony with others as priorities); and resolution of conflicting interests (through self-interest or commitment to others). Further, ethnopsychological and ethnographic studies in African, Asian and indigenous societies have additionally offered a more nuanced and varied specificity to the cultural norms and aims of different cultural groups. These frames of reference shape experiences of suffering and healing [9]. The implications of these forms of ethnographic studies are highly relevant to child-rearing and individuation aims and hence for transcultural family therapy work.

Often in child psychiatry or cultural consultation clinics, resilience promotion and protection issues arise in our assessment process of refugee or migrant clients [20]. Vulnerability versus resilience is often presented as a spectrum of functioning. Rutter [21] and Werner [22] based their work more on individual attributes interacting with protective factors than systemic models. These frameworks somewhat minimized the complexity of wider dimensions of family, cultural, social and environmental factors. Schemas of resilience as developed by Ungar et al. [23] propose a broader internal and environmental framework that may be more relevant both to diversity and the context of growing up with adversity. Ungar suggested that adolescents and youth in all cultures resolve and manage seven tensions that might present in different ways across local contexts and that inform our advocacy work in family therapy (Ungar et al., 2007, p. 295 [23]). The seven tensions of resilience for promoting mental health and growth include: access to material resources (availability of financial, educational and medical resources, employment, essential food, clothing and shelter); relationships (access to significant others, peers and others within family and community); identity (personal and collective sense of purpose, self-appraisal of strengths, weaknesses, aspirations, beliefs and values, spiritual and religious identifications); power and control (experiences of caring for oneself and others, the ability to effect change in one's social and physical environment in order to receive health and support resources); cultural adherence (adherence to one's local and or global cultural practices, values or beliefs); social justice (experiences related to finding a meaningful role in community and social equality); and cohesion (balancing one's personal interests with a sense of responsibility to the greater good; feeling part of something larger than one's self socially and spiritually).

Rather than applying a western understanding of resilience promotion, these authors suggest that we remain more fluid and flexible in approaching aims of development rather than specific pathways. In contexts of diversity, families determine the routes best suited to them based on their unique collaging of their histories and experience. Refugees bring developing children and youth across borders, frequently on complex migration journeys, and may seek to cope in a range of possible ways. During our engagement and systemic approaches, we should remain open to appreciating the impact of cultural embedding and trauma, avoiding diagnostic certainty until we understand the family's lived experience or leaving spaces for the solutions the family might choose to create. From this perspective, resilience frameworks are crucial, inviting family therapists to develop spaces to clarify, explore, facilitate and overcome barriers to family coping.

Refugee clients often occupy a subaltern position in our social context and, in fact, as underserviced populations, rarely have access to family therapy. Intersectional theorists underlined the stratification of class, race, sexual orientation, disability and gender as some of the elements of oppressive categories that excluded patients from institutional care. The articulation of these marginal vulnerabilities emerged with Kimberley Crenshaw [15], who articulated political barriers and lack of equity on the basis of gender and race. Her contribution of intersectionality theory expanded our understanding of the systemic frameworks of power and social categories needed for ethical and equitable approaches to patient care. The structural, political and representational categories of these vulnerabilities had already been introduced in the writings of Franz Fanon [24, 25] on the black and colonial subject and Suman Fernando [26, 27] on the issues of stigma, racism and barriers to services. These issues are relevant to understanding forms of institutional racism and remain widely evident in current predicaments of clinical access and detention policies for refugees and minorities in Europe and in North America. In clinical practices, socio-cultural dimensions of personhood and identity are entwined with those of the therapist and their institutions, whose policies may present bias or unwitting discrimination which is seldom owned or challenged. These elements in refugee care are addressed in the therapist variables of the cultural formulation outline [27].

Acculturation and Identity: Expanding Therapeutic Frameworks

Identity formation and acculturation as part of developmental passages, identity shifts and life stages are relevant for developing refugee children and youth but also for refugee parents. Salman Akhtar's conceptualization of the third individuation [31] proposes that culture and ethnicity are a bedrock aspect of the self in formation. Cultural identity is already evident by the final stages of the first individuation phase of development, but acculturation evolves and shifts throughout the life cycle. Akhtar drew on Mahler's phases of the first individuation [32] and formation of the self, culminating by age four with the emergence or 'hatching' of the self as a significant developmental step of the individual or personhood formation marked by gender and culture. The significant lesson of Akhtar's concept of the third individuation concerning our cultural identities is its endless and unresolvable aspects throughout the life cycle, influenced by immigration and host society realities within social and cultural dynamics.

Immigration encompasses attachments to an adoptive country and natal culture as internal elements of identity for first generation parents and older children or youth, but also for subsequent generations. Akhtar [31] proposes a reciprocity of inner and outer realities that are part of identity as an ongoing dynamic and generational process. His formulation suggests that immigration and identity are constituted of four interlinked strands of identity formation: drives and affective states; interpersonal and inner psychic space; temporality; and social affiliations. The therapist and the patient are mutually influenced by the nuances and complexities of whatever cultural hybridities are omnipresent in their societies. Akhtar implies how vicissitudes and the evolution of the immigrant identity are ongoing processes including shifts of identifications of idealization and devaluation, adoptive versus origin culture, closeness and distancing, hope and nostalgia, transitional phenomena, superego modifications, emerging mutualities and linguistic transformations, all fundamental to both immigrant identity and the therapeutic encounter.

Winnicott begins his chapter on culture in *Playing and Reality* [33] with a metaphoric line from Rabindranath Tagore's Gitanjali poems: 'On the seashore of the endless worlds, children play.' His classical paper *On the Location of Culture* is resonant with Akhtar's model of cultural and ethnic identity as an endless, lifelong agenda. Winnicott was writing in a post-colonial London flooded with migrants when he introduced the terms *transitional phenomena, transitional objects* and *transitional space* as fundamental to identity, culture and cultural hybridity. His premise on identity begins with the early capacity for play and symbolic transformation as a lifelong and evolving project of being in the world. He begins with the baby before the stage of individuation, where a symbiotic bond between mother and child eventually transforms as the baby differentiates with movement, speech and play and establishes its own private inner world. Attachment and healthy individuation are part of establishing a sense of self and continuity of personal existence with a capacity for play and a capacity to engage with cultural hybridity.

Winnicott states that he was exploring *cultural experience* as an extension of the idea of transitional phenomena and of play 'without being certain I can define the word "culture"' (Winnicott, 1971, p. 99 [33]). He does refer to cultural life as including historical, collective and intragenerational memory, or what he calls 'inherited tradition', 'something in the common pool of humanity to which individuals or groups of people contribute [...] *it is not possible to be original except on the basis of tradition*'. The formation of a separate identity remains for Winnicott really a space or a phenomenon between outer and inner realities 'in the potential space between the individual and the environment [...] the same as playing' (Winnicott, 1971, p. 100 [33]). The capacity to use spaces and the resilience to create within the potential or transitional space rest on individual strengths and unique capacities of confidence or security but also on contextual opportunities, including family therapy spaces. The internalized bits of cultural values, social identities and environmental conditions will eventually be the material for promoting resilience, hybridization or acculturation. In transcultural practice, shaping possibilities of transitional space and play in the creation of identity is a central condition of the therapeutic space.

Using the perspectives of Akhtar, Mahler and Winnicott, play and hybridity simultaneously progress as part of processing exile and the refugee experience to generate coherence and global functioning despite the attachment disruptions and breaks inherent to displacement. In post-migration resettlement, many mothers who are homebound or not working may have less exposure than children at school to opportunities to acculturate, or they may have constraints of gender values or language limitations. Traumatic intrusions, whether acute, chronic or cumulative trauma, also limit or change the possibilities of coping with or mastering the challenges of culture change, mourning and engaging with the stress of migration.

Indigenous Maori in New Zealand, interacting with primary care providers including nurses [34], introduced the concept of cultural safety as an essential aspect of therapeutic frameworks for engaging with cultural others. Systemic therapists are usually aware of the necessary conditions for cultural safety in the therapeutic setting [35], aiming to create a space for displaced families or individuals to work on issues of pre-migratory trauma, uncertain status, institutional racism [36] and social suffering [37]. Furthermore, since children and youth are often referred in collaboration with institutions preoccupied with protection and resilience promotion, therapy may equally embrace an advocacy role [38], which remains essential in any systemic assessment.

In addressing these complexities, we are challenged in the task of distinguishing distress versus diagnosis or disorders [29], especially in assessing difficulties in parenting capacity in refugees or recently displaced families. Paul Steinhauer [30] has cautioned us to reserve judgement as a fundamental approach in his guidelines for parenting capacity. It is difficult to assess strengths and resourcefulness under circumstances of disorganizing and uncertain conditions. Pre-migratory trauma, the uncertainty of immigration status, unresolved grief, poverty, illness and the reception of the host society contribute to the pathways of these regressions and strengths in family global functioning. Here, Steinhauer's guidelines for assessing parenting capacity (Steinhauer, 1991 [30]) are often cited in deciding whether parents fall below the minimal standards compatible with normal development in order to decide whether intervention is likely to sufficiently improve the parent's capacity. He outlines what the family therapist may need to consider for refugees or displaced populations in order to properly assess or realistically evaluate the adequacy of parenting and parents' potential for change in response to our interventions. His first guideline advises that the ethnicity and cultural context of the family, as well as the unresolved adjustment issues of refugee and migration experience, impede a fair or objective assessment of mental health and functional capacities. As family therapists, we first engage with alliance-building before making a definitive assessment of parenting capacity.

Clinical Case Examples

The Anorexic Boy and a Medea Response

The following case history spans a period from this refugee family's arrival, when Rakib was a preschooler, to his adolescence. The themes of acculturation shift over the course of his maturation from early childhood to adolescence and include events within peer groups, political gestalts, school environments and legal processes as well as the disorganizing impact of his mother's trauma, poverty and unresolved mourning. His role as a parental child may have secured a meaningful role in his precocious development, which strengthened him at the same time as it burdened him and accelerated his shift to youth agendas.

His narrative involved several crisis points (a few are presented here), while the continuity of his therapeutic network offered the family and the boy the possibility of entering, leaving and re-fuelling with the available consultants and social work supports. These continuities may have functioned as a holding environment which was supportive without the engulfing pressures that were part of his parent-child affective bonds.

A primary care setting was following a refugee woman and family for several years using medication (multiple anti-depressant trials), home visiting, therapy, social work interventions and school support while monitoring and developing a relationship with her two sons. At the time of an initial Cultural Consultation Service (CCS) consultation, the sons were aged four and eight in day care and school. After her refugee board hearings had been refused on appeal, her lawyers embarked on a humanitarian appeal process. At this point of marked uncertainty, the mother had become very distressed, threating to kill herself and to murder both of her sons rather than be deported back to the detention site in the US. This regression was triggered by memories of the detention setting where she had been raped (the existing laws of deportation routed refugees back to the last country from which they had entered Canada, the so-called third country law). The older son, Rakib, had been a witness of the rape and possibly knew that his brother was a product of this traumatic rape. His mother had escaped to North America, after domestic violence and marital rape in their country of origin, with the support of his maternal grandparents before he was of school age. His mother reported that her husband had been anti-social and had kidnapped and raped her in adolescence. She had not told her son these stories, but he was aware of her fear and dread of returning and of his father's violence towards his mother.

After the refugee board's refusal of the appeal, the school social worker noted that Rakib was now withdrawn, refusing to talk with professionals with whom he had had a previous warm bond. He was also refusing to eat and losing weight. Rakib had been his mother's protector and a parental child early in his development. He had acculturated quickly in a francophone school, refusing any connection with his ethnic group. His mother had a command of her native language and some English, limiting employment opportunities.

At the time of the crisis of their refugee board refusal, she had been seen at CCS by a male consultant and refused to speak. By the time of her second consultation with a female consultant, we had engaged in a systemically oriented session with her social worker. In the interview, it was clear that she had a good rapport with her referring therapist. Our focus became her suicidal crisis, which had escalated to threats to jump with both the children onto a freeway in front of her home. The mother revealed how the acute grief triggered by the refusal was also reviving festering wounds that had been present since the death of her parents. She had been unable to attend their funerals, and the current crisis had triggered the same sense of derealization as the parental deaths. She was unable to believe they had died. Their 'ghosts', however, inhabited her psyche; they were present and circulating as a dreamlike presence. Her threats to enact a Medea act appeared to be evoking a reunion fantasy embedded in unresolved mourning compounded by her distress, isolation, loss and fear.

The family meeting became a dialogue with the 'ghosts', which awakened a history of good object relations within her family of origin. In our fantasized dialogue with empty chairs in the therapy space representing her parents, they extended kindness and good wishes as the grandparents of Rakib and their wish for her to re-settle in a safe country. Without Rakib present, she shared the rape trauma that had overwhelmed her and that had been re-awakened with the deportation threat without discussing the tenuous bonding with her younger son. She shared her anger and distress that she had become very isolated from her small ethnic community. After sharing this secret with a woman she trusted, the story of her rape was spread through her ethnic group. She had also been traumatized when a community leader had accosted her, stealing money from her and threatening her. Rakib had been aware of her outrage and depressed states as well as their ongoing poverty and isolation.

The individual and family interventions were focused on processing grief, including creating a funeral ritual to honour his grandparents and displaying their photos at home. These themes of working through grief and establishing safety for her family emerged as a focus. We decided that the team would build supervision and sustaining resources around the family system to manage them during the period of uncertainty and legal processes. Rakib was enrolled in camp and after-school programs so that he could play and be with peers rather than feel the burden of the mourning at home. His mother's depressive and agitated states remitted and her moods stabilized.

When Rakib was aged 11, the family achieved their immigration status, their poverty diminished and the network around the mother improved as she was eventually able to find work. However, as he entered adolescence, Rakib began to have increasing social difficulties, with periods of school refusal. He encountered increasing racism in the post-9/11 period and eventually tried to join a gang. He became more precocious in his sexuality (his mother's engulfing moods may have been a factor) and there were enactments of anger in the street with bullies. By the time he entered high school, he was afraid of some of his host society peers. His marginality and subaltern positioning infuriated him while also provoking fear. His mother was seen in family sessions with him but found it hard to re-negotiate the structural reversals that put him in a sibling relationship with her rather than a parent-child hierarchy.

Eventually, he had an older girlfriend who came to live in the home when he was about 16 years old. His mother tolerated this relationship choice, as he was also available to watch his brother while she worked. She was not able to adjust the longstanding hierarchical parental child expectations. We supported a plan she was considering – to send him to her family in their country of origin, who had offered in a Skype consultation to have him schooled there, as he was in danger of engaging in anti-social activity and dropping out of school. This period of a boarding school education in his country of origin and his reunion with a family he had not known changed Rakib's previous ideas and fantasies about his family. He began to see positive aspects of their country of origin, his religious origins and their family's positive welcoming reparation attitude. He returned at age 17 with transformed ideas of his original ethnic identity and his host culture identifications. While formerly he had had an ambivalent or negative alienation about his ethnicity, he now felt internally more positive about his ethnicity. Rather than striving to only be identified with his host society and engaging from a marginal position, he began to see himself as embracing several identifications simultaneously. He returned to school and to his role as a parental child, but he also engaged in his education and business enterprises while his mother continued to work. Our last consultation was by phone. He was seeking resources as a parent would normally do for his younger brother, who had a learning disability, as he wanted to help him complete his high school education.

The acculturation and cultural hybridity process of this boy is only partially represented in this vignette but suggests some of the complexity of his familial, environmental and internal processes. His experience included his mother's stabilization after a series of cumulative trauma, poverty and intrusive emotional states with her sons. Much of the support she was given involved the progressive mastery of several aspects of her mourning. Additionally, she was challenged by cultural aspects of gender identity and the impact of multiple rapes, detention, poverty, language isolation and stigma.

The work of Carlos Sluzki [8] in his book *The Presence of the Absent: Therapy with Families and Their Ghosts* relates many clinical stories of ghosts and unresolved family mourning or inconsolable grief. He relates these vignettes not only to mourning and loss relevant to refugee work on the lost country and states of exile but also to his experience with the Argentinian political events of the 'disappeared'. These case histories offer a systemic view of working with grief that would be syntonic with the approach I have presented on working with the shadows of 'ghosts' in Rakib's family. His mother's culture is also conversant with djinn who occupy the nether worlds between life and death and which are described so well in Michael Dol's classic historical document *Majnun: The Madman in Medieval Islamic Society* [39], which outlines the long cultural antecedents for culturally embedded idioms that would have been common in the mother's cultural spaces.

The acculturation of each member of this family was situated at a different psychological distance from the mother's country of origin. Rakib's return to his parents' country also presents a re-alignment of the native county as perceived by his peers in the west, and of his family, as aspects of internalization and cultural hybridization. This process of creolization or hybridization is an internal and external positioning of transnational and transcultural belonging, which sustained his mother's sense of hope that her family's sacrifices and her own trauma had been the sacrifice foundational to these two sons having other worlds. Rakib returned from exile to find his family of origin, shifting from his self-denigration and alienation to a fuller integration of cultural possibilities. Edward Said [40] and Franz Fanon [24, 25], as well as many other scholars, have explored these distorted views of colonial or post-colonial worlds of otherness, and particularly the host society gaze upon the other. Immigrant children begin an acculturation process which will be shifting throughout their life cycle. However, early stages of identity in this internalization process are significantly influenced and constructed by the gaze of one culture upon another, and they are also complicated by host country uncertainties, as an adoptive parent, over offering refuge or membership.

The issues of resilience promotion and protection are often core agendas in referrals for refugee families with children at risk. The institutional agendas of the many primary, secondary or tertiary care clinical partners and the legal and school partners all contribute to supporting a coherent plan for care and therapeutic shifts that allow children to function optimally. Occasionally, parenting capacity and cultural agendas are complicated by context and institutional or clinician attitudes towards ethnic minorities, even though the premises of cultural safety may be understood by our mandate.

In Quebec, following the language law named Bill 101, immigrant families were mandated to have French-language schooling to support acculturation into a francophone province. Parents of refugee or immigrant families – especially mothers, as in Rakib's case study – who were not working outside the home often lagged behind their children in acquiring these skills and identifications with the host society cultural space.

In the case of refugees negotiating the legal process of attaining citizenship, decisions on parenting capacity with youth protection involvement can also cause great distress, as these situations have refugee, legal and custodial implications. In the case of Rakib, we decided to work with the primary care therapists, who had a good enough alliance and network approach, rather than introducing the agenda of placement, though we had made the mother aware of our legal obligations to maintain the objects of both care and protection at all times in such fragile situations.

The Boy Who Was Referred to as 'an Animal'

Amani, a 12-year-old refugee boy from the Caribbean, presented with his mother after expulsion from an elementary school French immersion class (i.e., a transitional setting for newcomers to support the acquisition of sufficient French skills to be fully integrated into the regular classes) for admission to intensive treatment milieu (4 days per week) in a child psychiatry day hospital. The referring teacher described Amani as a 'monkey and an animal': his description to the mother of her undersocialized and disorganized child.

Explosive dysregulation was often precipitated by humiliation in the classroom. Amani was English speaking and did not complete his work: 'I couldn't understand,' he reported in the intake interview, while his mother responded, 'I can't help him with French work.'

His mother had had an unresolved refugee status for more than five years and was re-united with him in Canada only when his caretaking arrangements had disintegrated in her country of origin. His biological father had never been involved with his care, and his mother's numerous siblings had refused to care for him. His mother had a toxic relationship with both her parents and had in fact left him at the age of six with a teacher who had offered to care for him in return for payment. However, this arrangement had soon dissolved and Amani was left with her mother. The maternal grandmother was rejecting and harsh. She had beaten him often, broken his arm and kept him in the house naked when she found him unmanageable. He had difficulty learning and many conduct issues but had always idealized his mother while longing to be re-united with her.

During our initial family therapy meeting, his mother was clearly angry that Amani's conduct at school within months of his arrival had caused her such distress and interrupted her work commitments. She stated that he was completely compliant with her and demanded to know why he was explosive, aggressive and oppositional at school, beha- viours that recurred in the initial weeks of day hospital admission. Amani appeared frozen and apprehensive and wept silently. The initial session was focused on beginning an attachment process between mother and son by gently asking the mother to model for him how to tell a story of her own life. In the initial family sessions, she reluctantly recounted to her son for the first time her own complex narrative of abuse, rejection, beatings and struggles as the 'blackest child' and the least favoured by her mother, 'though I was good at school, not like Amani'. She also conveyed her positive work ethic, her experiences of racism, her religious Christian life and her guilt and loneliness without her son. She reluctantly acknowledged that Amani was in a fragile state after a disrupted attachment and trauma as she recounted the trauma of her early life.

Reunification after absence for economic migration is a common inevitable stressor for many children left behind, the so-called 'barrel child' [41] who receives material goods from their absent parents in shipped barrels. His mother felt hurt that he was not adjusting, recounting that she had made 'sacrifices for you' and was 'ashamed' of his disruptive conduct, so she had sought the help of church and pastor. She also felt stigmatized to be in a mental health setting. Amani added, 'I am not crazy person . . . why does it say mental at the entrance?' As our working alliance progressed, both Amani and his mother re-aligned their feelings of dread and stigma related to colonial oppression and racism compounding their fears of psychiatry, shifting to mental well-being as a model of care.

Amani and his mother engaged in a year and a half of weekly family therapy to work on attachment and to mourn many years of absence. His violent aggressive episodes sub- sided as he formed a bond with the staff, becoming especially close to two male childcare workers. While he both feared and longed for closeness to his mother, the male childcare workers and pastor addressed some of his sense of 'father hunger'. He was able to progressively define and own his precipitating stressors and triggers, partly related to his previous abuse and humiliations, which erupted in displaced rage at strangers. Our assessment confirmed that he was severely learning disabled, which allowed him to eventually obtain English eligibility for schooling and an appropriate special needs class on discharge from the day hospital.

The pastor of their church, the lawyer pursuing humanitarian grounds for refugee status and the army cadet corps who later took him in training were allies in our work to create safety. He loved to sing, both in the church choir and with our theatre group. When his uncle, who was a talented musician, was murdered by a gang in the Caribbean, we prepared a memorial service with Amani which our staff, our child patients and his mother attended, playing the uncle's music. Mourning for this lost uncle was one of the most important bonding experiences within our day hospital milieu that allowed Amani to recover some dignified way to mourn his own sense of loss and sadness for many life events.

The process of family therapy shifted the mother's parental perception of Amani as 'bad' and 'mad' or 'hopeless' and gave a focus to re-framing identifications, losses and traumas to generate realistic goals, acquire social skills, acknowledge learning problems and build new capacities. The family continued to consult us until Amani reached age 19, when he completed high school and when the family was successful in gaining immigration status. His acculturation process was embedded in the black church congregation, within the black community and with his mother's relations in distant cities. His singing was part of a connection to his favourite deceased uncle, and his army training gave him a sense of pride and belonging, reinforcing a positive way for him to validate self-control.

A Refugee Girl Looking for a Safe House

At the time of this adolescent referral, there had been media coverage of three first generation Afghani Islamic sisters aged 19, 17 and 13 and the first wife of their father, who had all been drowned in 2009. Gender hierarchies and forced marriage were implicated, and youth protection had been marginally involved. There had been a widely reported catastrophic outcome where the parents and an adolescent son were charged with murder and incarcerated. The social climate in Quebec was also uneasy with the cultural values of others. A public discourse with two Quebec scholars as a government commission entitled 'Reasonable Accommodation' had provoked discussion on cultural minorities and raised concerns that some immigrants may be resistant to acculturation to Quebec values.

Rani was a refugee girl who arrived at the age of eight from a Middle Eastern country, though her parents came from the Indian subcontinent. She had arrived with her mother and with two siblings; one was three years older, the other was four years younger. Another elder brother had sought asylum in the UK as an unaccompanied minor. Her father had apparently been sought as a terrorist on the subcontinent and remained in the Middle East. Rani idealized her father, with whom she had had minimal contact, hated her mother – 'too old-fashioned, too strict and doesn't speak French' – and accused her brother (on behalf of her mother) of locking her in her room and hitting her when she wanted to go out at night. Youth protection had taken her into protective custody and was considering criminal charges against her brother, then in his late adolescence. Rani was later referred at age 16 to CCS for a consultation by youth protection after she ran away from a group home with 2 other adolescent girls.

Her mother had previously been a patient in CCS for several years. Her mother had been referred during the preparatory phases of her refugee board hearings, as she collapsed and dissociated, delaying completion of her hearings. She had had severe somatic distress, PTSD and depression for many years, which raised the concerns of her primary care physicians. Her treatment involved many medication trials, including anti-depressants and neuroleptics. The refugee declaration recorded that she was a religious woman whose husband had escaped the subcontinent. She had been tortured by police and possibly raped, though the patient refused to speak about sexual issues. Rani insisted that her mother had lied and that she had never had PTSD or depression, and she denied that she knew her father's history or the circumstances of their refugee status on her arrival in Canada.

At the first consultation with a large primary care team and youth protection, Rani did not attend, as she had not yet been found after leaving her group home with other peers. Her mother wept through the entire interview, with her son looking helpless beside her. Later, when Rani returned to youth protection custody, she revealed that she had visited her mother's home before our first consultation and warned her mother that if her family co-operated with youth protection she would fabricate more lies and never see them again.

At a second consultation, the mother was seen with her son separately. She was clearly upset with Rani's conduct, including her affiliation with other youth who were taking drugs and dating while she had quite conservative values. Her son said that there had never been locks on bedroom doors and that they had invited youth protection to visit. They both denied that Rani had been beaten. They had gone back to their immigration lawyer, as these charges had serious implications for both the application of their son to migrate to the UK and for their other son who was currently in Canada. They felt that Rani was often with a young woman whose immigrant family had advised her that youth protection would offer her a safe house. She told her mother that she did not have to adhere to traditional or 'village' values, and this family invited her to live with them before taking her to the police to make a complaint which became a youth protection issue.

The third consultation visit included the family and the group home therapists. Rani was not interested in speaking to her mother or her older brother, nor did she ask about her younger sibling, who was apparently very distressed that she had left. She was pleased with her new group home placement, where the attendants described her as a model Quebecois adolescent oppressed by her family's culture. She related that her interest in meeting me was to see whether I would like to purchase her crafts, as she needed some money (which I declined). The attendants praised her for being enterprising.

While we tried to engage in parent-child dialogue, Rani ignored everyone but the group home attendants, with whom she spoke in French, hence excluding her mother. Her mother was clearly annoyed by her behaviour. At the closure of the short encounter, her mother commented to her in her native language: 'You are accountable in the end only to yourself and your God.' Her brother attempted to speak to Rani about the gravity of the situation and asked her to tell the truth about the incidents she had reported. She had recently told youth protection that she had gone to the temple of their faith and was threatened by some men, 'a kind of Mafia' sent by her brother. She refused to discuss this story when the brother denied all knowledge of this event. When I asked whether she generally went to the temple, she said she particularly wanted to have the food: 'I miss it; it's part of my culture.'

In responding to the consultation, I suggested to youth protection that it did not seem plausible that Rani was denying any awareness of maternal depression prior to the granting of immigration status to the family. Her mother had been a patient for many years and her treating physicians did not feel that she had fabricated somatic injuries, PTSD or major depression. The agency questioned me about the 'Indian mafia' and asked if I knew members of this group. They suggested that I may not be objective, as I may be overidentified with the parent, given our ethnic match. My assessment concluded that Rani's narrative was unlikely to be truthful given her attitude suggestive of 'la belle indifférence' and a history of earlier incidents consistent with bicultural identity strains, family conflict and adolescent differentiation issues. Youth protection decided that a safe house in a distant part of the province would be the only way to ensure her safety, as she was positively acculturating as a francophone and, in their view, her family appeared to be assimilating 'poorly', further obstructing Rani's positive Quebecois assimilation.

Some years later, a youth protection delegate present during the process approached me with a follow-up that Rani had left care with a young Caucasian man and was living in another province as a single parent with a young child. She had contacted them and asked to be reconciled with her mother and was seeking a reparation process.

These case history narratives indicate complex aspects of acculturation and family process complicated by institutional and socio-political agendas. Adolescents and youth seek a sense of belonging as they differentiate from their families, while they may also rehearse identities and choices that allow them to enact difference and hybridity. The acculturation process progresses through many iterations of these stages while they consolidate their hybridization paths and establish a secure sense of their identification. Institutions and therapists are often mediators in negotiations of these processes and need to reflect on their empathy for both parents and children and avoid stereotyping, identifications and ethnocentric value biases. As in any process of family systemic work, therapeutic teams must balance positions that are empathic to each family member.

In Rani's case, no one may know objectively which family member may be presenting denial or authenticity of emotional or factual aspects of events. Nonetheless, the narratives of institutions are more likely to be balanced when multiple team members and culture brokers are involved in reflecting on the symptoms and phenomenology of the patient presentation. Institutions whose members represent only the host society and no members of the ethnic groups for whom they provide services may be more prone to a bias in dealing with otherness.

Conclusion

The agendas of identity, cultural hybridity and acculturation are a major aspect of clinical work in a multi-ethnic society and within its institutions [42]. Working with refugee families requires flexibility and reflective capacity and for therapists to monitor their assumptions and premises of health, aims of development, ideologies and cultural differences. Provided cultural safety remains a parameter, therapists and families are co-constructing approaches to advocacy, alliance, assessment and intervention.

Forced exile, pre-migratory trauma, separation from families of origin, war and conflict trauma, collective meanings attributed to these traumas, and marginalization once they arrive or cross borders all contribute to the adversity variables. Appreciating the cultural embedding of personhood, especially where collectivist or culturally specific frameworks of self are operating [9], is crucial, while multiple influences remain fundamental to unpacking issues of identities and roles.

The ethnographic literature on the developmental paradigms of childhood underlines the ethnocentrism of western psychological literature, which is largely biased towards a motif of individuation with an emphasis on local context and autonomy or individualism-driven paradigms. Hence, cultural metaphors and meanings of distress and adversity are another variable that emerges in family and systemic therapies as well as institutional responses to minorities at risk, and they remain topics of careful negotiation within therapeutic interaction.

References

1. L. J. Kirmayer, L. Narasiah, M. Munoz, M. Rashid, A. Ryder, J. Guzder et al., Common mental health problems in immigrants and refugees: A general approach in primary care. *CMAJ*, 183(12) (2010), 1–9.

2. L. J. Kirmayer, D. Groleau, J. Guzder, C. Blake and E. Jarvis, Cultural consultation: A model of mental health service for multicultural societies. *Canadian Journal of Psychiatry*, 49(3) (2003), 145–53.

3. R. Lewis-Fernando, N. Aggarwal, L. Hinton, D. E. Hinton and L. Kirmayer, *DSM-5 Handbook on Cultural Formulation Interview* (Washington, DC: American Psychiatric Association, 2016).

4. R. Williams, Cultural safety. *Australia and New Zealand Journal of Public Health*, 23 (22) (1999), 213–14.

5. M. McGoldrick, J. Pearce and J. Giordano, *Ethnicity and Family Therapy* (New York: Guilford, 1982).

6. M. McGoldrick, R. Gerson and S. S. Petry, *Genograms: Assessment and Intervention* (New York: W. W. Norton & Company, 2008).

7. J. Cleveland, C. Rousseau and J. Guzder, Cultural consultation for refugees. In L. J. Kirmayer, J. Guzder and C. Rousseau, eds., *Cultural Consultation: Encountering the Other in Mental Health Care* (New York: Springer, 2014), pp. 245–68.

8. C. E. Sluzki, *The Presence of the Absent: Therapy with Families and their Ghosts* (New York: Routledge, 2016).

9. L. J. Kirmayer, V. Dzokoto and A. Ademole, Varieties of global psychiatry and constructions of the self. In S. Fernando and R. Moodley, eds., *Global Psychologies: Mental Health and Global South* (New York: Palgrave Macmillan, 2018).

10. H. R. Marcus and S. Kitayama, Culture and the self: A cycle of mutual constitution. *Perspectives in Psychological Science*, 98(2) (1991), 420–30.

11. A. Roland, *In Search of Self in India and Japan: Towards a Cross-Cultural Psychology* (New Haven, NJ: Princeton University Press, 1988).

12. S. Kitayama, M. Karasawa, K. B. Curham, C. D. Ryff and H. R. Markus, Independence and interdependence predict health and wellbeing: Divergent patterns in the United States and Japan. *Frontiers in Psychology*, 1 (2010), 163.

13. S. Kakar, *The Inner World: A Psychoanalytic Study of Childhood and Society in India* (Oxford: Oxford University Press, 1978).

14. G. Obeyesekere, *The Work of Culture* (Chicago, IL: University of Chicago, 1990).

15. K. Crenshaw, *Demarginalizing the Intersection of Race and Sex: A Black Feminist Critique of Antidiscrimination Doctrine, Feminist Theory and Antiracist Politics* (Chicago, IL: The Chicago Legal Forum, 1989), pp. 139–66.

16. S. Akhtar and P. Tummala-Narra, Psychoanalysis in India. In S. Akhtar, ed., *Freud along the Ganges* (New York: The Other Press, 2005).

17. T. G. Vaidyhanathan and J. J. Kripal, *Visnu on Freud's Desk: A Reader in Psychoanalysis and Hinduism* (New Delhi: Oxford University Press, 1999).

18. T. Doi, *The Anatomy of Dependence* (Tokyo: Kodansha, 1971).

19. V. L. Vignoles, E. Owe, M. Becker, P. B. Smith, M. J. Easterbrook, R. Brown et al., Beyond the 'East-West' dichotomy: Global variations in cultural models of selfhood. *Journal of Experimental Psychology*, 145(8) (2016), 966–1000.

20. C. Rousseau, T. M. Said, M.-J. Gagne and G. Bibeau, Resilience in unaccompanied minors from the north of Somalia. *The Psychoanalytic Review*, 85(4) (1998), 615–37.

21. M. Rutter, Psychosocial resilience and protective mechanisms. *American Journal of Orthopsychiatry*, 57 (1987), 316–31.

22. E. E. Werner, High-risk children in young adulthood: A longitudinal study from birth to 32 years. *American Journal of Orthopsychiatry*, 59(1) (1989), 72–81.

23. M. Ungar, M. Brown, L. Liebenberg, R. Othman, W. M. Kwong, M. Armstrong et al., Unique pathways to resilience across cultures in adolescence. *Roslyn Heights*, 42 (166) (2007), 287–310.

24. F. Fanon, *Black Skins, White Masks* (New York: Grove Press, 1967).

25. F. Fanon, *The Wretched of the Earth* (New York: Grove Press, 1963).

26. S. Fernando, ed., *Mental Health in a Multi-ethnic Society: A Multi-disciplinary Handbook* (London: Routledge, 1995).

27. S. Fernando, *Mental Health, Race and Culture*, 2nd ed. (London: Palgrave, 2010).

28. D. C. Jack and A. Ali, eds., *Silencing the Self across Cultures: Depression and Gender in the Social World* (New York: Oxford University Press, 2010).

29. A. V. Horowitz, Distinguishing distress from disorder as psychological outcomes of stressful social arrangements. *Health*, 11(3) (2007), 273–89.

30. P. Steinhauer, *The Least Detrimental Alternative: A Systematic Guide to Case Planning and Decision Making for Children in Care* (Toronto: University of Toronto, 1991).

31. S. Akhtar, A third individuation: Immigration, identity and the psychoanalytic process. *Journal of American Psychoanalytic Association*, 43 (1995), 1051–84.

32. M. Mahler, The first three sub-phases of the separation-individuation process. *International Journal of Psychoanalysis*, 53 (1972), 333.

33. D. W. Winnicott, *Playing and Reality* (London: Tavistock Publications, 1971).

34. R. Williams, Cultural safety: What does it mean for our work practice? *Australian and New Zealand Journal of Public Health*, 23(2) (2008), 213–14.

35. L. De Haene, C. Rousseau, R. Kevers, N. Deruddere and P. Rober, Stories of trauma in family therapy with refugees: Supporting safe relational spaces of narration and silence. *Clinical Child Psychology and Psychiatry*, 23(2) (2018), 258–78.

36. J. Guzder, Institutional racism as a seminal concept of cultural competency training. In R. Moodley and M. Ocampo, eds., *Critical Psychiatry and Mental Health: Exploring the Work of Suman Fernando in Clinical Practice* (New York: Routledge, 2014).

37. A. Kleinman, V. Das and M. Lock, eds., *Social Suffering* (Berkeley, CA: University of California, 1997).

38. L. Kirmayer, R. Kronick and C. Rousseau, Advocacy as a key to structural competency in psychiatry. *JAMA Psychiatry*, 75(2) (2018), 119–20.

39. M. W. Dols, *Majun: The Madman in Medieval Islamic Society* (Oxford: Clarendon Press, 1992).

40. E. Said, *Orientalism* (London: Routledge, 1978).

41. M. Lashley, The unrecognized social stressors of migration and reunification in Caribbean families. *Transcultural Psychiatry*, 37(2) (2000), 203–17.

42. L. J. Kirmayer, J. Guzder and C. Rousseau, eds., *Cultural Consultation: Encountering the Other in Mental Health Care* (New York: Springer, 2014).

Working with Spirituality in Refugee Care
ACT-Buddhism Group for Cambodian Canadian Refugees

Kenneth Fung, Mony Mok, and Vireak Phorn

Introduction

Canada is often known as the country of immigrants, with the latest 2016 census indicating that about one in five Canadians are born elsewhere [1]. This includes almost 860,000 refugees who were admitted since 1990 and who are still living in Canada [2]. The source of refugees has varied over the years, with about 18,602 Cambodian refugees arriving in Canada between 1980 and 1992 [3]. In this chapter, we will focus on our experience of providing mental health care for Cambodian Canadians in Toronto and the use of Acceptance and Commitment Therapy (ACT) as a group intervention to improve their mental health and wellbeing. This therapeutic approach, appropriately adapted and incorporating Cambodian cultural and spiritual beliefs and concepts, also helps to address family issues that are embedded in everyday concerns and struggles. To understand Cambodian Canadians' cultural context, we begin with an overview of Cambodia, its culture, family relations, and the relevant political history and war that continues to affect generations of Cambodian Canadians.

Background on Cambodia

Cambodia, officially known as the Kingdom of Cambodia, is located in Southeast Asia with an area of approximately 181,000 square kilometres, bordered by Thailand to the northwest, Laos to the northeast, Vietnam to the east, and the Gulf of Thailand to the southwest [4]. Its population is about 16,204,486 (est. 2017). It has a tropical climate with a rainy monsoon season from May to November and a dry season from December to April, with relatively little seasonal temperature variation. Leaving behind this tropical climate is one of the many challenges faced by Cambodian Canadians.

Traditionally, Cambodia is an agricultural country, with rice being the main crop. During the harvest season twice a year, community members help each other and work closely together, building a strong sense of community. In fact, Cambodians rarely feel socially isolated because of the strong social support network from close family members and the community. Families and community members often get together to socialize or go to the Buddhist temple together. The temple is not only a place for worship, it is also a place for the community to gather and support each other.

The family bond is particularly strong and is a lifelong commitment and obligation in Cambodian culture. Traditionally, two or three generations of the family reside together. The elders are well respected by all age groups. Parents look after their children closely and, in reciprocation, when children become adults, they care for their parents and elders. There are strong gender and role expectations, with the husband bringing home income, providing shelter and food, and making decisions, the wife taking charge of the family budget, chores, and childcare, and the children listening, obeying, and honouring the parents.

When a family member gets sick, support from the family is very important in the recovery process. Quite often, other community members will be involved as well. This has obvious implications for the mental health, wellbeing, and recovery of Cambodian Canadians, many of whom have lost family members as refugees and are separated from other family members back home.

When a person dies, the care of the body is undertaken by the family. The body is brought home, washed, dressed, and placed into a coffin. The organs are not to be removed because it is believed that this affects one's re-birth, as there is a belief rooted in Buddhism that all beings evolve in a successive cycle of birth, old age, sickness, death, and re-birth. Traditionally, the body is kept in the house for a few days before cremation. The Buddhist monks go to the home and recite a sermon for the body. On the third or the seventh day, a funeral procession is organized, carrying the body to the temple for cremation. It is believed that cremation allows the soul to part from the body and go to hell or heaven in order to wait for reincarnation. After cremation, the ashes (bones) are collected, cleaned, and usually kept in a taupe at the temple compound. There, it is believed that the deceased is close to Buddha and to the monks, and the soul is able to be re-born sooner next life cycle. It is common for Cambodian Canadians to arrange the seventh- and the one-hundredth-day funeral ceremony at the local temple for their parents, children, or relatives who have died in Cambodia. The ritual ceremony done after one year is believed to honour the dead and promote re-birth. The inability to carry out these rituals for those who died during the war compounds the unresolved grief for many refugees. In some cases, ghosts are understood as the wandering souls of those who have not been honoured properly [5].

Khmer is the official spoken language. As in many Asian cultures, Cambodians often use indirect and highly context-dependent communications [6]. For example, when people are offered food, they may say 'no,' but a 'no' may mean 'well … maybe … let's see …' If the offering person insisted, the food would eventually be accepted. Nuanced tone and the implications of words and statements are often carefully considered, especially if they may invoke a negative affect socially. Thus, if Cambodians disagree with an idea, they may remain silent or neutral rather than make any negative comments, especially towards elders and other authority figures such as teachers, doctors, lawyers, etc. A gentle communication style is preferred over a more assertive style, such as a loud voice or a perceived pushy demeanour, which actually risks shutting down communications.

In context-dependent cultures, non-verbal behaviour is especially important in communications. Smiling is situational and can mean happiness or agreement. However, it can also be a signal of not understanding, embarrassment, being nervous, feeling irritated, or even sadness. Showing overt negative emotions is often considered inappropriate. Ideally, expressions of anger, impatience, or frustration are kept hidden, as they may lead to a loss of face. Silence when people are gathered together can be quite acceptable. Head-nodding may be perceived as impolite among Cambodians, but is often deemed acceptable coming from non-Cambodians.

War and Trauma

In 1975, the communist Khmer Rouge, led by Pol Pot, reached the capital, Phnom Penh, and took power. They changed the official name of the country to Democratic Kampuchea and immediately evacuated the cities, sending the entire population on forced marches to rural work projects. The Cambodian genocide was carried out by the Khmer Rouge regime between 1975 and 1979, during which an estimated 1.2 to 3.4 million Cambodians perished [7]. Persecution, atrocities, and trauma included forced re-locations from urban centres to rural areas, the prohibition of Buddhist practice and ceremonies, torture, mass executions, forced labour, malnutrition, and disease, leading to the death of an estimated 25 percent of the population. The genocide ended in 1979 following the Vietnamese invasion of Cambodia. As of 2009, 23,745 mass graves have been discovered [8].

Hundreds of thousands of Cambodians fled across the border into refugee camps in neighbouring Thailand after 1979, hoping to find a safe place to settle. Many Cambodians subsequently migrated to Canada, the USA, France, and Australia. Most Cambodians in Canada arrived during the 1980s as part of the large Indochinese refugee flow [3], including about 55 per cent government-sponsored and 45 per cent privately sponsored refugees. Most did not have close relatives or kin in Canada. The majority were from rural areas with little education or knowledge of urban life. About 92 per cent could not speak either of Canada's official languages of English and French. According to the 2016 national census, Canada has recorded a Cambodian Canadian population of 38,490, one of the smallest minority groups among the 6,095,235 Asian Canadians [9]. They have escaped war and chosen Canada as their land of hope. However, leaving families behind and settling in Canada often proves to be challenging physically, mentally, and emotionally, as they face the daunting long cold winters, the lack of community and social support, unprocessed trauma, unresolved grief – especially over family members who were separated, missing, or killed – and the adjustment process to a new language, culture, and way of life.

Meeting Mental Health Needs of Cambodian Canadians

Due to limited English proficiency and the lack of community resources, Cambodian Canadians had tremendous difficulty accessing mainstream mental health services after arrival in Canada. Hong Fook Mental Health Association, a community mental health agency providing and facilitating access to mental health services for the East and Southeast Asian communities in the Greater Toronto Area (GTA) since 1982, has been providing the only ethnospecific mental health service to Cambodian Canadians in the GTA.

In 1987, the Cambodian community first began to approach Hong Fook to get help in understanding mental health and mental illness. Social isolation, lack of informal support, strong stigma against mental illness, language and cultural barriers, and fear of gossip among the small Cambodian community are among the major barriers to accessing care. Over time, as Cambodian Canadians started to establish trust in receiving culturally competent services at Hong Fook, they have been able to reconnect with their own community members, reducing their social isolation and fears about getting help. Once connected, many have been able to disclose and share their personal traumatic experiences with service providers and other Cambodians at Hong Fook and in their own community, including the torture and starvation they went through, the losses and deaths from the communist regime, and their unique refugee experiences prior to coming to Canada.

Hong Fook plays an important role in the recovery journey of many clients from the Cambodian community, and word of mouth has become one of the major sources of referrals in addition to outreach events. Currently, Hong Fook meets the mental health needs of clients and enhances their quality of life through a diversity of services, including intake, case management, an Asian Community Psychiatric Clinic, supportive housing, and self-help programs. The programs see clients presenting with a wide variety of common mental illness, from depression and anxiety to primary psychotic disorders. From the Cambodian clients' cultural perspective, they often suffer from 'thinking too much (with no reasons)', 'worrying too much', ongoing nightmares about life during the communist regime, somatic complaints including pain, and insomnia. This may be related to trauma as well as unresolved grief related to the loss of family members.

In addition to addressing trauma and mental illness, the underlying social determinants of health, the process of acculturation, and the sociocultural context are all an integral part of many clients' problems. Many experience marital problems, intergenerational cultural gaps, discrimination at work, and the basic struggle to maintain an adequate income, especially in view of limitations due to language barriers and educational background. Further, it is common among Cambodian Canadians to feel burdened by guilty feelings caused by not being able to directly care for their family members or relatives in Cambodia or to adequately financially support them by sending money back, out of a strong cultural sense of duty to kin. Addressing these sociocultural issues become a core part of our work with Cambodian clients. Not to be neglected also is the key role that Buddhism plays for many clients.

Buddhism in Cambodia

Buddhism is the main religion of Cambodia, with about 90 to 95 per cent of the population being Buddhists [10]. It is deeply integrated socioculturally into Cambodian society, including major national holidays such as Vesak Day, celebrated on the full moon day of the Vesak month according to the lunar calendar. There are many Buddhist monks, temples, and schools in each city and province. In accordance with traditional Buddhism, practising Cambodians strive to take refuge in and worship the three gems, the Lord Buddha, the Buddhist teachings known as the *Dharma*, and the religious communities known as the *Sangha* [11].

Buddhism has a primary role in Cambodian culture, philosophy, and moral guidance. There are many television channels and radio stations that broadcast dharma talks for people of all generations to learn the Buddhist teachings so that they can adapt them and put them into practice in daily life. The Cambodian people believe in the philosophy of *Karma* as a principle in Buddhism; they believe that their whole lives are shaped by a powerful energy/force that is the product of their actions from their previous life in combination with their actions in the present life.

Cambodians highly respect and honour the Buddhist monks, who serve important roles as spiritual leaders. It is believed that bad luck or bad effects in life will come as a result of disrespect to Buddhist monks. Buddhist monks give spiritual guidance as well as special blessings for peace and prosperity. They are often invited to give dharma talks or advice as Cambodians strive to become good citizens. Every day and everywhere, people can be seen celebrating events in Buddhist ways led by blessings from Buddhist monks. These blessings are important in all major life events, such as the birth of a baby, housewarmings, weddings, funerals, etc. It is believed that through these powerful blessings, bad luck, bad effects, bad Karmic energy, sickness, and evil spirits can all be dispelled.

A Buddhist Holy Monk's Perspective on Mental Health and Trauma

There are many kinds of mental health issues and trauma. Some people are born with mental issues; some have mental issues due to their experiences through life. Buddhism offers the path towards the ultimate calm, peace, and bliss. Those who have mental issues or any trauma due to their experiences in life are known not to understand and not to practise Buddhism. They have a high attachment to worldly things, and they do not accept the reality of nature or do not let go of all things that happen, based on the Buddha's teaching that all beings have the three characteristics of life which are: everything is impermanent, suffering, and non-self [12].

There are many examples, stories, and anecdotes in Buddhism that people can take as examples to apply in their own lives, such as the story of Patachara, who experienced the loss of her sons, a husband, parents, and a brother. She became crazy. With the help of the Lord Buddha, she became conscious of the understanding of the law of karma and the law of life. She wholeheartedly accepted life the way it was and no longer had attachment toward her late relatives as she became enlightened [13].

People can heal their mental health issues and trauma by diligently practising Buddhism, understanding the law of karma, accepting changes in life, and conducting wholesome deeds in life.

Use of Acceptance and Commitment Therapy

Acceptance and Commitment Therapy (ACT) is one of the third wave psychological interventions that incorporates principles of mindfulness and acceptance [14]. Further, more explicitly than many other mindfulness-based therapies, ACT has close correspondence with Buddhism, from its underlying philosophy, *functional contextualism*, emphasizing the importance of context, to the overall formulation of suffering being over-attachment to thoughts, which bears a resemblance to the Four Noble Truths and the Buddhist perspective outlined above [15–17].

In brief, ACT attempts to reduce suffering by enhancing one's psychological flexibility through enhancing six underlying processes: (1) *defusion* describes the capacity to relate to one's thoughts as merely thoughts, rather than being caught by their literal contents; (2) *acceptance* describes the willingness to experience our internal thoughts and feelings rather than to avoid them; (3) *present moment* describes the capacity to stay in experiential contact with the present rather than being stuck ruminating about the past or worrying about the future; (4) *self-as-context* describes the capacity to experience the self as an observer (the context), rather than being defined by various ideas and concepts about ourselves (the content); (5) *values* describes the capacity to clearly be in touch with the values we really care about, which can then provide us with a sense of direction in life; and (6) *committed action* describes the capacity to remain consistent and persistent in aligning our actions with our values [14].

ACT has been applied effectively in diverse clinical populations, including those with depression, anxiety, psychosis, chronic pain, substance abuse, and trauma [18, 19]. As ACT is a non-pathologizing model, it has also been used in non-clinical populations, such as to increase resilience to prevent burnout, to increase coping among parents with children with autism [20–22], and to decrease stigma [23]. Given its congruence with Buddhism and its efficacy with mood, anxiety, and trauma-related issues, which are common in this population, we have been applying the principles of ACT both in individual work and in group work. We will emphasize how this form of intervention can allow some work on important family issues: absence and grief, relations to those who are dead, duty towards family, and honouring family relations.

ACT-Buddhism Group

Building on our previous work [15], we held the third ACT-Buddhism group with 1 male and 10 female Cambodian Canadian participants in summer 2017, led by the authors, a psychiatrist (K. F.), a Holy Monk (V. P.), and a mental health worker (M. M.). All participants had been receiving services at Hong Fook for mood or anxiety disorders and did not have a primary psychotic disorder. The group consisted of six sessions of about two hours each. Often it ran over time, as most participants wanted to stay longer to have snacks together. The overall structure and content of our group is found in Table 11.1. For illustrative purposes, below is a brief description of five of the group exercises conducted.

Present Moment with the Apple

In addition to conventional ways of discussing mindfulness in our previous two groups (e.g., through a raisin-eating exercise [24]), we explored different ways of conveying this concept, which was at once culturally familiar but by no means fully grasped by our patients. In the first session, we began with a discussion on the experience of touching the table that they were sitting around. They had been leaning on the table and using it to complete the pre-group questionnaires. Attention was brought to the tactile sensations of the table. This was continued the following week, with everyone attempting to peel an apple in a spiral without a break. The continuous apple skin represented the stream of concentration, which, when broken, could be redirected to continue. It was pointed out that practice would increase the focus and hence the skills in contributing to success both in this exercise and in mindfulness meditation. The participants were able to engage in this exercise much better than the raisins exercise, especially since raisins are not a common food in Cambodia. The concrete action of peeling an apple became a touchstone that was revisited throughout the group when people commented on their difficulties with mindfulness meditation.

Acceptance as Non-avoidance of Emotions and Ghosts

To discuss emotions in the group, we had to develop an easier way to communicate this than using pure emotional words, which were not in common usage culturally. For our participants, emotions were often embedded in and inseparable from thoughts, somatic connections, and the situational context. We printed a card with circles and invited them to draw simple facial expressions on them. We were then able to discuss making room for the acceptance of emotions, allowing all of the faces on the card to be 'uncovered' and present, as if they were children with different emotional facial expressions. When the group shared the emotions that they would like to avoid the most, an emergent topic of discussion was their common fear of ghosts. Everyone had a very strong interest, opinion, or experience to share about this. Several patients talked about their experiences with ghosts; many insisted

11.1 ACT-Buddhism group: Content and structure

	ACT process	ACT exercise/discussion	Related Buddhist concepts
1	Present Moment	• Touching the table	• Mindfulness meditation
2	Acceptance	• Peeling an apple • Drawing emoji faces and covering them up	• Suffering • Wisdom • 10 Perfections (equanimity, acceptance)
3	Defusion	• Acceptance of various faces – as like children • Fears and thoughts vs real experiences (e.g., fear of ghosts vs real ghosts, shadow of a rope vs snakes)	• Impermanence

4	Self-as-Context	• Lego exercise:
		  - Last summer
		  - War experience and trauma
		  - Happy childhood experience
			• Emptiness and no self

5	Values	• Honesty vs pleasing someone (e.g., reacting to shared food that does not taste good): preference, feelings, actions from both perspectives • Video clip on values – man demonstrating persistent actions in giving, though he is poor and others disapprove; no conditions or evaluation of who deserves it • Birthday cake and candle: values as birthday wishes	• Eightfold Path • 10 Perfections (giving, morality, honesty, compassion, loving kindness) • Karma
6	Committed Action	• Bus driver	• Eightfold Path • 10 Perfections (energy, determination, renunciation) • Nirvana/enlightenment

on their existence, and all wanted to know our thoughts about them from both a scientific and a spiritual perspective. Our monk co-facilitator was able to discuss the nature of spirits and ghosts from a Buddhist and a metaphysical perspective. This helped to address their present fear of ghosts and their existential concerns about their own mortality, as well as facilitating them to make peace with their loss and grief over their deceased loved ones during the war. Drawing on the Buddhist parable of the rope and the snake, the psychiatrist co-facilitator discussed how avoidance might perpetuate the fear of illusions. Just as light may enable us to clearly perceive a rope as a rope rather than as a snake, mindfulness may help us to see more clearly through illusions; that is, there is an opportunity to experience and deal with the situation at hand rather than imagined fears if we mindfully face our own fears instead of avoiding them. This exercise and ensuing discussion helped not only to evoke the absent members of the family but provided an appropriate cultural and spiritual vehicle to mourn them [25].

Exploring Traumatic Moments with Construction Blocks

A group exercise using toy construction blocks (Lego) was designed to explore self-as-context [23], and in this group we also used it to explore traumatic experiences while invoking the concepts of defusion and acceptance as well as self-as-context. Participants were each given a paper plate and were instructed to write their name on the paper plate. Each participant was then given some Lego pieces. In three stages, the participants were asked to use the pieces to re-construct scenes of the past followed by mutual sharing and discussion. The three scenes were: something that happened to them last summer, which served as a warm-up to this exercise; a traumatic memory, which gave them a chance to share their war experiences; and finally, a happy childhood memory, which allowed the exercise to end on a wholesome note. Almost always, the participants related stories that involved their family members in all three scenarios. During the sharing of traumatic memories, the participants each shared different aspects of their own experiences and fears with varying degree of emotional attachment. Some discussed these events as being in the past and as though they were already able to let them go, while others discussed these memories as still painful and causing them fear. One particular participant laid a small Lego window flat on her plate among other pieces, which represented a pile of dead bodies that she had seen, and she expressed intense fear about this. The nature of fear and avoidance were explored and she was gently encouraged to use her finger to touch this empty toy window frame. She was extremely hesitant at first, but was eventually able to embrace her projected fear and put her finger into the window frame. This helped the entire group to grasp the concept of acceptance in the face of traumatic memories. She noted that she had less fear after the exercise, although she admitted that she would not be able to poke real corpses. We discussed the fact that we all have realistic fears of actual war and death, while we can learn to face our past memories and representations of war (e.g., Lego pieces). For the final revelation, participants were asked to find their self-representation in the exercise. We had a discussion of the sense of conceptualized self as particular Lego pieces versus the sense of self-as-context as being the plate on which they had already written their names. Their sense of self as the plate would allow them to have a stable platform on which to experience and let go of past traumatic scenes, which were literally deconstructed along with the Lego blocks following each re-telling of the traumatic story.

Values: Do You Like My Cooking?

The discussion of values as an abstract quality was difficult for participants to grasp. We began to embed this in everyday examples. We discussed the quality of being honest and kind with one another. While they initially agreed about the obvious importance of honesty, most – though not all – shared that they would not say something that would be critical of another person, even if it was the truth, in interpersonal contexts, such as commenting on someone's new haircut or the food that they made. We explored how participants might differ in their relative valuing of honesty versus caring for others' feelings. They were then invited to share how they might react if they did not like a family member's cooking or conversely if a family member or friend criticized the food they made in a rude way, such as spitting out their food. Many women in the group thought that the latter was the ultimate insult. In this case, we discussed the challenge of persisting in the values of staying open, friendly, and kind to someone who was overtly critical of their cooking. This became such a striking and humorous example that they spontaneously quoted this example frequently for the remainder of the group. We also discussed how these considerations might improve their everyday family interactions, including intergenerational issues, which was one of the core life domains that they highly valued.

The Bus Driver Learning English

For the values and commitment group exercise, a role-play version of the bus driver metaphor was used [23]. In this exercise, a person role-plays the bus driver and the other participants role-play the passengers. The bus driver first articulates an area of their lives in which they struggle to take committed actions and lists a number of negative thoughts as barriers. When the role-play starts, the passengers line up to enter the bus one by one. Each passenger takes turns to step in front of the bus driver and say discouraging things based on what was shared, and the bus driver is physically pivoted to avoid facing the challenging passenger, after which the passenger lines up behind the bus driver. By the end, the bus driver has been turned around 180 degrees with the passengers lined up behind them, and we discuss how the passengers have successfully distracted the bus driver from their mission to drive towards the originally desired destination. This role-play would be replayed with the bus driver coached to welcome the passengers on board while persisting in physically facing the same way throughout the exercise.

For this particular group, the group member role-playing the bus driver chose to focus on the challenge of living in Canada, specifically the language barrier. She felt that she would not be able to do anything about this as an elderly person, given her previous difficulties in English as a Second Language (ESL) classes. She outlined a number of negative thoughts as barriers (e.g., 'I can never learn English', 'I'm too old', 'I'm too busy', etc.), and these were role-played by other group members as unruly passengers. She was coached to use ACT skills to 'welcome' these passengers onto her bus while envisioning her persistence in pursuing a valued goal – in this case, learning English. This exercise resonated with the entire group, as they all struggled with this as a major acculturative barrier in Canada.

In this last session, the monk sang an epic poem which focused on a specific form of values and commitment – parents' love and filial piety, a core Asian cultural and family concept that espouses the virtue and obligation of loving, honouring, and caring for one's parents. Regardless of age, the role and bond between parents and children among Asians are traditionally quite entrenched and immutable to change. This became the quintessential value that the group ended on.

Buddhist Teachings

Each session included a component of mindfulness meditation led by the monk. This included both sitting and walking meditation. The dharma talk in each session covered a wide range of topics, including mindfulness, defilements, perfections, and impermanence.

The importance of interacting with each other with loving kindness was also discussed. The dharma talks complemented the ACT exercises and discussions.

Response and Group Feedback

Preliminary pre- and post-group results demonstrated that group participants had significantly reduced depressive symptoms as measured by the Patient Health Questionnaire and increased psychological flexibility as measured by the Acceptance and Action Questionnaire II. Qualitative feedback was also obtained from the participants. All participants expressed their appreciation of the group and felt that it was a valuable opportunity to reflect on their difficulties, increase their understanding of their problems, and increase acceptance of their struggles. They enjoyed the group despite the long commute, including a participant who travelled 2.5 hours one way to the group. The participants formed their own social support network by reminding and supporting each other to attend the group. During the sessions, they felt safe and a sense of mutual trust as they shared their war experiences as well as personal struggles.

All participants remarked that they forgot about their problems while attending the group. Seven of the 11 participants said that after the group their sleep problems and bodily pain subjectively decreased by around 40 percent and their 'thinking too much' problem reduced by about half. Seven participants used the emotional faces on a card, which they kept after the group, to identify their own feelings and laugh about them to help them cope with stress. When struggling with problems or making decisions, nine participants would recall the bus driver role-play and position themselves as the bus driver to overcome their problems. Five participants stated that they had been continuing with meditation exercises, such as walking meditation and deep breathing exercises, while others said that they would need more time to incorporate mindfulness into their daily routine. Four participants said that they increased their focus by practising mindfulness when preparing meals. Four participants stated that if they missed meditation before bedtime, they felt restless and guilty. Five participants wanted to repeat this ACT group experience in order to deepen their learning. Some of the outstanding issues that they hoped to address in the future included forgetfulness due to ageing, ongoing difficulty learning English, and the sense of guilt over not being able to financially support their family or relatives in Cambodia.

Discussion

Overall, the ACT-Buddhism group appeared to have some benefits in increasing the patients' resilience to help them cope with stress, both from the traumatic past as well as from the present, including family relations. There was more active engagement incrementally in this recent group compared to previous groups. In addition to factors that might have been related to the specific composition of the group members, the group exercises had been further simplified and culturally adapted, which appeared to have successfully increased the participants' capacity to understand the exercises, reflect on the concepts, and contribute to mutual discussion. Focusing on everyday common examples helped participants to grasp ACT concepts and apply them to their daily lives. In the intervention, family relations are not a topical focus in and of themselves, but rather a naturally recurrent theme as we work through and apply each of the ACT processes to their everyday life experiences and struggles, which are often inextricably linked with family relationships present or past.

It is evident in this group, as well as in our experiences of providing mental health care, that recovery from mental illness and trauma is inextricably linked to the patients' psychosocial and cultural realities, from family conflicts to spiritual beliefs to financial stress to acculturation challenges. Our case management service addresses many of these issues with psychosocial interventions, while the psychotherapy group complemented this by addressing the psychological and spiritual needs.

In this unique therapy group, the dharma teachings were helpful in reinforcing ACT concepts from a cultural, religious, and metaphysical perspective. It also opened up rich discussions around ghosts, spirits, and karma, which were fundamental to their experiences and yet which would have been difficult to address merely from a scientific or a 'neutral therapist' perspective. Trauma and grief were thus addressed both through ACT principles and from a broader spiritual perspective.

While preliminary evidence suggests that the group appears to be effective and highly rated, there are limitations to the group. All participants appear to have benefited to varying degrees, and yet for some, this represents the opening of a dialogue and the beginning of a therapeutic journey which needs to continue with further individual sessions along with appropriate interventions to address the complex intertwined psychosocial and familial issues. As skills like mindfulness and defusion need to be continually encouraged, reinforced, and practised, follow-up sessions are needed in order to support and maintain ACT concepts and skills in the face of ongoing stressors.

Some Cambodian patients were not suitable for the group, such as patients whose mental illnesses were not yet symptomatically stabilized enough to attend the group; those who had very low motivation and were unwilling to commit to a group; and a very small minority who disliked or felt unready to engage in mindfulness, a Buddhist group, or group psychotherapy in general. Other culturally appropriate interventions would need to be developed to meet the needs of these patients.

The principles of ACT and Buddhism can also be flexibly applied in individual or family sessions. For example, we were treating an elderly single woman with refractory depression who had recently started living with her younger sister and her family. One of the main perpetuating factors of her depression turned out to be related to her feeling of subtle disrespect culturally from her younger sister, resulting in her suppressed anger and feelings of uselessness. Through a family intervention session involving both the patient and her sister, we were able to work through their latent conflict. The patient was able to hear how much her younger sister still loved and respected her, even though the elder sister was no longer working or living independently. As we all reflected on her younger sister's own disappointment with the lack of respect in the younger generation, she became more keenly aware of her older sister's hurt ego. Drawing on ACT, the clarification of core family values of love and respect to which they were both committed, the use of mindfulness principles to become grounded in the present to facilitate letting go of past losses, the defusion of their unmet expectations in Canada, and the acceptance of changes in family roles and scripts ultimately facilitated their mutual reconciliation and the patient's recovery from depression.

As a caveat, it is important not to essentialize or overgeneralize cultural information. Culture itself is dynamic, and its influence on any given individual needs to be understood in its complex interactions with the individual's personality and experience as well as the current and past sociocultural context.

Conclusion

Surviving trauma and tremendous losses, refugees are often remarkably resilient, and many Cambodian Canadians readily exemplify this. While trauma leaves an indelible impact, it is important to not over-pathologize or focus solely on the traumatic experience in isolation. It is equally if not more important to understand their suffering from a sociocultural perspective and address the multiple needs arising from issues and struggles in their psychosocial context. Drawing from the rich Cambodian cultural and spiritual beliefs, especially Buddhism, can be tremendously helpful to augment conventional psychological approaches to address the complexity of the human experience and suffering and to identify culturally appropriate values in living a good and meaningful life. Further, addressing the grief over lost loved ones, the guilt of not being able to carry out familial duties of caring for family and relatives back home or financially supporting them, and the everyday family tensions that are evoked by sociocultural and acculturative stress is of paramount importance to the recovery and maintenance of the mental wellbeing of individuals as well as of their families. As we continue to explore and synthesize wisdom from diverse cultural, spiritual, and psychological perspectives, therapeutic developments may continue to broaden the capacity and reach to help more people in their recovery journey from trauma.

References

1. Statistics Canada, *Immigration and Ethnocultural Diversity: Key Results from the 2016 Census* (Ottawa: Statistics Canada, 2017).

2. Statistics Canada, *Gateways to Immigration in Canada* (Ottawa: Statistics Canada, 2017).

3. J. McLellan, *Cambodian Refugees in Ontario* (Toronto: University of Toronto Press, 2009).

4. Central Intelligence Agency, Cambodia. In *The World Factbook* (Internet). (Washington, DC: Central Intelligence Agency, 2017). www.cia.gov/library/publications/resources/the-world-factbook/geos/cb.html

5. R. Rechtman, Stories of trauma and idioms of distress: From cultural narratives to clinical assessment. *Transcultural Psychiatry*, 37(3) (2000), 403–15.

6. K. Fung and T. Lo, An integrative clinical approach to cultural competent psychotherapy. *Journal of Contemporary Psychotherapy*, 47(2) (2017), 65–73.

7. D. de Walque, *The Long-Term Legacy of the Khmer Rouge Period in Cambodia* (Washington, DC: The World Bank, 2004).

8. T. B. Seybolt, J. D. Aronson and B. Fischhoff, *Counting Civilian Casualties: An Introduction to Recording and Estimating Nonmilitary Deaths in Conflict* (Oxford: Oxford University Press, 2013).

9. Statistics Canada, Census Profile. 2016 Census. (Internet). (Ottawa: Statistics Canada, 2017). www12.statcan.gc.ca/census-recensement/2016/dp-pd/prof/index.cfm?Lang=E

10. J. Hays, (2008). Buddhism in Cambodia. (Internet). http://factsanddetails.com/southeast-asia/Cambodia/sub5_2e/entry-2880.html

11. H. Saddhatissa, *Buddhist Ethics* (Somerville, MA: Wisdom Publications, 1997).

12. S. H. Sugunasiri, The Buddhist view concerning the dead body. *Transplantation Proceedings*, 22(3) (1990), 947–9. http://eutils.ncbi.nlm.nih.gov/entrez/eutils/elink.fcgi?dbfrom=pubmed&id=2349713&retmode=ref&cmd=prlinks

13. P. Epasinghe, (2012).The tragic story of Bhikkhuni Patachara. *Sunday Observer*. http://archives.sundayobserver.lk/2012/12/23/spe02.asp

14. S. C. Hayes, J. B. Luoma, F. W. Bond, A. Masuda and J. Lillis, Acceptance and commitment therapy: Model, processes and outcomes. *Behaviour Research and Therapy*, 44(1) (2006), 1–25.

15. K. Fung, Acceptance and commitment therapy: Western adoption of Buddhist tenets? *Transcultural Psychiatry*, 52(4) (2015), 561–76. http://tps.sagepub.com/content/early/2014/08/01/1363461514537544.abstract

16. K. P. L. Fung and J. P. H. Wong, Acceptance and commitment therapy and Zen Buddhism. In A. Masuda and W. T. O'Donohue, eds., *Handbook of Zen, Mindfulness, and Behavioral Health* (Cham: Springer, 2017), pp. 271–88.

17. K. Fung and Z.-H. Zhu, Acceptance and commitment therapy and Asian thought. In R. Moodley, T. H.-T. E. Lo and N. Zhu, eds., *Asian Healing Traditions in Counseling and Psychotherapy* (Los Angeles, CA: Sage, 2018).

18. F. Ruiz, A review of acceptance and commitment therapy (ACT) empirical evidence: Correlational, experimental psychopathology, component and outcome studies. *International Journal of Psychology and Psychological Therapy*, 10 (1) (2010), 125–62.

19. J. G. L. A-Tjak, M. L. Davis, N. Morina, M. B. Powers, J. A. J. Smits and P. M. G. Emmelkamp, A meta-analysis of the efficacy of acceptance and commitment therapy for clinically relevant mental and physical health problems. *Psychotherapy and Psychosomatics*, 84(1) (2015), 30–6.

20. K. Fung, J. Lake, L. Steel, K. Bryce and Y. Lunsky, ACT processes in group intervention for mothers of children with Autism Spectrum Disorder. *Journal of Autism and Developmental Disorders*, 48 (8) (2018), 2740–7. http://link.springer.com/article/10.1007/s10803-018-3525-x

21. K. Fung, Y. Lunsky, L. Steel, K. Bryce and J. Lake, Using acceptance and commitment therapy for parents of children with Autism Spectrum Disorder. In K. Guastaferro and J. R. Lutzker, eds., *Evidence-Based Parenting Programs for Parents of Children with Autism and Intellectual or Developmental Disabilities* (London: Jessica Kingsley, 2018).

22. Y. Lunsky, K. Fung, J. Lake, L. Steel and K. Bryce, Evaluation of Acceptance and Commitment Therapy (ACT) for mothers of children and youth with Autism Spectrum Disorder. *Mindfulness*, 9(4) (2018), 1110–6. http://link.springer.com/article/10.1007/s12671-017-0846-3

23. K. P. Fung and J. Wong, *ACT to Reduce Stigma of Mental Illness: A Group Intervention Training Manual on Acceptance and Commitment Therapy* (Toronto: Strength in Unity, 2014).

24. J. Kabat-Zinn, Eating meditation. In J. Kabat-Zinn, *Mindfulness for Beginners* (CD) (Louisville, KY: Sounds True, Inc., 2006).

25. G. Obeyesekere, *The Work of Culture: Symbolic Transformations in Psychoanalysis and Anthropology* (Chicago: Chicago University Press, 1991).

Collaborating with Refugee Families on Dynamics of Intra-family Violence

Kjerstin Almqvist

Domestic Violence (DV) or Intimate Partner Violence (IPV) is a major public health problem, and worldwide almost one-third (30%) of all women who have been in a relationship have been exposed to IPV. Although a global curse for women, the prevalence rate varies and lifetime exposure to IPV of between 15% and 71% has been shown in women across different countries [1].

Abused women have been shown to be at increased risk of a variety of health problems, such as chronic pain, gynaecological problems, depression, post-traumatic stress disorder, anxiety and sleep disorders [1]. Exposure to parental IPV has also been shown to increase the risk of adverse health outcomes for children, such as post-traumatic stress symptoms, depression, anxiety and aggressive behaviour [2, 3]. Children who are exposed to parental IPV risk developing an increased awareness and mistrust of others, causing relationship problems and affecting their social development in a negative way [4]. In addition, exposure to parental IPV has been shown to be associated with decreased cognitive functioning, causing problems with school performance and language development [5, 6]. The risk of child abuse in families where the mother is exposed to violence has also been shown to be high [7]. Not being able to rely upon either the abusive or the abused parent for protection, support and emotional regulation may undermine the child's confidence in the parents' availability [8]. This is especially detrimental for a refugee child, as the forced migration often separates them from the extended family, crystallizing children's dependency on their parents. The high risk of negative outcomes in the developing child makes early recognition of IPV an urgent preventive matter.

Refugee families are in no way at less risk of IPV than others. On the contrary, women from refugee backgrounds seem to be particularly at risk of exposure to IPV [9, 10], and there seems to be a higher prevalence of IPV among refugee and immigrant families in western countries than within the native population [11, 12]. There are several plausible explanations for this; differences in the prevalence and acceptance of domestic violence in different cultures, migration stress affecting both individuals and family dynamics, increased aggressive behavior due to previous exposure to organized violence, and post-traumatic symptoms causing increased relationship tension and decreased emotional and behavioral regulation abilities. In this chapter, we explore the dynamics of IPV within refugee families resettled in western host societies and address the process of collaborating on IPV in clinical practice with refugee family members. We begin by describing different processes that contribute to increased stress and adverse dynamics in families in exile and continue with a discussion, illustrated by a case example, on how to support refugee parents and children exposed to family violence.

Normative Notions of Intimate Partner Violence in Transcultural Perspective

Legislation on IPV, as well as the predominant opinion about IPV in the population, varies between countries. In some societies, it is legal for men to use corporal punishment against their wives, and their behavior is accepted by the majority, such as in Ethiopia and Afghanistan [13, 14]. In western countries, such as in Sweden or Germany, IPV is defined as a crime in the legislation, and using violence against an intimate partner is behavior that is despised by the majority of the population.

When studying the international variation in cultural beliefs and values, such as in studies developed by the World Value Survey Association (www.worldvaluesurvey.or), countries can be described as more or less traditional or secular in their values. Gender equality is one of the topics that varies most between traditional and secular countries. Protestant countries like Sweden, Norway, Germany and the Netherlands have populations with high levels of secular-rational and self-expression values, while the African-Islamic region is characterized by the opposite, cherishing traditional values and values based on the need for survival [15]. To use violence within a family is in a traditional context seen as the husband's right and responsibility, while in a secular context domestic violence is a crime against wife or child [14, 16]. Most refugees who escape from organized violence are not challenged in their cultural core values, as they stay as close to their homes as possible for safety reasons, displaced in their own country or in a refugee camp close to the border. Some, however, have the chance and wish to try to reach a more permanent place of safety. Today we find refugee families resettling in countries far away from their homeland; in countries such as Canada, France, Norway, Germany, the Netherlands and Sweden. During the first decades of the twentieth century, the major flows of refugees have been from countries with civil war or political upheaval in the Middle East and the northern parts of Africa. Refugee families from countries such as Afghanistan, Iraq, Syria and Somalia who migrate to western countries such as Sweden or Canada have lived in societies where it is legal and accepted (when deemed rightful) for husbands and fathers to use corporal punishment against their children and wives and moved to societies where this is a crime and despised by the majority. To live according to the laws of and integrate within the resettling society, the family dynamics will need to change.

In most cases, the families are informed about the ban on violence within the family soon after their arrival in the resettling country, but competence for handling conflicts in the family without physical violence tends to take time to learn. When the refugee family belongs to a community of people from the same country living in a segregated neighborhood, the values of their home country concerning IPV may continue to dominate, or even to grow more conservative. As shown by Sullivan and colleagues [13], there is a risk that the migrant community might continue to respond to domestic violence as in the country of origin, minimizing the significance of the abuse and supporting the abuser over the abused. Moreover, if integration within the resettling society is hampered by racism or public prejudices against foreigners and Muslims, the risk of such processes within migration communities increases. In addition, the marginalization of migration communities contributes to distancing people from the resettling society and facilitates rumors such as those about social services taking children from their families if the authorities learn about domestic violence or the corporal punishment of children [17].

Cultural Change and Gender Roles in Exile

Adjustment and integration in the resettling society tend to take different periods of times for different individuals. Younger people find it easier to change and adjust to new circumstances than older ones, and children find it easier to learn new customs than adults [18]. If a new cultural value is beneficial for you it is easier to accept it than if you are adversely affected by it. In the process of acculturation, different family members tend to be more or less prone to adjust to the resettling country and its predominant cultural values, and the differences frequently cause tension within the family [18]. Children who settle in secular countries such as Norway, Canada or Sweden soon learn in school and from their friends that their parents are not allowed to spank them, and they dispute their parents if they continue to use corporal punishment. The same applies to the women, who more easily adjust to values that support gender equality than their men do [19]. For many men, however, the new cultural expectations of how to be a good father and a good husband constitute a real challenge, invoking complex questions on how to disconnect from cultural notions of male gender roles without experiencing the loss of fulfilling, deeply rooted expectations of what constitutes a protective, providing spouse and father [20]. They must give up their patriarchal position in the family and learn to negotiate with their wife on important things. Especially if their adjustment in society – such as learning a new language, getting a job and finding a decent place to live – seems to fail, men can find it hard to let go of their role as the one in charge of their family, and they become provoked by their children's and wives' demand for equality and equity. Raised in a society where male superiority is unquestioned, and unaccustomed to a relationship characterized by the need for the agreement of both parties, many men find it hard to change and feel like they are losing everything in exile [20]. The process of cultural change challenges male dominance and the existing power hierarchy in the family, which seems to increase the risk of male aggressive behavior and the abuse of women [21, 19]. As a result, the divorce rates are high among refugee families who have resettled in secular countries, sometimes even higher than in the native population.

When you are accustomed to a family dynamic where the hierarchical order is an aspect that defines who you are and how you are treated by your family, it can be hard to orient yourself in a society where the ideal family is characterized by the ability to form relationships that are not superior or subordinate but equal. Even if the demands of the wife concern the right to be listened to, to be respected and to be treated as an equal, the husband may conceive her quest as a challenge about power. In some cases, it may also be that wives or children take the opportunity to swing the positions around, keeping the hierarchical dynamic but improving their own position.

> When we left Afghanistan, I arrived first to settle with the children, as my husband stayed and tried to sell our house. I got my own name on the door to the apartment, and I got my own money for the first time in my life. When he arrived a year later, I told him that it was the custom in this country that it was the wife's name outside on the door, not the husband's. And that it was not possible to change who the money from the social insurance was sent to.

Oppression of women and girls is not only a question for the nuclear family. In many traditional societies, the norms in the extended family and in the community of people from the same country have a strong impact on the family dynamics. In so-called honor cultures the oppression of women, especially young women, is strong, and their behavior and relationships are controlled by the men in their family to keep them pure in the eyes of others. If they want the same freedom as other women in the resettling society, such as the freedom to spend time with friends outside the home, date and choose a husband by themselves, they risk abuse and even being killed [22].

As shown by Nilsson and colleagues [19], the risk of exposure to IPV and DV seems to increase for women who become more integrated within society and who learn to speak the new language. This may be explained by their increasing acculturation and awareness of their rights.

The stress provoked by acculturation and gender role changes risks increasing conflicts within the family, and the lack of a supporting social network may worsen the situation. When living together in an extended family, many conflicts in newly wed couples are handled with the contribution of other important relatives, such as parents and grand-parents [13]. When parents arrange the marriage, maybe with a cousin, the whole extended family has a responsibility for the marriage to work out. In well-functioning extended families, many conflicts are resolved in this way. When left on their own, conflicts between husband and wife risk accelerating in another way. The stress of acculturation may therefore contribute in different ways to an increase in conflicts and the use of violence against a spouse. On the other hand, the use of violence to control an intimate partner cannot solely be blamed on cultural practices or on acculturation stress. The use of violence in intimate relationships is a behavior that can be found globally, but never in every relationship in a society. It is always the perpetrator who is responsible for their actions. We need to discuss how cultural values and migration stress may contribute to triggering or aggravating IPV without losing the perspective of individual responsibility.

Another risk when discussing the prevalence of IPV among refugee families is that of strengthening the stereotypical prejudiced view of the aggressive Muslim male, a representation of "the other" that is spread through the media and the Internet. Describing an increased risk of using violence is, however, not the same as accusing all fathers and husbands from the Middle East or North Africa of abusing their wives and children. In most refugee families, even in families with relationship conflicts, the men are not abusing their wives. But we need to recognize that IPV constitutes a problem in many refugee families, and we need to be able to talk about it in order to help both individuals and families in the best way.

Post-Traumatic Stress and Post-Traumatic Family Dynamics

Finally, and obviously, previous exposure to organized violence is another factor that risks triggering or aggravating IPV in refugee families. War-related trauma exposure has been linked to aggression and increased levels of both community and family violence [23]. Many refugees suffer from post-traumatic stress symptoms, such as hypervigilance, increased irritability and mood dysregulation, that increase the risk of aggressive behavior. An increased prevalence of aggressive behavior and a positive association between PTSD symptom severity and reactive aggression has been shown repeatedly in studies of war survivors [23, 24]. We need, however, to note that post-traumatic stress seems to develop different predominant patterns in symptomatology in women and men. Men show an increased tendency towards aggressive behavior, while women predominantly show depressive and emotional symptoms [23]. Another adverse consequence for psychological health from taking part in organized violence has been recognized: the development of appetitive aggressive behavior. In some situations, being a perpetrator of violence may foster the development of fascination and a taste for violence. In a violent environment, this may be an adaption to a situation of constant threat and high levels of stress. This appetitive aggressiveness seems to be associated with lower levels of post-traumatic stress. In a dangerous environment, this adaptation may be protective, as has been shown by surviving child soldiers, but when returning to family and community it may cause major problems for rehabilitation [23]. Appetitive aggressiveness is rare compared to aggressive behavior associated with post-traumatic symptoms, but it is important to be aware of the phenomenon when working with refugees who have been soldiers or members of paramilitary groups.

Recognizing Intimate Partner Violence in Refugee Families

Despite the adverse impact of IPV, women are unlikely to disclose the abuse unless directly asked, and many have argued that there is a need for health care professionals to routinely ask about exposure to IPV [25]. Currently, the World Health Organization (WHO) recommends screening for IPV in vulnerable or at-risk groups [26].

IPV is a taboo behavior in many societies; something you do not talk about. Even in western countries where IPV is high on the political agenda, such as the Nordic countries, recognizing women and children who are exposed to IPV is a challenge due to professionals' reluctance to ask questions about exposure and victims' reluctance to admit exposure. Lack of concrete protection, stigmatization and fear of leaving the perpetrator are different causes that may contribute to the difficulty in disclosing IPV, despite living in a societal context where legislation prohibits it. When someone is an asylum applicant, revealing IPV may also cause difficulties in the asylum process, and may even risk counteracting the goal of receiving a legal permit to stay in the country. IPV, therefore, is rarely detected during the asylum process unless the violence is so brutal that the police get involved or injuries are recognized by health care or other authorities. For refugees without a legal permit to settle in a country, the situation is the same; women who are abused fear that contacting authorities may lead to their family being forced to leave the country.

As IPV is usually hidden by family members and unknown to the surrounding community, violence is not often seen as a possible explanation for adverse health outcomes, either in women or in children. Most times it is not until a long period of time has passed, when the parental relationship has been ended by a divorce or the child has grown up and left the family for a life of their own, that the IPV is acknowledged.

During the last decade, different initiatives have been taken within the health and social care systems around the world to increase the chances of recognizing women exposed to IPV. Routine questions (screening) about exposure to violence in health care settings have been shown to increase the possibility of recognizing exposed women and children, and this is now recommended in many countries. With reference to the WHO recommendations, the health care systems in many western countries have implemented screening for IPV during pregnancy [26]. Still, many refugee women are excluded from these interventions, either because of lack of resources such as interpreters, or because of health care professionals' misdirected adherence to the family's cultural values.

Another arrangement which has been shown to be essential in enabling women to reveal exposure to IPV is an individual and confidential dialog with the health care professional without the partner's presence [27]. In many cases, health care assessments of children as well as assessments by social services are made with both parents present, making it impossible for them to speak about sensitive topics such as IPV and substance abuse in the family. Professionals may be aware of the necessity for individual and safe interviews when addressing IPV, but despite that they may fail to offer this to refugee women. It may be the case that the wife needs an interpreter to be able to express herself and that her husband is the one who interprets for her. Another common situation is that the husband does not accept his wife being alone, especially not if the professional in question is a man. It is necessary to plan resources to avoid such situations and give refugee women similar opportunities to speak for themselves as those offered to other women in society. In every case when a child has shown some deviant behavior, in school or in another place, it is relevant to investigate whether violence within the family is a problem. To make that possible, individual dialog with both parents is needed, as well as with the child themselves. Otherwise there is a high risk of not recognizing an ongoing traumatic situation. The need for assessing individual dialog does not replace the need for joint family sessions where acknowledged problems are addressed.

The following case study illustrates how a history of interpersonal violence and wartime rape may be unveiled when collaborating with refugee parents looking for support for a child with severe behavioral problems.

A Four-Year-Old Boy Referred for a Neuropsychiatric Investigation

A mother from Kosovo is asking for help with her son, as the staff in the daycare center at the refugee camp has demanded that she do something about his behavior and recommended her to contact a child psychologist. The boy is 4 years old, living together with his family, asylum applicants in Sweden for 10 months. He is aggressive and restless, hits both children and staff at the daycare center, and has many times tried to destroy toys and furniture. He arrives with his mother and aunt at a refugee mental health service unit, his father being unable to attend. The mother describes the boy as totally out of her control. She is not able to calm him down, but is herself afraid of him and describes how he hits her when he does not get candy or other things that he wants. She has learnt that she is not allowed to use corporal punishment on children in Sweden, and she knows no other way to stop his aggressive behavior. His aunt has a better relationship with the boy, but the mother says that this may be explained by her giving the boy toys and candy without trying to deny him anything. The mother describes her young son as a dangerous and threatening tormentor. The child psychologist, recognizing several possible explanations for the boy's aggressive and hyperactive behavior beyond what was suggested in the referral (namely a neuropsychiatric disorder), starts building an alliance with the mother and family, trying to understand their history. The mother eventually describes how she and the other female members of her family, her sister and their mother, were all raped and assaulted by a group of men when they had escaped from their village and were on their way to the border to find safety in Macedonia. Her son witnessed the brutal incident, but without being hurt himself. When they finally arrived in Macedonia, they spent a week on a field without protection, sanitary resources and other things that they needed. The women decided never to tell anyone what had happened to them, but the mother describe how she still has nightmares of the gang-rape and cannot forget what happened. She also thinks that her son changed after the traumatic event, becoming more distant from her and more aggressive. Her husband, who had left the family to fight with the liberation army, was not aware of her trauma. He arrived in Sweden a month later. The psychologist invited her to bring her husband to discuss their son and his problem together. After several sessions without bringing her husband as she had promised, she told her therapist about the abuse he had exposed her to both in Kosovo and after their arrival in Sweden. She was now living together with her sister and mother, and she had forced her husband to move and live with one of his friends. She did not want his abuse to be known by the authorities, as she wanted him to be able to receive his legal permit to stay in Sweden, but she did not want to live with him. He had had a drinking problem since before the war, and his violence had increased over the years. In Kosovo it was not possible to do anything about this, but she understood that she had other opportunities in Sweden if they could receive a legal permit to stay. When working with the family to support the young boy to change his aggressive behavior, the previous trauma needed to be addressed, but more important was to address the current situation where the boy had taken on the role of his father. As violence had been the only way to handle conflicts in the family, the boy had failed to develop an emotional regulation capacity and his mother had been too scared to give him comfort and safety. In collaboration with the family to restore the mother as a psychological shield, someone able to give the young boy both protection and comfort, the support from the aunt and grandmother was essential. The psychologist eventually succeeded in inviting the father to individual meetings, addressing the boy's need to learn to regulate his emotions without using aggressive behavior if he was to have a good future, and the focus was on how his father could contribute to this goal. Although the father denied his own responsibility and aggressive behavior, he could see the need for safety and stability for his boy's further development. Eventually the father was able have regular visitation with his boy without aggressive behavior and conflicts with the other family members.

This case illustrates some principles that may guide therapeutic work with refugee families. Aggressive and hyperactive behavior in young children is a frequent cause for referrals, as such behavior in children causes problems in school and daycare. A combination of vulnerability in the child, previous or current environmental stressors and family dynamics which contribute to or maintain the symptoms calls for a thorough assessment of every case to identify different factors, including post-traumatic stress, that may contribute to the problem. In the presented case, the maternal description of her child signals that the mother-child interaction is characterized by an aggressive-punitive controlling attachment in the child with mirrored helplessness and fear for the child in the mother [28]. The mother-child interaction signals that the child has been left without support to cope with toxic stress of some kind and that the mother's capacity to offer comfort and safety has been negatively affected. Initially, the mother did not describe any possible explanation for her child's behavior, but silencing traumatic events is a predominant behavior in traumatized families [29]. To facilitate traumatized refugees describing their experiences, we need to ask initiated questions about frequent kinds of traumatic exposure and to explain the rationale for doing so. Explanations of how traumatic experiences risk affecting your mental health negatively and how post-traumatic stress in parents may affect children are helpful interventions. To learn that aggressive behavior is a common reaction in children traumatized by violence in different forms helps parents to describe experiences they might otherwise have preferred to leave unmentioned. To ask routine questions about frequent traumatic events, after explaining the rationale for this, makes it easier to reveal traumatic exposure, such as the rape in this case. It is important that clinicians are well informed about the kinds of atrocities that are committed in societies plagued by organized violence in order to be able to ask initiated questions [30].

For many women, a rape is something that feels shameful and it is hard to talk about. In a society in which female sexuality is associated with the family honor, public recognition of a rape may even be a threat to your life. For men, being raped may be equally stigmatizing. Many soldiers or imprisoned men have also been exposed to (or have themselves committed) atrocities they do not intend to let their wives or children know about. It is therefore necessary to always do the anamnestic interviews with each parent alone, offering a secluded environment [27]. In the initial meeting with the family, when informing the family about the procedure to come, we describe the need for individual interviews with each of them, explaining that family members otherwise tend to protect each other from their experiences, symptoms and worries.

In the presented case, the additional trauma of long-term intimate partner violence was eventually revealed as the psychologist continued to insist on meeting the father. The mother was even more reluctant to reveal the IPV than the gang-rape, as she was anxious not to risk the chance of getting a legal permit to stay as refugees in Sweden for the whole family. In addition, if the family was denied asylum they would have to return to Kosovo together, and consequently there was a strong motivation for her not to bring the IPV into public view. It is not unusual for there to be layers of traumatic experiences in traumatized refugee families, some more easy to access than others. When collaborating with traumatized refugee parents, we need to respect their difficulties being open about their history as they try to navigate in the best way for themselves and their children. Changes in and additions to their stories are understandable in their delicate position, and IPV is frequently something that they will not bring up unless directly asked about it.

To address symptoms displayed by a child, we wish to collaborate with both parents or all primary caregivers. In the presented case, it was not possible to have the parents collaborate as a couple, but it was possible to mobilize them as parents supporting the best for their child. Although the father denied the abuse, he accepted that it would be beneficial for his son if he was able to collaborate with his wife without violent conflicts. The psychologist's insistence on the importance of him as a father also made him commit to not drinking alcohol during the days he had his son with him. The aim in this case was to improve the child's safety and parental support, accepting that the family history and current situation as asylum applicants gave restricted options.

It has been shown to be difficult to motivate abusive husbands to change. To address the needs of their children seems, however, to be a more possible way of motivating behavioral change [31, 32]. In refugee families, and especially during the asylum application period, the first years in the country of resettlement is a period when women who are exposed to IPV, for several reasons, feel a need to keep the family together. When health care or social service professionals recognize that violence is a problem within a family, there is a risk that they will choose to back off due to a mixture of respecting the family's cultural norms, the complexity in approaching the violence when a family may be denied asylum and forced to return, and the general reluctance to acknowledge IPV. How to act when faced with IPV in a family is always a challenge, and the transcultural and exile perspectives add to the complexity and increase barriers among professionals in the resettling country to addressing it and intervening to protect the victims. Acknowledging the difficulties in recognizing domestic violence, both Intimate Partner Violence and child abuse, in families previously exposed to organized violence and traumatized by this multiplicity of adverse experiences is a first step to working and collaborating with refugee families. Getting to know the family and their particular history and value system is the next step to making a grounded intervention possible.

With the growing awareness in society of the adverse outcomes for women and children exposed to Intimate Partner Violence, different interventions have been developed, both community based and within mental health care. Although the need to develop more effective preventive, supportive and treating models remains, several programs and methods have shown promising results in decreasing psychological symptoms and strengthening coping abilities in women and children [33–35].

Conclusion

When working with refugee families who need support and treatment for psychological symptoms in one or several family members, a thorough assessment of the family history and functioning is needed. The family history is seldom one and united. Every member, adult or child, has their own experiences and fears. Symptoms in the individual, child or adult, may be explained by a range of experiences and traumatic exposures. As part of the assessment and before working with the family together, individual interviews need to take place. And the interviews need to address not only things in the past that have happened before the exile, in their homeland or on the way. It is also necessary to ask about the current family functioning and the context in the resettling society [36].

When wishing to support a vulnerable family, it is easy to avoid questions that feel as though they undermine the family stability or accuse the husband or the parents. But to avoid asking, or neglecting signs of IPV, is not a proper way to support anyone. For a child currently suffering from abuse in the family, it is not supportive to talk about family suffering before the forced migration and their arrival in the resettling country. The child needs the current situation and parental functioning to be addressed, not to feel betrayed or abandoned by the authorities. Otherwise the risk of future marginalization and psychological disturbances in the child increases [37]. To avoid recognizing a woman exposed to violence by her husband risks in a similar way worsening the situation for the family in the future, both for the adults and for the children.

It is necessary for professionals who collaborate with refugee families to have knowledge about the increased risk of family conflicts posed by migration and acculturation in both individuals and the family dynamics, as well as knowledge about the adverse consequences – such as increased aggressive behaviour – of post-traumatic stress. Knowledge about the increased risks of family violence in exile facilitates a dialogue about how the individual's symptomatology is expressed within the family. Knowledge about different societal opinions and legislation about domestic violence and corporal punishment may help a professional to discuss these issues in terms of how to change parental behavior when living in exile and how to handle conflicts within the family without violence.

References

1. World Health Organization, *Global and Regional Estimates of Violence against Women: Prevalence and Health Effects of Intimate Partner Violence and Non-partner Sexual Violence* (World Health Organization, 2013). www.who.int /reproductivehealth

2. Y.-C. Chan and J. W.-K. Yeung, Children living with violence within the family and its sequel: A meta-analysis from 1995–2006. *Aggression and Violent Behavior*, 14(5) (2009), 313–322.

3. S. Evans, C. Davies and D. DiLillo, Exposure to domestic violence: A meta-analysis of child and adolescent outcomes. *Aggression and Violent Behavior*, 13(2) (2008), 131–140.

4. A. Levendosky, G. Bogat and A. Huth-Bocks, The influence of domestic violence on the development of the attachment relationship between mother and young children. *Journal of Psychoanalytic Psychology*, 28 (2011), 512–517.

5. K. Kitzmann, N. Gaylord, A. Holt and E. Kenny, Child witnesses to domestic violence: A meta-analytic review. *Journal of Consulting and Clinical Psychology*, 71(2) (2003), 339–352.

6. G. L. Carpenter and A. M. Stacks, Developmental effects of exposure to intimate partner violence in early childhood: A review of the literature. *Children and Youth Services Review*, 31(8) (2009), 831–839.

7. E. M. Annerbäck, L. Sahlqvist, C. G. Svedin, G. Wingren and P. A. Gustafsson, Child physical abuse and concurrence of other types of child abuse in Sweden: Associations with health and risk behaviors. *Child Abuse and Neglect*, 36(7–8) (2012), 585–595.

8. C. Zeanah, L. Berlin and N. Boris, Practitioner review: Clinical applications of attachment theory and research for infants and young children. *Journal of Child Psychology and Psychiatry*, 52(8) (2011), 819–833.

9. J. Perilla, (2003). Domestic violence in refugee and immigrant communities. Tapestri Inc., Refugee and Immigrant Coalition Against Domestic Violence. www .tapestri.org/article_Domestic_Violence_I mmigrant1.html

10. H. Al-Modallal, I. Zayed, S. Abujilban, T. Shebab and M. Atoum, Prevalence of Intimate Partner Violence among women visiting health care centers in Palestine refugee camps in Jordan. *Health Care for Women International*, 36(2) (2015), 137–148.

11. J. Annan, K. Falb, D. Kpebo, M. Hossain and J. Gupta, Reducing PTSD symptoms through a gender norms and economic empowerment intervention to reduce intimate partner violence: A randomized controlled pilot study in Côte D'Ivoire. *Global Mental Health*, 4 (2017), e22(1–9).

12. C. Jernbro and S. Janson, (2017). *Våld mot barn 2016. En nationell kartläggning.* Rapport från Stiftelsen Allmänna Barnhuset (*Violence against Children. A National Survey Report from Allmänna Barnhuset Foundation*).

13. M. Sullivan, K. Senturia, T. Negash, S. Shiu-Thornton and B. Giday, 'For us it is like living in the dark': Ethiopian women's experiences with domestic violence. *Journal of Interpersonal Violence*, 20(8) (2005), 922–940.

14. R. K. Biswas, N. Rahman, E. Kabir and F. Raihan, Women's opinion on the justification of physical spousal violence: A quantitative approach to model the most vulnerable households in Bangladesh. *PLoS One*, 12(11) (2017), e0187884. https://doi.org/10.1371/journal .pone.0187884

15. P. Norris and R. Inglehart, *Sacred and Secular: Religion and Politics Worldwide*, 2nd ed., Cambridge Studies in Social Theory, Religion and Politics (Cambridge, UK: Cambridge University Press, 2012).

16. H. Al-Modallal, Patterns of coping with partner violence: Experiences of refugee women in Jordan. *Public Health Nursing*, 29(5) (2012), 403–411.

17. C. West, African immigrant women and intimate partner violence: A systematic review. *Journal of Aggression, Maltreatment & Trauma*, 25 (1) (2016), 4–17.

18. J. Phinney and J. Flores, 'Unpackaging' acculturation: Aspects of acculturation as predictors of traditional sex role attitudes. *Journal of Cross-Cultural Psychology*, 33(3) (2002), 320–331.

19. J. Nilsson, C. Brown, E. Russell and S. Khamphakdy-Brown, Acculturation, partner violence, and psychological distress in refugee women from Somalia. *Journal of Interpersonal Violence*, 23(11) (2008), 1654–1663.

20. M. Darvishpour, Immigrant women challenge the role of men: How the changing power relationship within Iranian families in Sweden intensifies family conflicts after immigration. *Journal of Comparative Family Studies*, 33 (2002), 271–296.

21. C. Fisher, Changed and changing gender and family roles and domestic violence in African refugee background communities' post-settlement in Perth, Australia. *Violence Against Women*, 19(7) (2013), 833–847.

22. B. Hayes, J. Freilich and S. Chermak, An exploratory study of honor crimes in the United States. *Journal of Family Violence*, 31(3) (2016), 303–314.

23. T. Hecker, S. Fetz, H. Ainamani and T. Elbert, The cycle of violence: Associations between exposure to violence, trauma-related symptoms and aggression – Findings from Congolese refugees in Uganda. *Journal of Traumatic Stress*, 28(5) (2015), 448–455.

24. C. Catani, N. Jacob, E. Schauer, M. Kohila and F. Neuner, Family violence, war and natural disasters: A study of the effect of extreme stress on children's mental health in Sri Lanka. *BMC Psychiatry*, 8 (2008), 33.

25. R. Dagher, M. Garza and K. Backes Kozhimannil, Policymaking under uncertainty: Routine screening for intimate partner violence. *Violence Against Women*, 20(6) (2014), 730–749.

26. World Health Organization, (2013). *Responding to Intimate Partner Violence and Sexual Violence against Women: WHO Clinical and Policy Guidelines*. www .who.int/reproductivehealth/publications/ violence/9789241548595/en/

27. K. Almqvist, Å. Källström, P. Appell and A. Anderzen-Carlsson, Mothers' opinions on being asked about exposure to intimate partner violence in child healthcare centres in Sweden. *Journal of Child Health Care*, 22 (2) (2017), 228–237.

28. E. Moss, J. Bureau, D. St-Laurent and G. Tarabulsy, Understanding disorganized attachment at preschool and school age: Examining divergent pathways of disorganized and controlling children. In J. Solomon and C. George, eds., *Disorganized Attachment and Caregiving* (New York: The Guilford Press, 2011), pp. 53–79).

29. N. Dahlgaard and E. Montgomery, Disclosure and silencing: A systematic review of the literature on patterns of communication in refugee families. *Transcultural Psychiatry*, 52 (2015), 579–593.

30. K. James, Domestic violence within refugee families: Intersecting patriarchal culture and the refugees experience. *Australian & New Zealand Journal of Family Therapy*, 31 (3) (2013), 275–284.

31. S. Aaron and R. Beaulaurier, The need for new emphasis on batterers intervention programs. *Trauma, Violence & Abuse*, 18 (4) (2017), 425–432.

32. S. Meyer, Motivating perpetrators of domestic and family violence to engage in behaviour change: The role of fatherhood. *Child and Family Social Work*, 23(1) (2018), 97–104.

33. C. F. Rizo, R. J. Macy, D. M. Ermentrout and N. B. Johns, A review of family interventions for intimate partner violence with a child focus or child component. *Aggression and Violent Behavior*, 16(2) (2011), 144–166.

34. C. Bourey, W. Williams, E. Bernstein and R. Stephenson, Systematic review of structural interventions for intimate partner violence in low- and middle-income countries: Organizing evidence for prevention. *BMC Public Health*, 15 (2015), 1165.

35. M. Ellsberg, D. Arango, M. Morton, F. Gennari, S. Kiplesund, M. Contreras et al., Prevention of violence against women and girls: What does the evidence say? *The Lancet*, 385(9977) (2015), 1555–1566.

36. L. Elliot, M. Nerney, T. Jones and P. D. Friedmann, Barriers for screening for domestic violence. *Journal of General International Medicine*, 17(2) (2002), 112–116.

37. R. Saile, V. Ertl, F. Neuner and C. Catani, Does war contribute to family violence against children? Findings from a two-generational multi-informant study in Northern Uganda. *Child Abuse & Neglect*, 38(1) (2014), 135–146.

Chapter 13

Supporting Refugee Family Reunification in Exile

Nora Sveaass and Sissel Reichelt[†]

Introduction

When Sara first contacted the Psychosocial Center for Refugees, she was waiting for her husband, Hassan, to arrive in Norway after many years apart. He had been in prison for 10 years, and she expected that it would be good but also a very difficult situation. We agreed that she should call back on his arrival; she did and she told us, "I got back a corpse." He was alive, of course, but had serious pain following torture, and was in all ways strongly affected by the years in prison. It was hard for him to reintegrate into the family. He had had little contact with his wife during these years and had not seen their two daughters since they were very small. They had been looking forward to finally being with their father again, and they were disappointed at his inability to engage in what they wanted to include him in.

Ahmed was referred to individual therapy because of a growing depression. He had functioned well in the new society during the first period he was here, and he was expecting that his wife Fatima and their son, then five years of age, would be able to join him quickly. Unfortunately, this period lasted longer and had more stumbling blocks than he had expected. His wife, temporarily while awaiting reunification, had settled in a country close to their country of origin together with their child. As time went by, she became both impatient and depressed and started mistrusting her husband, living in this country so far away. Was he doing anything to enable them to come? Perhaps he did not want them to come. Ahmed became deeply concerned about his wife's suspicions, and, not being in any condition to do something to make reunification happen, he became increasingly depressed. During sessions, he cried and explained how he had tried to communicate that the only thing he wanted was to be with them again and that he was completely unable to influence the process from where he was. Finally, after having secured the information that was needed, the family was reunited. Before this happened, Ahmed asked for conversations with himself, his wife and their child present, to explain how difficult it had been for him – he knew that, even with the prospect of coming to join him, she was not a happy woman.

In both these case examples, to be united again was the dream that had kept them going. Hassan would one day be free from prison and from the pain he had endured. He would live with his wife and two lovely daughters again, that he had not seen for so many years. He

[†] At the end of this chapter, the reader finds a tribute to Sissel Reichelt, who passed away when finalizing this book.

Acknowledgments: We want to thank our colleagues in Trondheim for their contribution to the project on conversations with families reunited in exile, in particular professor Berit Berg (NTNU), Vigdis Ledal, Tove Buchmann, Anne-Britt Johansen (Refugee Health Team in Trondheim Municipality), Solveig Gravråkmo and Jorunn Gran (Regional Team for Violence and Traumatic Stress, Mid-Norway). Warm thanks also to Trondheim Municipality and the Directorate of Integration and Diversity (IMDi) for their important support in developing this work.

212

knew that they would hardly recognize him, but they would be happy to live with their father again. Sara would finally be with her husband again, and they would become the family they had once been.

Ahmed was dreaming of the day he could have a life in Norway with his wife and son. The vision of her being with him again, safely, their son attending school and finding friends and he himself back to his work and studies, had been with him day and night for the almost three years they had been apart. Fatima wanted to live with her husband again, there was no doubt about this – they loved each other and had been there for each other, but now, after such a long time apart, she often felt that she had lost trust in him, and most of the time she felt very sad and lonely. Nevertheless, being reunited, seeing father and son together again, gave her some hope.

Both of these families had their dreams fulfilled, and the relief experienced was strong, but both families were faced with a difficult and challenging process.

In this chapter, we will approach these separation and reunification experiences of refugees through a family lens. Hereto, we focus on the need to strengthen work with refugee families in general, and in particular with families that have been separated and that are living through the process of reunification. From a legal perspective, the right to be together with close family members and the right to be reunited in situations related to flight and protection are addressed in several international human rights conventions and agreements. The Universal Declaration of Human Rights from 1948 (16.3) states: "The family is the natural and fundamental group unit of society and is entitled to protection by society and the State" [1]. The UN Convention on the Rights of the Child (1989) defines the right of children to be with their families, the right to have parents as their primary caregivers and the right not to be separated from them unless very specific conditions make this necessary (CRC, art. 7, 9, 10) [2]. The UN High Commissioner for Refugees, in a document from 2008 on evaluation and determinations of the best interests of the child (BID), states: "Family reunification, whenever feasible, should generally be regarded as being in the best interests of the child. Once the family is traced, family relationships verified and the willingness of the child and the family members to be reunited has been confirmed, the process should not normally be delayed by a BID procedure" (2008, p. 31 [3]).

The Geneva Convention of 1949 (IV, art. 24–26) highlights the right to know the whereabouts of missing family members and to obtain help to track and find them [4]. The International Committee of the Red Cross (ICRC), since its establishment in 1883, performs as one of its major activities the tracking of persons missing and separated from family as a consequence of war and armed conflict. *The International Convention for the Protection of All Persons from Enforced Disappearance* is also relevant here [5], defining the right to protection against being forcefully disappeared and the responsibility of states to track missing persons and to hold those responsible to account. This obligation also includes the opening of mass graves and the identification of victims. The *EC Directive for Family Reunification* is particularly relevant in Europe and its member states: "Measures concerning family reunification should be adopted in conformity with the obligations to protect the family and respect family life, as enshrined in many instruments of international law" (2003, para. 2 [6]). It further notes in paragraph 4 that "Family reunification is a necessary way of making family life possible. It helps to create socio-cultural stability facilitating the integration of third country nationals in the Member State, which also serves to promote economic and social cohesion, a fundamental Community objective stated in the Treaty" [6]. This means that part of its work as a helper of families can be to ensure that these rights are in fact enjoyed by families in situations of separation and uncertainty.

This chapter addresses the provision of therapeutic support to refugee families that are reunited in exile after social, political or cultural events have kept them forcefully apart. Hereby, we develop a particular focus on families with one or more family members who were exposed to severe human rights violations, such as long-term detention and torture, and explore how these families can be supported in the process of reunification. First, we describe what is meant by family reunification and highlight some relevant research in relation to refugees, stress and families. Second, we discuss the specific challenges faced by reunited families, such as establishing new patterns of communication and finding ways to live together again. Third, we present a possible way of assisting families based on an ongoing project. Here, the newly reunited families are invited to family conversations, aiming at assisting them to deal with the many challenges that may follow in the wake of reestablishing life in exile. Finally, we will discuss these experiences and how such an approach may be useful in work with families, in particular in situations that may give rise to conflict, misunderstandings and disappointment, often combined with high expectations of reunification. This specific focus emerged in the context of our therapeutic work with refugee families. We saw that many of the challenges the families were struggling with were rooted in their experience of separation and all that had happened when the family was apart, as well as by the challenges encountered when reunited [7–10].

Developing a Family Perspective on Refugee Family Reunification

Family reunification refers to families being united again after a period of involuntary and undesired separation. The form of reunification discussed in this chapter is about families who have fled their country of origin in order to seek protection elsewhere in the face of armed conflict, forced migration and severe human rights abuses and who are reunited in a country other than their own.

The rights regarding family reunification are usually related to the kind of residence permission the family has in the host country, whether they are refugees transferred through the UN system who have been accepted as refugees protected under the Geneva Convention or whether they are individuals applying for protection who have been granted either asylum or subsidiary protection. Those who have been denied a legal stay have meager chances of being reunited, whereas those obtaining refugee status, and on certain conditions subsidiary permissions, have better reasons to expect reunification to happen.

Research on family reunification has focused both on the experiences of families that have been reunited and on the difficulties of prolonged separation, sometimes evoked by restrictive immigration policies in host countries [11]. Rousseau and colleagues [12, 13] argue that the many painful processes related to reunification in exile are frequently overlooked and forgotten. They further argue that whereas armed conflict and war trauma are seen as the violence of others, looking into the prolonged separations that families experience is to highlight Western administrative violence, and, as such, this receives little attention [14]. Bragg and Wong have likewise addressed the impact of changes in Canadian immigration policy, in particular how this negatively affects separated families (2015, p. 60 [11]).

Host societies contribute to holding people apart and separated through a set of complex and thorough rules. This happens in combination with a reluctance to reevaluate rejections of reunification, even in the light of previous serious human rights violations experienced by

those involved. Studies by Choummanivong et al. [14] have further highlighted the importance of family reunification for successful resettlement and discussed how lack of
reunification affects mental health and wellbeing, representing significant obstacles to the
process of resettlement. Another study by Rousseau et al., comparing traumatized refugees
from Latin America and Africa reunited in Canada [12], highlighted that those who were
reunited showed less problems in their daily lives than those who were denied reunification.
The study further suggested that those who were reunited still struggled with insecurity and
fear of being separated again, and concerns regarding challenges and negotiations over new
roles and responsibilities in the family and in the host society [12]. In other words, they
found that family reunification, and thus the presence of family, had important effects on
lives in exile.

In his articles on families, migration and political oppression, Sluzki [15, 16] describes
stresses that families encounter when confronted with human rights violations and long-
term political oppression, including the dynamics in families with a missing family member
and the problems involved in such complicated losses [15–17]. Sluzki compares the situation of families with a missing or forcedly disappeared member to that of a tortured person,
where the truth has been shattered and cannot be reassembled.

Given the numerous studies documenting family relationships as a vital source of
support in refugees' wellbeing and adaptation, family separation may form a pervasive
stressor and family reunification may operate as a source of stabilization and restoration. In
research on resilience, social support and the presence of significant others are referred to as
important and positive factors. Network and family constitute protective factors, and
a frequent strategy is to mobilize the network surrounding persons under stress. Studies
of soldiers returning from war show that acceptance and a sense of relationship and
belonging to family or close others have important implications for how they deal with
traumatic experiences in their aftermath [18]. From what we know about protective factors,
both in relation to coping with prior stressors and dealing with present burdens and
changes, family plays an important role [19, 20]. It has nevertheless been suggested that
families in and of themselves do not always function in protective ways. If a person
returning from war or other stressful events is met with rejection and/or indifference,
family may be more of a problem than a resource [21]. It is important that the family or
network is accepting and gives room for emotional support.

Some studies have explored the significance of family when new life is reestablished in
exile. While Krupinski and Burrows [22] did not find any differences in the level of
psychological illness in refugees arriving alone compared with those who came together
with their families, other studies indicate that loneliness and the absence of family and
meaningful activities are highly relevant factors in relation to psychological wellbeing in
exile. Beiser [23] concluded in one of his studies that refugees who arrived with their spouses
were less depressed than those who came alone, both 10 and 12 months after arrival.

The role of family is especially relevant in the case of child refugees. A study by
Montgomery [24] concluded that stressful life in exile seems to be the most problematic
factor affecting their ability to recover from earlier trauma, and that quality of family life
seems particularly important in order for children to cope. A study by Gorst-Unsworth and
Goldenberg [25] of Iraqi refugees living in Germany suggested that lack of social support in
exile seemed to be a stronger predictor of depression than preflight traumatic events. The
researchers also concluded that the quality of social relationships was important and that
experience of emotional support was vital with regard to the reduction of the development

of trauma-related distress and depression, in particular in those subjected to serious traumatic events. A Norwegian study of the role of family and work or activity in a large refugee sample found that having close family in Norway had a positive impact on traumatized refugees, and that this effect was stronger the more exposed the refugees had been [19, 26].

Family Consequences of Separation

Refugee families are frequently exposed to a large number of serious human rights violations and threats prior to leaving their country of origin. These range from long periods of insecurity and fear, including persecution and hiding, to experiences of loss, brutality, detention and torture. For many families, the flight itself may be the worst experience. There may be serious dangers involved in the journey – in some places immigrants risk detention after having crossed the border – and it may also involve the possibility of family members becoming separated from each other.

Family separation is often due to armed conflict, abduction, detention or having to go underground, but it may also be due to disasters of different kinds. In such situations, family members are exposed both to great uncertainty regarding each other's conditions and to different forms of extreme stressors themselves. Women who are left alone with children may be at risk of economic problems and the fear of violence against their children or of sexual assault on themselves. Likewise, for children and adolescents, separation from their parents or parent constitutes a very serious threat to their present situations and future possibilities. Not knowing where the rest of their family is or in what situation they are living represents to most people a serious stressor, and their possibility of dealing with other daily challenges is often seriously reduced. The difficulties involved in mobilizing help to find missing family members are also sources of serious stress. Life during such periods may be extremely distressing. Family members are often faced with very different life conditions and experiences. For example, while some members may be exposed to detention, abduction or other forms of limited liberty, others may be in camps or even in safe places such as shelters. Some family members may not know anything about the situations of the others. Some of these experiences – that is, different forms of stressors while living through separation – may constitute problems that are difficult to deal with when they are reunited. It is important for those trying to help in the new country to recognize the major changes in family relations that must necessarily have occurred at the point of reunification of the family and which may be confusing and disturbing for the family members.

The stresses related to life in a host country may include the prospect of not being accepted for protection reasons, the fear of expulsion and even separations within the family [27, 28, 11]. The challenges involved in life in exile have been described in various studies [29, 30], and refugee families' need for support may be comprehensive and at times difficult to deal with. In the hope of support, refugees will often present claims for allowing their family to come and stay with them. They may be youngsters who have arrived as separated minors, but after some time they may communicate their need and wish for their family to join them in the host country. Adults, as well, will often request reunification with close relatives. Administrative delays and hindrances may make reunification a very difficult, often almost impossible, project [12]. Families often have little information regarding the whereabouts of other family members – they may be abducted, possibly disappeared or missing in conflict. The hardships involved for families that live with family members who have been forcibly disappeared are, as already referred to, well described by Sluzki in his articles on family therapy and political disappearance [15, 16].

A period of waiting can give rise to uncertainty and even distrust among family members. There may be serious doubts as to when and whether they will meet again and return to the family life they once lived. Family members in exile have described their problems related to understanding the system and conveying this to those waiting somewhere else. Particularly, young people who are hoping that their parents will arrive have often been expected to do more to obtain reunification, and they often feel that the responsibility put on their shoulders has been difficult to deal with [30]. Lack of information is difficult for all parties involved, and mutual expectations and doubts as to whether something could be done better and more effectively often emerge between family members.

The family that is waiting for the chance to travel and reunite with their loved ones may fear that they have been forgotten – that those in exile are fine without them, meeting new people – and have the idea that they have not undertaken sufficient efforts to keep in contact or ensure that reunification happens. It can be difficult to understand that there is, in fact, little the family member(s) in the host country can do to influence this process in any way. Because of this, it seems particularly important that those in contact with the waiting family outside the host country, first of all embassies, delegations and consulates, provide relevant and adequate information about the process and prospects of reunion.

Intrafamily Dynamics during the Reunification Process

High expectations regarding reunion is a natural part of the picture. Many have lived for years with the wish that this will happen one day. They may have pictured the moment that they finally meet again, and in their dreams this may be an almost perfect situation. Many families refer to the first period together as a "honeymoon," but difficulties can soon arise, often related to issues that are hard to share or talk about. Thus, having some help available to deal with such situations may be of value, and, if possible, as soon as possible. Difficulties can arise in relation to child-rearing, and the person who has been in charge of childcare may find it difficult not to be in full charge anymore, leading to disagreements. How to reestablish oneself as a parent after a long time away from family life is not easy and may require both time and negotiation. One part of the family may have been through an acculturation process and the newly arrived ones may find that there have been major cultural changes in the family, and they may not approve of this. In some families where the woman has been alone with the children, and where she has adapted herself to gender roles and ways of parenting more in line with the host society, conflicts may arise, both in relation to parenting and spousal roles. Also, children who have integrated into the new culture may find that the newly arrived and longed-for family member disapproves of such a development and resists it, either openly or more indirectly. Such experiences can be interpreted as if the family members have drifted apart from each other. In their study of reunited Congolese refugee families, Rousseau et al. [13] refer to family separation as an ambiguous loss (p. 1095) because of the many uncertainties and risks involved and the impossibility of knowing about future options to be together again. The study discusses the need for support and finding ways of dealing with the reunification, an observation that inspired the work described here. These authors highlight the need to recreate balance, belonging and continuity, and in this process, traditions, memories and experiences are described as important ways of reestablishing the thread in the family after an often long and painful rupture [13].

Families that reunite in exile may have lived through long periods of harsh experiences, and this may affect them in ways that make them different. Returning to everyday family life after years of detention and torture, or after active life as a soldier in war, or as a civilian in a war zone may be extremely difficult for all family members. Both spouses and children may be changed, and these changes may not be easy to speak about in open conversations, and experiences may not be easy to share. Shame and guilt may be experienced in such situations, and in some families, family secrets develop.

The Development of a Family Therapeutic Project: Main Therapeutic Approaches

A family therapy project with the aim of exploring family therapy approaches in work with refugee families [7–10] significantly informed us about the effects and challenges related to serious traumatic events prior to leaving the country of origin, as well as the many stresses involved in separation and reunion. In half of the 50 families involved in the family therapy study, 1 or 2 members had been exposed to serious violence such as torture or imprisonment. Twenty of the families had been reunited in exile and were struggling to find a good way of living together now. The many stressors refugee families have been exposed to and the many challenges they face in exile make it paramount to develop adequate therapeutic approaches in work with refugee families and find ways to assist them in their daily lives.

Recent perspectives in family therapy, based on social constructionism, seemed highly relevant for the issues involved in work with refugees. Social constructionist viewpoints stimulated explorations of how the world is understood and interpreted differently by participants in the same systems [31–33]; the introduction of the reflexive stance in family therapy [34–36] provided a solution- and possibility-oriented perspective [37] and the active use of narratives and alternative stories for families to live by [38], all therapeutic positions that seemed especially challenging to explore within a context of therapy with refugee families. Throughout the development of the family therapeutic service, we identified core dynamics in establishing a therapeutic relationship with refugee families.

First, developing a "common ground" for our cooperation was a vital aspect of family therapeutic work. The families had strong concerns about practical and economic difficulties, which they experienced as much more urgent to cope with than the relations between them. They frequently attributed relational problems to such issues, in contrast to the referring agents, who considered emotional and relational difficulties to be rooted in psychological distress, often due to former traumatic experiences. The challenge of establishing a common ground or shared platform for our collaboration was vital. Our main strategy to establish a common ground was to undergo a thorough exploration of the concerns of the clients and to metacommunicate about the usefulness of discussing them with the therapist. This often led to a change of focus, bringing in psychological and family difficulties as well, and an agreement that these issues should be the central ones in our session while other instances should deal with practical issues. This agreement was often precarious, as practical issues were experienced as so urgent. At times, we would help them to contact other professionals or care providers; we might write letters of recommendation or we might invite other helpers to the sessions. The process of establishing a better life situation was, however, slow, and one very helpful maneuver was to ask what they wanted to do "in the meantime." This question increased their motivation to work with psychological issues: "We have to start changing immediately; we can't live together like this."

Refugee families often have a rather comprehensive network of helpers assisting them in their acculturation process. We were interested in exploring this system, with special focus on the referral process [39, 40]. The idea of close collaboration with the larger system surrounding the families, as described by Imber-Black [41], seemed highly relevant. And it also seemed to be a good way of establishing a common ground, not only for the family therapy work but for the collaboration between the family and the larger system.

Second, another challenge consisted of the feelings of hopelessness, caused by a high degree of past and present stress, that taught us to work with small steps that could increase their experience of mastery. Nevertheless, therapeutic experiences that inspired us were studies by Bemak [42] and Ganesan, Fine and Lin [43] with a focus on cultural sensitivity and culture-informed approaches, as well as experiences described by Arredondo et al. [45], emphasizing the importance of having a focus also on the here and now; that is, the present situation for the family, including their legal status [45]. A respectful approach to working with the families is one that balances the pain, suffering and even hopelessness they have struggled with on one side and the resources, hopes and future possibilities for the family on the other [46, 47]. Establishing a relationship between care provider and family where there is room for exploring the many stories, the many voices and the different positions is needed, and this may also allow for new stories to be told and problem-solving conversations to evolve [45, 32].

A third challenge is related to cultural aspects. We found it useful to have a general attitude of "not knowing," which helped us to explore the issues in question thoroughly, making their cultural expectations and attitudes explicit and working on "their ground." This was particularly important when dealing with conflicts, because the exploration additionally clarified the viewpoints of the parties to each other. Exploring cultural notions and coping strategies of the families was particularly important as part of a "not knowing" approach. Nevertheless, when conflicts are particularly destructive, we might leave the "not knowing" position and become more authoritative.

In exploring approaches with refugee families, including families that had been separated and reunited in exile, we experienced the importance of early assistance for families that were reunited. These experiences triggered our interest in exploring more carefully ways to deal with the challenges and natural stresses implied in reunification in exile and to develop approaches to avoid such situations resulting in critical situations and possibly separation again. Ways of approaching these issues will be elaborated in the following.

Developing a Family Therapeutic Approach to Supporting Refugee Families during Reunification

Refugees have left oppressive, unjust and unsafe predicaments, and through the refugee process they are confronted with systems that influence and form their lives, especially when settling in new countries, often very different from what they are accustomed to. Developing the family system and adjusting to new forms of living represent challenges both to the arriving family and to the receiving society. In situations where the family has been divided and reunited, within a larger context that may be totally new to some in the family and more familiar to others, understanding the dynamics of the systems, and of families in such systems, is called for. Below, we identify core perspectives underpinning our family therapeutic approach to working with refugee families during the process of reunification.

Working with Extended Systems

Within systemic thinking there is an interest in the extended or larger system, which also includes professional helpers and others in the communities that families are part of. Such systems may contribute to establishing, upholding and even reinforcing problems in the family [33, 41]. Most reunited families become part of a larger helper system quite rapidly. In order to establish oneself as a family, together and in a new environment, often following a multitude of challenges on many different levels, the needs may be many and complex, requiring contact with different helpers. This may of course be smooth and unproblematic, but there are many examples of the relationship between the families and the helper networks becoming problematic and stressful. At times there are also serious tensions and conflicts within the helper network itself due to differences in perceptions of the families' situations and evaluations of their needs [9]. Helpers may align themselves with different members of the family and even at times work against each other, even if this is not the intention.

Supporting Family Communication

Family therapists generally have a good understanding of and suitable ways of dealing with the problems that families struggle with in a family context. When looking into families reunited in exile, we would like to focus on the following issues:

Working with different aims and objectives

Families often have quite different ideas regarding what may be useful or helpful to them. The wife may perhaps want the husband to adapt to the new norms that the family has developed during their time in the host country, whereas the husband and father wants the family to return to "where they were." In other families, the husband may be quick to move into working life and as such the new society, whereas the wife may continue to live the traditional role she is used to and possibly be isolated and somewhat on the margins of the new society. The children may be split between the positions of their parents and struggle to find their role. Relevant family therapeutic competences that seem useful in work with reunited families are described. Such methods and strategies may be something that the family can accept and work with in order to move ahead as a family.

Supporting the reestablishment of parental collaboration

It is not easy to collaborate as parents when one of them has had the main responsibility for years, and the other may easily feel set apart from the family. This pattern may also be seen in regular families; for instance, differences in parental roles related to developmental phases in families or crises may occur in the process of children's development or during family crises such as spouses finding new partners, etc. Such challenges are often well known to therapists and may be very useful when working with parents who are polarized in relation to each other. The ability to be culturally sensitive in a way that enables the therapist to, in spite of conflictive attitudes between spouses, find something that they nevertheless may share and that can lead them through elaboration of the conflict may be a highly useful approach. One such idea could be to explore the positions carefully, understand their approaches and thoughts – and, perhaps, find that the wife has more respect for her husband than is shown in a tense situation, and that this can be used in order to elaborate a common perspective for the parents to work from.

Working with conflict and conflict resolution

This is a central part of family therapists' work, and many of the conflicts that they encounter in reunited families are not very different from the ones that other families struggle with. Some of these conflicts may nevertheless have a somewhat different character due to the fact that the families are from different countries and traditions and have different trauma-related experiences [48].

Opening perspectives in conversations

One of the challenges in relation to family reunion is the question of how the family can deal with and relate to what can be called "tacit" or "silenced" topics. One of the challenges in relation to family reunion is how to deal with these. Such issues may be linked to experiences that have happened to family members while they were apart and that are difficult to talk about now. One example may be traumatic experiences. Should one choose silence about these or should they be spoken about? Family therapists are trained to deal with family secrets and situations that seem stuck.

Focus on Resources and Possibilities

A salient aspect of family therapy and family-oriented approaches is the focus on resources. This is particularly important in work with families that may have lost hope and belief in any form of future. The adults may feel that they have been destroyed by very painful experiences and lack the trust in their own ability to use skills and capacities from their country of origin. As a very resourceful father said in the session, "Here I am a zero" – and he added, "Like a zero on the right side of the comma." Many parents express that they have given up a life of their own, but what they are now aiming for is to secure a good future for their children. In such cases it can be very useful to engage in a thorough exploration of what may exist in terms of resources and possibilities in the family and in the spousal relationship.

A Narrative Approach

Narrative approaches give emphasis to having a story about oneself and the family; that is, a story that one can live by and with. When families are being reunited, the shared history has been broken and will in addition have elements that are painful and difficult to deal with. To find good enough stories together with the families may be a special challenge. Family therapists are used to family members having different versions of the same story, and the therapist has ways of dealing with this. This understanding of multiversity and even at times paradoxes, adversities and lack of consistency in the family stories thus represents important knowledge when working with families who again need to create a story and an understanding that can be shared and cherished by all of them.

Psychoeducation as Integrative to Family Counselling in Exile

Living in a new society may mean different things for the family members, and this is something that can be highlighted and explained. Using joint family conversations as a vehicle to explain and comment upon "local" ways of looking at things, highlighting local ways and traditions – including child-rearing practices, collaboration between husband and wife and problem-solving strategies – can be useful for families that have not experienced the new society together before and who may be afraid of or bewildered by what they see, experience and are informed about in the new country.

Something which can also be dealt with in a psychoeducational way is talking about reactions after trauma and severe stress – about how a lot of what they are experiencing are reactions and situations that are to be expected and that must be understood in terms of post-traumatic reactions and reactions to the stressors they have been faced with over long periods of time.

In Dialogue with Refugee Families

Initiating Family Conversations

When families reunite in exile, they are often provided with practical assistance and support, but there is less focus on their emotional needs in such situations. Developing voluntary and preventive family conversations with recently reunited refugee families aiming at strengthening the family's own capacity to deal with new and challenging situations may be an important way to go. Through regular contact with the families, especially during the first critical period, one may contribute to useful ways of dealing with problems and enabling adequate communication. We see such conversations as an offer to deal with transitional periods, aiming at reducing some of the tension and apprehension that families may struggle with following a dream that has come true. In particular, assisting in creating a shared understanding of what happened in relation to separation (i.e., how was it? What happened? How was the time apart?) and then developing a family narrative that the family finds adequate may be of value. Being together again is of course what the family has wanted to happen, and the first period is often a very good one. There is no meaning in entering a family and telling them that problems will arise, but rather that experience shows that, after a long time apart and with difficult events in their lives, there are certain stumbling blocks that normally arise in such situations, and that dealing with them in an early phase seems to be a good idea. Offering families that reunite, regardless of any given or defined problem, family conversations as a kind of welcome and preparatory initiative to discuss present issues as well as issues that may arise seems to be a good initiative, but also one that needs further elaboration.

One point that may frequently give meaning to families is to ask them about their own experiences and ways of coping during separation and hardships in order to learn from them. Exploring families' experiences and ways of coping, with the perspective of sharing their lessons learned in work with other families in a generalized way, often makes sense to the families. Most families are willing to talk about this. This may enrich our approaches as professionals in working with reunited families and developing preventive approaches in this context.

Finally, exploring expectations may be a good way to start. What were their thoughts, dreams and ideas with regard to getting together again? This, of course, is a conversation that requires sensitivity and prudence on the part of the clinician.

In our work, we basically provide family conversations where the family is together and reflects and explores together. Nevertheless, there may be situations where family members are offered conversations separately as well. It may be clear in the first conversation with a family that one of the family members has a story of serious human rights violations such as torture or forms of ill-treatment that do not seem suitable for joint conversations, especially with children. One can agree that such topics may be dealt with in other types of conversations, or at least that we will help to find ways to prepare such stories should the family want them to be shared. At times it may be the right thing to do to invite parents or children for a separate session, or even to give those who have been together the chance to speak together alone first.

Themes in Family Conversations on Coping with Reunification

Conversations with families may take different forms, but in the following, we describe more systematically an approach developed in collaboration between the Department of Psychology at the Universities of NTNU and Oslo, RVTS Midt and the refugee health team in the municipality of Trondheim. These approaches have been systematized and presented in a booklet, representing a guide for conversations with reunited families [49]. This work was first published in 2016, and training and implementation of the conversations have taken place in many different municipalities in the Trøndelag region. An evaluation of this work is not yet completed, so the approach described in the following is based on clinical work and numerous conversations with families as well as on informal evaluations and summaries of these experiences, based on both clinicians' and families' comments after the conversations. At this point, the strategy seems promising and includes knowledge and approaches that have been used and implemented in other forms of work with families in general, refugees and reunited refugee families in particular. Below, we delineate core themes addressed during family conversations.

A Transitional Ritual

Creating a good context for the reunion is something which can be done in a simple way but which can nevertheless be quite effective. When we see the family for the first time together, they have recently been reunited and we do not know how this event has been celebrated or marked, either by themselves or by others. To say some words about this, perhaps even treat the family with soft drinks or sweets, can be a way of celebrating and highlighting the event. Performing a kind of ritual, like standing together holding hands or just talking about how it was when they first saw each other again, is a possible approach. The idea is to give a lot of attention to and "lift" these experiences and mark the reunion as something very special in their lives. Then, talking in general terms about years and months that have been difficult but also about how a new morning is arising and possibilities lie ahead of them. This may be a way of focusing on the essentials without getting into complicated details at the start. The therapist is thus presenting themselves as a "master of ceremonies," welcoming the family and inviting them to enter into conversations about this transition, and also as a person who may be of some help and assistance.

Acknowledging Suffering during Separation

It is important to listen and to acknowledge the variety of experiences that family members have had and have struggled with during their time apart. This can also be a way of communicating the need to be seen and acknowledged between family members themselves. Each family member has their own story that it is important for them to share with the rest of the family, at least to a certain extent. It is not easy to talk about such difficult matters, and an outside helper may start a process of talking about them, acknowledging their sufferings and facilitating their acknowledgement of each other. This process is of great significance in preventing feelings of loneliness and bitterness.

Mobilizing through Activity

Joint activities and tasks to be done during the sessions may be relevant; they may also make it easier and more attractive for the children and for parents and children together. Initiating drawings that can mark the start of stories to be told about who they are and what happened can be a useful thing to do. Even more structured assignments can be used, such as drawing the "river of life," where the family can sit together around a large piece of paper and draw their lives as a river that flows and bends, is stopped and thwarted but then continues to flow. This allows family members to share events that they can and want to share in a way that may create a better understanding and communication between them. Here, the clinician may locate how and where they place separation, time apart and struggle for reunion, and then finally being reunited in real life. Also, thoughts about the future can be integrated into this drawing.

Various forms of activities can be used, such as family figures, sandbox material and even organizing cuttings in magazines to illustrate the path from then to now and into the future, engaging the family in something that may be the beginning of a family narrative. Furthermore, jointly drawing genograms can contribute to the family commemorating and talking about families and important relations. Such conversations may allow family members to speak to each other about what happened in a new way and help them to better understand what has happened during the separation. But again, there is often a lot of tension and problems in these stories, and it is therefore important that the therapist has a good hand in developing and encouraging such activities with the family. But, done with care, some of the material that emerges based on this can be valuable in future conversations with the family.

Focus on Strengths and Cohesion

In conversations aiming at preventing conflict and opening up for collaboration and mutual support in the family, it seems particularly important to focus on strengths and resources in the family, underlining and shedding light on ways in which family members, together or apart, have coped with difficulties. Being very attentive to the family's own coping and problem-solving strategies and the potential that they may have but which they are not necessarily fully aware of is important. Eliciting stories about the nonproblematic aspects of their lives, good examples and even exceptions to problems are good ways of entering into a more positive and resource-oriented mood. The capacity of family therapists to look for exceptions and alternative stories and also to redefine what may seem difficult as something promising and good constitutes a very valuable strategy in this work. Furthermore, it gives the therapist the possibility of acknowledging what the family members have done to support each other and the efforts and hardships they have gone through in order to be together. This may help the members to see and treasure the contributions of the others, even if these were not so obvious from the start. Their struggle to be together, their strength and perseverance, even the sacrifices and difficulties along the way, even if they have experienced these in very different ways, may be underlined. This may be a way of strengthening cohesion and mutual respect in the family, even if family members have experienced the process in very different ways. Such approaches may also allow some room for problems and future challenges to be brought up gradually and open up ways of dealing with them at a later point.

Working around Cultural Change and Cultural Continuity

To establish oneself in a new society, with all that this entails, is a complex endeavor, and both the individual and the family will have to find ways of managing this. Talking about present experiences in the light of migration and acculturation may be useful to the families that often find themselves at different stages in the process of adaptation and acculturation. Sometimes exploring the meaning of acculturation, not as a one-way process but as something that happens between the newcomer and society at large, can create a positive tone. Going into the experiences of the families, examples and episodes, including those that may be humorous or a little embarrassing, can create good conversations about difficult topics. In families where the children have stayed longer than one or two of their parents, the children's cultural knowledge may be seen as a threat to the adults. Exploring this, also in a resource-oriented way, can be a way of cherishing and feeling proud of their children's expertise rather than being threatened by it or denying it.

Knowledge about Systems

The opportunity to inform the family about existing systems of support and health services can be of good use to families who have recently arrived. Who one can approach, with what kinds of questions, and what one can expect, is not obvious to individuals who have only recently settled in the host country. The part of the family that has been in the host society for a while may perhaps have its own network of helpers, but certain things may not be as evident to those who have recently arrived. Giving some space for these kinds of discussions may create a feeling of having a better overview and understanding of a new and often seemingly complex system of public services.

A Possible Outline for Family Reunification Conversations

As described above, the aim of family reunion conversations is to strengthen communication in the family and to establish an understanding that being apart and uniting again after separation naturally implies challenges regarding readaptation and the reorganization of family life.

Before Reunification

It may be wise to have regular contact with the part of the family that lives in the host country already, preparing for the reunion and the possibility of joint sessions. In addition to practical issues, it is important that the therapeutic system also touches upon the emotional preparations, fears, concerns and hopes. These conversations can include exploring expectations, preparing for the reunion and talking about what has been done to obtain reunion, what kind of contact they have had during their time apart and any major concerns in relation to being reunited.

First Conversation with the Family Together

The first conversation can be held shortly after reunion. The clinician should introduce the idea with such conversations and spend some time ensuring that the whole family understands what it is about and accepts the invitation. Sometimes it may be relevant to leave some space for practical issues at the beginning, such as things they are struggling with, understanding the responsibilities of the family itself in relation to resettling as a family and what kind of support and assistance they can expect from the host society. Then, when moving into a conversation about the family and family history, it seems important to clarify if there are specific issues the family wants to talk about or issues that they do not want to talk about when they are all together. The family members can be invited to give a quick overview of their past as a family, of their present situation and of their perspectives on the future. It is important to engage all present members and adapt to the fact that children may be small or any other special conditions that are relevant in order for the conversation to flow well.

It may be useful to draw a timeline and define certain events or dates worth special attention. At this point, employing the "river of life" described above is a possibility, and even if there have been a lot of problems "down the river," it is essential to keep a focus on strengths and resilience, coping and problem-solving. After all, the family has managed to leave problematic places and situations and is united as a family again. There may be losses and experiences that cannot be included in the story of possibilities, and it may be useful to explore with the family how they handle such problematic events.

For the clinician, it may be useful to take notes in order to ensure that important points are not left behind or overlooked. It is a good idea to talk to the family about the next meeting and listen to their ideas and perhaps prepare some issues. Towards the end of the session, the family should have the opportunity to talk about urgent needs that have not been dealt with.

The Second Conversation with the Family as a Whole

Being open to and exploring what has happened since the last meeting is a good way to start, including talking about if and how the family have discussed their experiences with the first session. The therapist may go back to the drawings made the first time and engage the family members in exploring how these themes appear now. Concrete examples of episodes or experiences they want to talk about may be useful. Conversational themes may pertain to daily life and functioning and their possible stumbling blocks while simultaneously acknowledging their attempts to create a full family again. If the family appears stuck in conflictual patterns, it is useful to engage in ways of redefining them or looking at them from different perspectives, trying to loosen up such patterns. Using metaphors, stories or even situations brought into the room by the family itself, for instance, through their elaboration of the genogram or the "river of life," can be good ways of dealing with stuck situations.

There may be special themes or situations that have come up that seem important to talk about, including what the family's hopes and expectations are, both with regard to the other family members and to the community in which they live. How is life today seen from the point of view of earlier dreams and hopes about what being together would look like? Have apprehensions vanished or have new ones arrived? Are things better or more difficult now? Do the members of the family experience such matters differently? Do they want to split up the family for further talks? There is also the possibility that families may need more than three sessions. What are their plans for the future now, and what will they need beyond these conversations? Talking concretely about this may be useful, and may give the clinician a possibility of looking into wished-for or necessary help and assistance from the relevant parts of the supporting care system available in the host society.

The Third Conversation with the Family: 4–6 Months after Reunification

This conversation can be about the families' experiences today and give some time to whether and how the conversations have been helpful and what could have been different.

The helper should use all possible opportunities to support the family's efforts and constructive initiatives. If they report problems, it is important to look for how they have dealt with them and support and acknowledge solutions or attempts at solutions or, if required, what kind of help will be needed in order to reduce conflict. It is important to highlight that disagreements and even quarrels may be expected or even natural in such situations, and also that the aim is not to avoid problems but to learn how to deal with them.

It may be useful to explore the lessons learned in the families and ideas that can be shared with other families in similar situations.

Organizing Voluntary Conversations

The possibility of organizing conversations aimed at preventing conflict and strengthening communications in families reunited in exile is dependent on a willingness on the part of the system to engage in preventive work – not wait until conflicts and problems are so serious that something has to be done. There must be preparedness in the municipality or the system in which the family is settled and reunited, and those engaging in this should be well prepared to conduct these conversations. They should also have a strategically good position to enable them to refer families to other parts of the system or ensure that other agencies are brought onto the scene if this is wanted or necessary.

We have in this chapter often referred to family therapy and therapists. We would like to underline that helpers do not have to be trained family therapists, but clearly they must have a family focus in what they do and engage in methods that are family informed. It can be important to collaborate with others working with the family and have a dialogue with the families about their needs during the challenging process of reestablishing themselves in new territories after being apart, suffering and working hard to be together again. This is a situation that we know is risky, and which can easily be understood as a crisis, where the process may either move in a good or a bad direction, resulting in the worst case in a new separation. For many, this would be the most painful scenario, and in addition to being a loss, it may be humiliating and shameful.

Conclusion

The approach delineated above is not therapy as such, but conversations aiming at preventing the kinds of problems that would require therapy or other more intensive help. They are meant to support and collaborate with families that are making efforts to get together. Many will, through a new separation, experience that the only person who knew them from before – who was there when things were more normal – is no longer in the family or in the daily relationship, and this in itself constitutes a loss and a source of grief.

With this background, investing in this model of assistance for families in these particular situations seems to be the right thing to do based on both mental health understanding – family psychology, trauma psychology, humanistic perspectives – and a human-rights-based approach.

Our hope is that this approach can be further developed, that experiences can be registered and evaluated, and that a body of knowledge can be established to document the impact of such conversations both through practical work and research. We also hope that the experiences described here can be inspiring to those who work with refugees and their families, and that more focus will be given to family approaches to refugees as part of enabling them to live to their maximum potential in a new society. We introduced the reader to two family stories at the beginning. Here is what happened.

In the case of Sara, Hassan and their two daughters, things were difficult at first. Disappointment combined with relief. The family came to sessions together and their idea of becoming a family again, the one "we once were," was explored. It was clear that the father had a terrible story to tell, but it did not seem right to present this in the joint sessions. He was therefore offered individual therapy with another therapist. The conversation could therefore concentrate on steps they had taken and steps that could be taken in order to get closer to each other, getting to know each other again. Simple drawings illustrating distance and proximity, and asking the family to score positive changes that had taken place on a scale from 0–10, enabled them to deal with their relationship in a different way. Some homework was given, and they reported that they had moved upwards on the scale of positive development. What seemed valuable afterwards was that the family could be engaged in sharing ideas and expectations about being together again in a rather simple and easy-to-grasp way. They all knew that there were problems ahead, but the conversations early after reunion permitted them to find room to approach each other again without expecting everything to be fine. The family later thanked the therapeutic team for this. The couple continued in spousal therapy after having had the number of joint family sessions that seemed necessary.

Ahmed and Fatima came with their child to the first conversation after reunion. There was no doubt that Fatima was both angry and anxious, and the trip to Norway had not helped her to overcome her deep mistrust of her husband and what she thought was his lack of will or action to get them there. He had asked for conversations on her arrival, and he expressed it in the following way: "Somebody needs to be my witness to the pain I have suffered." The family was invited to a session with the therapist and a representative from the local municipality. We brought sweets and soft drinks to the session; their little son was going to be present and we wanted to give them a positive time. Fatima entered the room with her husband and son, and there was no doubt that she was very skeptical of this encounter. She sat down reluctantly, observed that their son was happy with sweets and drinks, and accepted our warm welcome to them and saw how pleased we were finally to welcome them to Norway. Then we started talking about our work with him, what we had observed and how her husband had expressed sorrow and depression. We encouraged her to speak about her life while waiting and her thoughts about their relationship. It was only after quite a while that we noticed that she was taking in how depressed and sad he had been; he had cared, and somebody could "prove" it. When we finally closed the session, Fatima stood up, took our hands and said, "This is the most important conversation I have had in my life."

References

1. The Universal Declaration of Human Rights, (1948). (16.3). www.un.org/en/universal-declaration-human-rights/

2. The UN Convention on the Rights of the Child, (1989). (art. 7, 9, 10). www.ohchr.org/en/professionalinterest/pages/crc.aspx

3. UN High Commissioner for Refugees, (2008). *UNHCR Guidelines on Determining the Best Interests of the Child.* www.unhcr.org/refworld/docid/49103ece2.html

4. The Geneva Convention. (1949). Convention (IV) Relative to the Protection of Civilian Persons in Time of War (art. 24–26). www.icrc.org/eng/assets/files/publications/icrc-002-0173.pdf

5. United Nations. *The International Convention for the Protection of All Persons from Enforced Disappearance.* Adopted by the United Nations General Assembly on 20 December 2006; entered into force on 23 December 2010. www.ohchr.org/EN/HRBodies/CED/Pages/ConventionCED.aspx

6. European Council Directive 2003/86/EC, (2003). *On the Right to Family Reunification.* http://eur-lex.europa.eu/legal-content/en/ALL/?uri=celex%3A32003L0086

7. S. Reichelt and N. Sveaass, Therapy with refugee families: What is a 'good' conversation? *Family Process*, 33 (1994), 247–263.

8. S. Reichelt and N. Sveaass, Creating meaningful conversations with families in exile. *Journal of Refugee Studies*, 7 (1994), 124–143.

9. N. Sveaass and S. Reichelt, Engaging refugee families in therapy: Exploring the benefits of including referring professionals in the first family interviews. *Family Process*, 40 (2001), 95–114.

10. N. Sveaass and S. Reichelt, Refugee families in therapy: From referrals to therapeutic conversations. *Journal of Family Therapy*, 23 (2001), 119–135.

11. B. Bragg and L. L. Wong, 'Cancelled dreams': Family reunification and shifting Canadian immigration policy. *Journal of Immigrant and Refugee Studies*, 14(1) (2015), 46–85.

12. C. Rousseau, A. Mekki-Barrada and S. Moreau, Trauma and extended separation from family among Latin American and African refugees in Montreal. *Psychiatry*, 64(1) (2001), 40–59.

13. C. Rousseau, M.-C. Rufagari, D. Bagilishya and T. Measham, Remaking family life: Strategies for re-establishing continuity among Congolese refugees during the family reunification process. *Social Science & Medicine*, 59 (2004), 1095–1108.

14. C. Choummanivong, G. E. Poole and A. Cooper, Refugees' family reunification and mental health in resettlement. *Kotuitui: New Zealand Journal of Social Sciences Online*, (2014). ISSN: (Print) 1177-083X (Online) Journal homepage: www.tandfonline.com/loi/tnzk20

15. C. E. Sluzki, Disappeared: Semantic and somatic effects of political repression in a family seeking therapy. *Family Process*, 29 (1990), 131–143.

16. C. E. Sluzki, Deception and fear in politically oppressive contexts: Its trickle-down effects on families. *Review of Policy Research*, 22(5) (2005), 625–635.

17. C. E. Sluzki, Toward a model of family and political victimization: Implications for treatment and recovery. *Psychiatry*, 56 (1993), 178–187.

18. R. Rosenck and J. Thomson, 'Detoxification' of Vietnam War trauma: A combined family-individual approach. *Family Process*, 25 (1987), 559–570.

19. B. Lie, N. Sveaass and D. E. Eilertsen, Family, activity and posttraumatic reactions in exile. *Community, Work & Family*, 7 (2004), 327–351.

20. R. Schwarzer, M. Jerusalem and A. Hahn, Unemployment, social support and health complaints: A longitudinal study of stress in East German refugees. *Journal of Community & Applied Social Psychology*, 4 (1994), 31–45.

21. Z. Solomon and M. Waysman, From front line to home front: A study of secondary traumatization. *Family Process*, 31 (1992), 289–302.

22. J. Krupinski and G. Burrows, Psychiatric disorders in adolescents and young adults. In J. Krupinski and G. Burrows, eds., *The Price of Freedom: Young Indochinese Refugees in Australia*, Rushcutters Bay (Sydney: Pergamon Press, 1986).

23. M. Beiser, Influence of time, ethnicity, and attachment on depression in South Asian

refugees. *American Journal of Psychiatry*, 145 (1988), 183–195.

24. E. Montgomery, Trauma, exile and mental health in young refugees. *Acta Psychiatrica Scandinavica*, 124 (2011), 1–46.

25. C. Gorst-Unsworth and E. Goldenberg, Psychological sequelae of torture and organized violence suffered by refugees from Iraq. *British Journal of Psychiatry*, 172 (1998), 90–94.

26. M. Beiser, P. J. Johnson and R. J. Turner, Unemployment, underemployment and depressive affect among Southeast Asian refugees. *Psychological Medicine*, 23 (1993), 732–743.

27. G. J. Bjørn, P. A. Gustafsson, G. Sydsjö and C. Bertero, Family therapy sessions with refugee families: A qualitative study. *Conflict and Health*, 7 (2013), 7.

28. R. Sahal, (2015), *'Livet satt på vent': En studie om enslige flyktninger som har søkt om famliegjenforening* ('Life on hold': A study of separated minors who have applied for family reunification). Master's thesis at the Department of Psychology, University of Oslo.

29. D. Silove, The psychological effects of torture, mass human rights violations, and refugee trauma: Toward an integrated conceptual framework. *Journal of Nervous and Mental Disease*, 187 (1999), 200–207.

30. A. Sourander, Refugee families during asylum seeking. *Nordic Journal of Psychiatry*, 57(3) (2010), 203–207. www.tandfonline.com/loi/ipsc20

31. K. Gergen, The social constructionist movement in modern psychology. *American Psychologist*, 40 (1985), 266–275.

32. H. Anderson and H. Goolishian, Human systems as linguistic systems: Preliminary and evolving ideas about the implications for clinical theory. *Family Process*, 27 (1988), 371–339.

33. H. Anderson and H. Goolishian, The client is the expert: A not-knowing approach to therapy. In S. McNamee and K. J. Gergen, eds., *Therapy as Social Construction* (Newbury Park, CA: Sage, 1992), pp. 25–39.

34. T. Andersen, The reflecting team. Dialogue and meta-dialogue in clinical work. *Family Process*, 26 (1987), 415–428.

35. L. Hoffman, Beyond power and control. *Family Systems Medicine*, 3 (1985), 381–396.

36. L. Hoffman, The reflexive stance for family therapy. In S. McNamee and K. J. Gergen, eds., *Therapy as Social Construction* (London: Sage, 1992), pp. 7–24.

37. S. de Shazer, *Clues: Investigating Solutions in Brief Therapy* (New York: Norton, 1988).

38. M. White and D. Epston, *Narrative Means to Therapeutic Ends* (New York: Norton, 1990).

39. M. S. Palazzoli, L Boscolo, G. Cecchin and G. Prata, The problem of the referring person. *Journal of Marital and Family Therapy*, 6 (1980), 3–9.

40. L. Boscolo, G. Cecchin, L. Hoffman and P. Penn, *Milan Systemic Family Therapy: Conversations in Theory and Practice* (New York: Basic Books, 1987).

41. E. Imber-Black, *Families and Larger Systems: A Family Therapist's Guide through the Labyrinth* (New York: Guilford Press, 1988).

42. F. Bemak, Cross-cultural family therapy with South-East Asian refugees. *Journal of Strategic and Systemic Therapies*, 8 (1989), 22–27.

43. S. Gansan, S. Fine and T. Y. Lin, Psychiatric symptoms in refugee families from South East Asia: Therapeutic challenges. *American Journal of Psychotherapy*, 43 (1989), 218–228.

44. P. Arredondo, A. Orjula and I. Moore, Family therapy with Central American war refugee families. *Journal of Strategic and Systemic Therapies*, 8 (1989), 27–35.

45. L. De Haene, P. Rober, P. Adriaenssens and K. Verschueren, Voices of dialogue and directivity in family therapy with refugees: Evolving ideas about dialogical refugee care. *Family Process*, 51 (2012), 391–404.

46. K. Weingarten, Witnessing, wonder, and hope. *Family Process*, 39 (2000), 389–401.

47. C. Flaskas, Holding hope and hopelessness: Therapeutic engagements with the balance of hope. *Journal of Family Therapy*, 29 (2007), 186–202.

48. C. E. Sluzki, Migration and family conflict. *Family Process*, 8 (1979), 379–390.

49. NTNU, RVTS and the Department of Psychology, UiO. *Familiegjenforening i eksil: Forebygging gjennom familiesamtaler* (Family reunification in exile: Prevention through family conversations) (2016). https://samforsk.no/Publikasjoner/2016/Familiegjenforening_web.pdf

In memory of Sissel Reichelt

Sissel Reichelt died on March 18 this year. She was active in clinical practice and engaged in teaching and writing on family therapy and on the supervisory process, when she died unexpectedly. One of her last contributions was the chapter on refugee families and reunion in exile that we co-authored for this book, a work she was happy to share with an international audience. Sissel had a remarkable impact on clinical psychology in Norway, both as a researcher as a practitioner. In the early days of her career, approaches in clinical child psychology that she considered as too theory-driven and often remote from the contexts in which children lived and practiced. She suggested therapeutic interventions directed at children's behavior and their social relationships in families, schools, and day-care settings.

Sissel's contribution throughout a very long career was her ability to combine clear analysis with practical working methods, while never ceasing to ask questions. Her curiosity together with an explorative approach, never taking anything for granted, has inspired a large number of students and colleagues over the years. Her many publications and innumerous seminars have opened new doors in psychology. In many ways, Sissel brought modern family therapy based on communication theory and behavior observation to Norway. She learned and listened, and very quickly tried out new ways of working – always taking her team and students with her. Sissel opened up the therapy room and invited her team behind the one-way-mirror. She was a pioneer in working with reflecting teams, and was constantly looking for new and creative approaches to improve family communication.

Her ambition as a researcher was to demonstrate ways in which family therapy could be challenged by and subsequently adapted to new categories of clients. Sissel pioneered in applying family therapy in groups that were particularly vulnerable, such as families with drug-related problems, families marked by neglect or sexual violence, and refugee families, often exposed to severe trauma before arrival to the host country. She involved the families as active participants, with deep respect, engaging them in her never-ending quest for possibilities and ways out of locked circles and hopelessness.

With regard to clinical literature and new research in the field, Sissel was always in the forefront. She developed an impressive network, and worked closely with Tom Andersen, in developing the role of the reflecting teams in particular. Her regular contact with Harry Goolishian and Harlene Anderson developed over the years and was fruitful to all. In many ways Sissel was the embodiment of concepts such as "non-expert" and the "not knowing" approach, even before these were defined and explained. I had the tremendous privilege of working with Sissel over a long period of time – she was my highly respected teacher, then a close colleague, she was my creative and patient research supervisor, and we worked together with refugee families in therapy from the early 90ties. And she became a close friend. We are so many that will miss her, but her enthusiasm, warmth, insight, wisdom and explorative way of approaching the field, will always be with us.

Diagnosis as Advocacy
Medico-Legal Reports in Refugee Family Care

Debra Stein, Priyadarshani Raju, and Lisa Andermann

Introduction

Considerations around the dynamics of medicalization and social suffering are at the heart of working with refugees and refugee families. A self-reflective awareness of the "culture of psychiatry"[1] and the limitations of the medical model in mental health care are essential so as to avoid over-pathologizing and misdiagnosing vulnerable clients, who typically arrive in host countries with their own inherent resilience and coping strategies.

In the spring of 2017, the coauthors of this chapter were struck by reading an article by Rachel Aviv from the *New Yorker* on *Uppgivenhetssyndrom* or Resignation Syndrome [1]. None of us had had direct clinical experience of or even heard of such an extreme form of symptom expression as that which was described in refugee children in Sweden facing refugee hearings and possible deportation. We have assessed many refugee children and families in multicultural Toronto, Canada, yet have never encountered such a catastrophic reaction to migration stress. These intensely debilitating reactions have not been described anywhere but Sweden, leading to questions about the impact of the host culture on the illness.[2] Interestingly, Aviv wonders if physicians emphasizing the level of pathology in these children – intending to advocate for them – play a role in reinforcing their self-narrative of catastrophic suffering.

The clinical presentation often begins with social withdrawal, followed by an apathetic or passive response leading to a complete psychological shut-down of the child, including the inability to eat, often requiring tube feeding as a form of chronic treatment in the ER and a home setting [2, 3]. It was very clear from reading about these difficult cases that resolution of their immigration status was the only form of successful "treatment" for this expression of social suffering:

Acknowledgements: Thank you to our respective clinics, colleagues, and most of all to the children, youth, and families in our care, from whose trust and teaching we continue to grow every day. Thank you also to Raoul Boulakia and Clare Pain, who discussed certain aspects of the chapter with us during the writing process.

[1] These thoughts are partially derived from self-reflection in the classic "Culture of No Culture" article by Janelle Taylor, PhD (J. Taylor. "Confronting 'Culture' in Medicine's 'Culture of No Culture.'" *Academic Medicine*, 78 (2003), 555–559 [1].

[2] Interestingly, in the Russian refugee family described in the *New Yorker*, the boy had always been the most assimilated, "the most Swedeified," and had always communicated for his unilingual family, knowing the new language and culture better than his parents. With news of deportation, his "apathy" also made use of the local language and local idioms of distress.

In a seventy-six-page guide for treating *uppgivenhetssyndrom*, published in 2013, the Swedish Board of Health and Welfare advises that a patient will not recover until his family has permission to live in Sweden. "A permanent residency permit is considered by far the most effective 'treatment,'" the manual says. "The turning point will usually be a few months to half a year after the family receives permanent residence" [2].

Uppgivenhetssyndrom has been the subject of internationally published academic research [4, 5], and a search of Sweden's widely distributed medical journal, *Lakartidningen*, reveals no fewer than 12 articles on the subject [6].

This phenomenon has led us to reflect further on our own clinical practices with asylum-seeking and refugee families. As we grapple with dilemmas of diagnosis and medicalization, cultural differences in the presentation of distress, and the social context of our clinics, we often question how these shape our interactions with refugee children, youth, and families as well as their responses to pre- and post-migration stressors. These reflections have implications for our clinical practice as well as our approach to broader-scale advocacy. The latter was exercised in the spring of 2018 (even as this chapter was going through draft revisions), during the international outcry at the United States of America's policy of separating and detaining migrant families at the border, housing children in cramped facilities while prosecuting their parents. The advocacy coming from physicians and mental health leaders tended to use the language of trauma and "toxic stress" and predict dire future pathology in these children [7, 8]. Even more recently, we have seen reports of "traumatic withdrawal syndrome" (also dubbed "Resignation Syndrome," presumably due to the similarity of presentation with the Swedish cohort), described as an outcome of the desperate situation of children and families detained by the government of Australia on the island of Nauru [9]. We noticed ourselves balancing our own fears of these precise mental health consequences alongside our concerns about the impact of proclaiming such conclusions.

An article by Derek Summerfield on "Childhood, War, Refugeedom and Trauma" asks questions very relevant to this discussion [10]. He poses the question, "How can the predicament of refugee children be framed and when can their distress or suffering legitimately be seen as mental pathology?" and discusses post-migration stressors, insecurities, and the negotiation of "disrupted life trajectories" [10]. He explores the medicalization of distress as well as concepts of social suffering [11] and concludes that:

> Whatever their pain, the vast majority of refugee children seem competent to live on without breaking down, mourning or putting aside their losses and seeking creative accommodation with their present circumstances. It might be said that the imperatives of life leave little choice, that this is the lesson of history. With a few exceptions, these trajectories are scarcely visible from the clinic: tracking them is principally the work of historians, anthropologists, sociologists, political economists, poets, journalists, religious, political and community leaders, and via the verbal and written output of the actors themselves.
>
> (Summerfield, 2000, p. 430 [10])

Summerfield's thesis implies a risk of iatrogenesis in our work with refugee children and their families; we, too, wonder about the potential harm that might come of applying a psychiatric lens to these children's experiences. We are particularly interested in the way children crystallize and voice family distress through their symptomatic functioning and how we might, as well-meaning clinicians, be contributing to child-family narratives of dysfunction over resilience.

Social Stressors and Advocacy in the Psychiatric Clinic

Mental health professionals who choose to work with refugee children, youth, and their parents may eventually come to recognize that the medical model has poorly equipped them to help these families. Many of us have come to understand that the language of psychiatric disorder insufficiently captures their struggles and have moved away from a focus on diagnoses such as Posttraumatic Stress Disorder and typical "treatments" with medical/psychological technology. We note the Western origins of the psychiatric method and have learned to consider more holistic approaches that take into account the family's socio-cultural milieu. Writing about their experiences at the Canadian Centre for Victims of Torture, authors Pain, Kanagaratnam and Payne describe an evolution of their perspective as to what is truly helpful in fostering the wellbeing of asylum seekers and refugees, emphasizing the paramount role of strategies which support social participation and belonging:

> But working at this agency has taught us to look beyond the refugees' symptoms and explore and ameliorate the causes of distress in the "here and now" of the complexity of resettlement in Canada. We find a refugee's symptoms improve once they have been accepted as a convention refugee, and seldom find medications and therapy popular or useful options for the clients. Most usually English lessons, the pairing of a befriender (volunteer) with the refugee, homework club for refugee children, music and art groups, cooking club and other similar group activities form the most popular and useful "treatments." The routine employment of exposure techniques to desensitize the refugee to their experiences of war, torture and other atrocities seems, in our experience and in reading the literature on the subject, to have no role in their successful treatment. However, follow-up studies of distressed refugees, and community-based research on the long-term adjustment and mental well-being of accepted convention refugees are necessary, to evaluate current services. They would also identify the need for developing individual or collective approaches to further support the successful settlement and prosperity of convention refugees in their new home. (Pain et al., 2014, p. 58 [12])

This emerging sense of something different being needed in our support of young refugees is reflected in the development of cultural competence/safety/humility frameworks[3] and their incorporation into psychiatric training programs [16]. While these have been helpful, they are still insufficient, as refugee families tell us in no uncertain terms that social and settlement concerns are their biggest priority. Indeed, we ourselves have seen too many families felled not by the terrible events in their past but by the "everyday trauma" of living in an unfamiliar culture, often in conditions of poverty, insecurity, and marginalization.

---

[3] We are using the Terry Cross et al. definition of *cultural competence* as "a set of congruent behaviors, attitudes, and policies that come together in a system, agency, or among professionals and enable that system, agency or those professionals to work effectively in cross-cultural situations" (Cross et al., 1989, p. 166 [13]). *Cultural safety*, developed with Maori populations in New Zealand but now used widely in multiple settings, including by the Mental Health Commission of Canada, "builds on knowledge of historical and political experiences of oppression and marginalization to give explicit attention to structural and organizational issues that protect the voice and perspective of patients, their cultures and communities" (Kirmayer et al., p. 4 [14]). Finally, *cultural humility* also sets a tone of respect and seeks to redress power imbalances and iniquities in the doctor-patient relationship by placing expertise in the realm of the patient rather than the health care specialist, inviting "self-reflection and self-critique" (Fung et al., p. 168 [15]).

Some important post-migration stressors are known as the "seven Ds": detention, denial of employment, dispersal, denial of health care, destitution, delayed decisions on applications, and discrimination [17]. What psychiatrists need, now more than ever, are hard skills in improving the social environments of refugee families and in addressing social change [18]. The recent development of Structural Competency training programs in psychiatry [19] has been important in this regard, representing "one evolving approach that enables clinician practitioners to bridge the microprocesses of their interactions with patients with the macroprocesses of population-level inequalities that often determine their patients' mental health outcomes" (Hansen and Metzl, 2017, p. E2 [20]).

Given our position of power and privilege in society, we recognize that our most salient interventions may be in the form of advocacy for (and alongside) the children and families in our care. Indeed, advocacy has been argued to be a key aspect of structural competency [21]. Our practice regularly includes phone calls and letters of support to help families to access better housing in safer neighborhoods, social and community programs, inclusion in employment training initiatives, and so on. This particular type of advocacy draws upon one particular skill: the "rhetorical skill to present evidence and arguments in ways that are compelling" (Kirmayer et al., 2017, p. E1 [21]).

Asylum Claims and Medical Reports

Much like our Swedish counterparts, we have seen how highly stressful it is for families to be in limbo with respect to immigration status in their new country and the extent to which this state of uncertainty impacts negatively on their mental health. We have time and again followed families as they apply for refugee status, await hearings, and receive the decisions of our immigration system and been struck by the difference between before and after the family receives a decision of being granted refugee status. This phenomenon is described in the literature, with consistent reports of high rates of depression, anxiety, and PTSD during the asylum-seeking process which worsen over time as asylum seekers await the outcome, then improve when refugee status is obtained [22–24].[4] We are also aware of the damage inflicted on families by the experience of immigration detention, which has been discussed in detail elsewhere [25].

In our ongoing practice, we therefore extend our advocacy to providing medical testimony to support asylum claims. This occurs through a psychiatric consultation in which the clinician and the asylum-seeking family engage in a complex negotiation to describe events, emotional reactions, and bodily experiences – always in the context of the more powerful actor, the psychiatrist, having the ability to produce a report. The psychiatric report, which is intended to highlight for immigration adjudicators the psychological effects of exposure to traumatic events in the country of origin, has become a mainstay of clinicians supporting asylum seekers from at least the early 1990s [26]. It has developed into a genre of

---

[4] While many people do very well with regard to their mental health once the refugee process is settled, we note here the wide variety of trajectories possible. Even after asylum is granted, issues such as grief, loss, and trauma, separation from (and ongoing fears for) relatives left behind, and other post-migration factors discussed above can lead to the later development of psychological symptoms in some cases.

medical documentation in its own right, with guidelines being circulated to enhance this skill.[5] In Canada, we have incorporated teaching about refugee consultations and report-writing skills into our supervision of psychiatric trainees. We have seen increasing efforts to promote this learning widely, as evidenced by a recent workshop attended by lawyers and physicians in Toronto and broadcast nationally.[6] These are important developments which increase our capacity to deliver what has now become an essential skill within the sphere of refugee mental health.

It is not without discomfort, however, that we witness this increasing push to disseminate report-writing skills within the wider psychiatric community. Rachel Aviv's article serves as a cautionary tale in its depiction of the risks of using compelling medical language to advocate for families' rights to asylum. She tells the story of Georgi, a Russian boy suffering from *Uppgivenhetssyndrom*, and of the efforts of his treating physician, Dr. Elisabeth Hultcrantz, to advocate on his and his family's behalf. Hultcrantz's take on her role in the family echoes the way many of us have positioned ourselves with respect to the asylum-seeking families in our care:

> As Hultcrantz sees it, her most important task as doctor is to be a good writer, constructing a coherent narrative from her patients' physical symptoms, which she interprets as metaphors for psychic distress. In a letter to the Migration Board, Hultcrantz wrote that Georgi "suddenly fell into a deep sleep when he perceived that his final hope for the future was taken from him," a description that she recently applied to another patient. "If the boy can get secure residency with his entire family, the prognosis is good and you can expect a full continuous recovery within one year," she wrote. "If the boy does not have security, he will not wake up in whatever country he is in" [2].

The country-wide dissemination of *Uppgivenhetssyndrom*, a disease for which the only known cure is ensuring safety in Sweden, echoes Arthur Kleinman's original thesis that healers are invested by their communities with the power to shape both symptoms of and solutions to personal distress [27]. In this way, illnesses are coconstructed by healers and their patients, leading to local variations in mental disorder. Indeed, *Uppgivenhetssyndrom* seems to be a uniquely Swedish phenomenon which probably could not have developed or gained legitimacy elsewhere, even in other Scandinavian welfare states with robust historical commitments to refugee protection, such as Denmark [28]. Sweden's particular cultural context has been described in terms of its founding ethos of equality [29], its secular national identity, and, perhaps most significantly, the Swedish experience of WWII neutrality and postwar prosperity, which led to humanitarian action being made a prominent part of the government agenda, which Swedes draw on as a source of national pride [30]. Swedes themselves have noted the contribution of collective postwar guilt to their current moral and humanitarian values and to the development of *Uppgivenhetssyndrom* in particular. In the words of Swedish historian Karins Johannisson: "Never has the ethics of compassion had such power, fed by historical

---

[5] One example is the 2012 publication *Examining Asylum Seekers: A Clinician's Guide to Physical and Psychological Evaluations of Torture and Ill-Treatment*, put out by Physicians for Human Rights.

[6] Refugee Health: *Mental Health Reports and Evidence in Refugee Claims: An Interprofessional Workshop for Lawyers, Mental Health Professionals and Trainees* (September 25, 2017).

guilt. This was about the whole image of Sweden – a country dripping with wealth but prepared to deport the most defenseless" [2].

Rachel Aviv sees Sweden's physicians as reflecting and amplifying this zeitgeist. Dr. Hultcrantz, a professor emeritus at Linköping University and a volunteer for the charity Doctors of the World, is portrayed by Aviv as a passionate advocate for her patients who continually leverages the medical aspects of each case before the immigration authorities ("A chipper, gray-haired grandmother, Hultcrantz seems unaware of her power. She sometimes encourages families to 'get their tubing' – the feeding tube – as quickly as possible, in order to emphasize their suffering to the Migration Board") [2]. Aviv astutely highlights the risks attached to this type of advocacy:

> [T]he story [Dr. Hultcrantz] tells about her patients' illness is perhaps too compelling; she seems to inadvertently reinforce their symptoms. Like the medicine man, she has the authority to shape people's beliefs about their own biology. In more contemporary terms, she and other Swedish doctors create the conditions for a nocebo effect: the families expect that unless they are granted residency – the only medicine – their children will waste away [2].

This leads us to reflect upon the ways that leveraging psychiatric and biomedical paradigms to advocate for asylum-seeking families can potentially do harm. Does our focus on the signs and symptoms of psychiatric disorder – instead of on resilience and strategies for coping outside of the psychiatric model – inadvertently alter family discourse around a problem and negatively influence family dynamics and family functioning? Below, some case reflections emerging from our ongoing practices shed light on this question.

Case Examples

D. S. was asked to assess a 15-year-old girl in order to produce a report to accompany her application for Permanent Residence on Humanitarian and Compassionate grounds. The youth had been sexually abused by an ex-police officer in the family's home country, and her father had subsequently been assaulted and threatened with death. For a number of reasons, the family's original asylum claim had been rejected and they were facing deportation. The youth had recently been seen by a crisis team after she had voiced suicidal thoughts to her settlement counselor. Going into this particular assessment, D. S. acknowledged the high stakes at play, with family security and the youth's personal safety being foremost in her mind.

Over her first two encounters with the youth and her father, D. S. gathered information about symptoms and functioning, asked about the youth's sense of what could happen should she and her family be forced to leave Canada, and focused on safety concerns, as the youth continued to voice a wish to kill herself. It became clear during the assessment that the youth had many symptoms consistent with a diagnosis of Major Depressive Disorder, which was supported by her past personal and family history as well.

D. S. provided psychoeducation to the family about common symptoms of depression, including suicidal ideation, and described how significant social stressors, such as living in conditions of chronic insecurity, can worsen these symptoms. Then, in an effort to instill some hope in the client, D. S. concluded the assessment by voicing that she believed she could produce a compelling report from what the client had described to her thus far.

In her report, D. S. emphasized the extent to which her patient was vulnerable; she diagnosed Major Depressive Disorder and highlighted several of the youth's symptoms of Posttraumatic Stress Disorder, which included intrusive memories and nightmares of the sexual abuse, a strong avoidance of talking or thinking about the abuse, feelings of shame and culpability, and an erosion of her sense of the world being a safe and benevolent place. Referring to the academic literature, she noted that in children and adolescents, subsyndromal PTSD can be just as debilitating as the full-criteria disorder. D. S. expressed concern about the youth completing suicide should she be forced to return to her home country, and she addressed the potential psychological impact should her father be deported separately. She described the youth as a "very vulnerable child who does not have the resilience to cope with further separations and losses." Besides treatment with antidepressant medication and close psychiatric follow-up, D. S. recommended stepped-up psychological support with significant attention to her risk for suicide should she or her father receive a decision about deportation, suggesting that the youth might indeed need hospitalization in order to maintain her personal safety.

Over the course of their work together, the client's communication to D. S. about her distress became increasingly distilled into the mantra "If I am forced to return [to my home country] I will kill myself." This statement continued well beyond her achieving remission from her depression, and it seemed to be especially contingent on D. S.'s inquiries into news about the family's claims. D. S. wondered if she had somehow given her client the message that as long as the client continued to make unwavering statements about her suicidal intent, D. S. could be useful in portraying her as high-risk to the immigration review board. In response to the client's (rather vague) statements of suicidal intent, her family could not shed the image of the client as ill and fragile and dangerous to herself, even when she clearly appeared to be better. Her father would keep the client with him at all times; she did not return to school and he himself turned down work opportunities to remain on constant watch over her. The father's level of distress was palpable during office visits. D. S. wondered if she had inadvertently reinforced this young woman's language of suicide at the expense of family functioning. It became difficult to get the client to explore other ways of coping than being constantly by her father's side and other solutions to a potential deportation apart from suicide.

Another case illustrates pressures in the opposite direction: a psychiatrist needing to encourage a child to lower his adaptive defenses and acknowledge more of his symptomatology during an assessment for the sake of a report. P. R. was asked to assess and produce a report for a bright and athletic 11-year-old boy who had been kidnapped and beaten, as had his mother, by a powerful gang in their country. His mother informed P. R. that "something seemed off" about her son; he was doing well in school, but was not as chatty with the family as he used to be, which concerned her.

When P. R. saw the boy separately, he told her that his parents were struggling to cope with their own traumatic experiences. He was therefore reluctant to dwell on his own repeated awakenings at night and his general loss of interest in pleasurable activities. He was very hesitant to divulge any personal information (even his country of origin) to his classmates, and he was not making friends. Throughout the assessment, he minimized these and other posttraumatic symptoms, often qualifying responses with "but it's okay," "but it's getting better," etc. He emphasized what he was still able to do around the house to assist the family, his role in protecting his little brother, and other facts that supported his lifelong identity of high-performing and helpful son. Brief interactions with his parents were enough to elicit their pride in him and their reliance on his good function to reassure themselves about the health of their family as a whole. Any indication that their golden child might be struggling caused them worsened confusion and anxiety.

P. R. felt that the boy's determination to contain and overcome his symptoms for the sake of his family was a positive prognostic feature. However, this affected his reporting style to the point that it was difficult to clarify his true level of distress. Only after repeated probing did it become clear that this went beyond the "mild" level and well into the moderate range.

She therefore found herself in a dilemma: The boy's agenda was to protect his family (and probably himself) from his own difficulties, resisting giving information that could lead to a worrisome verdict of being "ill." Yet her psychiatric assessment – her agenda of outlining clear symptomatology in a report and possibly making a diagnosis – could serve a completely different version of "protection." She had to proceed carefully to encourage the boy's disclosure of problematic symptoms without destabilizing his identity, both for himself and in the eyes of his family, as a resilient and capable youth.

Case Discussion and Broader Implications

Diagnosis as advocacy is an outcome of doctors being "tasked with solving dilemmas that are not medical but social and structural, the responsibility of the government" [2]. It creates newer problems, drawing medical language further and further into a political discourse about a country's humanitarian policies. In the clinic, this translates into physicians emphasizing DSM diagnosis and dysfunction in order to help families to navigate an unjust system that clearly contributes to their distress. Families themselves, grappling with the power imbalance inherent to the clinical encounter, must also negotiate language and presentation – both consciously and unconsciously. The risk of both parties describing this suffering psychiatrically, emphasizing illness instead of resilience, is that the families might automatically reorganize around the sick role. The spectre of Georgi's family at the dinner table, with Georgi propped up in his wheelchair and being fed through a nasogastric tube [2], is an extreme example, but the cases described above show how our subtler exchanges with refugee families during the process of generating medical reports are also not without some risk.

In the first case, D. S.'s language around depression, PTSD, and suicide, which may not have been as pronounced had her assessment of the family been in the context of her usual practice, seemed to sway the family toward interactions which impeded the youth's potential expressions of resilience. In the second case, P. R.'s probing of symptomatology risked destabilizing the adaptive self-narrative of a youth and, by extension, the coping of an entire family who depended on him to present a strong front – this despite the fact that a "strong front" is arguably the opposite of what is needed for an immigration assessment report. We also acknowledge that in both cases, these youth were making their own conscious and unconscious choices about their discourse, which contributed to the outcome of the consultation.

The high stakes involved in medico-legal report-writing extend beyond families to the immigration system itself, where asylum seekers may increasingly need a rubber stamp of diagnosis to gain credibility as refugees. Vanessa Pupuvac's description of the transformation of the UNHCR from its 1951 mandate to uphold the rights of stateless persons to an agency that manages refugee flow, argues that this is the result, at least in part, of the transformation of the refugee from a political subject to a patient [31]. She describes how the exiles of postwar and Cold War Europe tended to be viewed as political heroes entitled to the rights laid out in the 1951 Convention, but that by the end of the Cold War there grew an increasing conceptualization of refugees as traumatized victims, spurred on in part by the changing demographic of the refugee population itself.[7] The notion of the refugee as political subject was still a force in play in the late 1960s and 1970s, when Latin American psychiatrists began treating victims of torture by repressive regimes; in this setting, therapeutic work was seen as complementing political resistance ("Interventions sought to resurrect a political subject and reintegrate the person into a political community" (Pupuvac citing Henrik Ronsbo, 2006, p. 17 [31])).

It was not until the American Psychiatric Association introduced, in 1980, the diagnosis of PTSD in the third edition of its Diagnostic and Statistical Manual of Mental Disorders (DSM-III) that professional interest in refugee mental health amplified. Pupuvac describes how with the "merging of the combat veteran, the torture victim and the refugee in the psychiatric literature of the 1980s there was a shift away from the idea of rehabilitating a political subject to managing a victim at risk" (Pupuvac, 2006, p. 18 [31]). The formation of physician-backed refugee centers (Denmark's Rehabilitation and Research Centre for Torture Victims in 1982, the Canadian Centre for Victims of Torture in 1983, and the Medical Foundation for the Care of Victims of Torture in the UK in 1985) and the growth of relevant academic literature into the turn of the twenty-first century reflect attempts to advocate for refugees' political rights through the language of psychiatry. Pupuvac notes that over time, more and more refugee advocates have invoked health paradigms to support refugee claims, to the extent that "a claimant's mental health has become an important component of substantiating claims to persecution in asylum cases" [31]. There have been stirrings of critique of the use of medical information in supporting asylum claims [31, 32] alongside a sense in the medico-legal community that we may be contributing to the very conditions we fear (i.e., the more we stress diagnosis and illness, the more we are *forced* to stress diagnosis and illness to achieve our goals of supporting the rights and wellbeing of these families).[8]

As two of the authors have elaborated elsewhere [33], this trend towards biomedical language has impacts beyond affecting a young person's self-narrative or reinforcing government expectations that only diagnoses can confirm the "truth" of traumatic experiences. A focus on individualized pathology pushes the *political* origins of the refugee's predicament – state abuse, persecution, increasing global disparity, other forms of systemic violence – into the background. The need to redress the person's political rights, as described by Pupuvac, is lost; states are absolved of their responsibility to act in the name of basic justice (rather than the more utilitarian goal of "preventing illness"). To use the recent example of the USA, we were struck by one

---

[7] Pupuvac also explores the role of colonialism and racism in the transformation of the refugee from political subject to medicalized "object"; this is a topic that deserves further unpacking.

[8] One very experienced and respected refugee lawyer, Mr. Raoul Boulakia, told us that the use of psychiatric reports in asylum claims has "created expectations" that these reports will be used for subsequent cases moving forward, leading to problem of "expectation build up" within the claims adjudication system to the point that it is taken for granted that lawyers should be able to obtain a psychiatric report. In cases where a claimant has endorsed distress or symptoms of trauma, without such a report, "the [judge's] question is always: 'Why don't you have one?'" (Raoul Boulakia, personal communication).

group's description of parents forcibly accepting criminal charges or being deported without their children as being examples of a "mental health crisis" being caused by government policy [34].

Psychiatrists advocating via diagnosis could be doing more than absolving states of their complicity in violence; as discussed in the Swedish context, we could be seeking absolution for ourselves as well. We are powerful members of societies that profit from the global disparities underlying refugee migrations, with laws that exacerbate immigration precarity. As "healers" who are often deeply uncomfortable inflicting harm on others, we may feel unconsciously reassured about our own morality by using language that allows us to "treat" the "wounded."

None of this is to discount the idea that there is indeed such a thing as trauma, toxic stress, and mental illness. We are not suggesting that "activist psychiatrists" are choosing to "invent" the notion of severe or even milder maladaptive reactions existing in refugee families. These phenomena certainly exist – we see them often, in fact, particularly in people forced to wait in limbo for years in a state of uncertainty about whether or not they will be protected. In these cases, our expertise can help refugees overcome extreme suffering and maintain some function, and we can engage in broader activism to mitigate such conditions. Inevitably, however, there *is* some clinical discretion involved in the complex mutual negotiation of interpreting a young refugee's experience. This exists in any field of medicine, but particularly in psychiatry. The current trend in psychiatry is to label an increasing swath of human emotions as pathology, as outlined in a vivid debate between the leaders of the DSM-IV and the DSM-5 in the last few years [35, 36]. There is, therefore, a broad acknowledgement that some clinical and institutional discretion is involved in the description of traumatic and other psychiatric pathology. These choices have consequences for the individual "patient" as well as for the direction of the field in general. The question is: how do we and the young refugees in our care exert this choice in the portrayal of psychiatric pathology, particularly when it seems that basic issues of safety are at stake?

Exerting Choice in the Dissemination of Medical Reports

One option would be to stop producing medico-legal reports altogether. We could refuse to add to the increasing medicalization of (particularly politically driven) suffering, hoping to stem the tide of expectations on psychiatrists to "validate" experiences via diagnosis. This would be the long game. However, in the current political climate, this hardly seems like a viable solution; the possibility of putting children, youth, and families who could have benefited from our expertise at considerable risk of deportation is certainly hard to stomach.

A less radical approach would entail promoting a new norm across the field of accepting only cases of severe and debilitating traumatic reactions or of preexisting severe and persistent mental illnesses such as schizophrenia. While doing this, we could concurrently work to legitimize the efforts of nonmedical experts (community leaders, agency managers, social and settlement workers, etc.) to bear witness to the experiences of asylum seekers, for example, by writing letters validating nonmedical reports and by providing education to immigration review boards about the importance of these others as experts – particularly in the absence of such severe pathology.

Unfortunately, this approach carries a risk of reinforcing a belief of the public – and immigration board members – that any suffering *not* captured by a psychiatrist is merely trivial. We have seen asylum-seeking children and youth who have traumatically fragmented memories, disorganized narrative styles, or presentations of distress that might be unusual in the Canadian cultural context, as well as other situations that are psychoemotionally grounded but less obviously linked to severe psychiatric illness. Our refusal to assess these "less severe" cases might result in reduced chances for them of succeeding at immigration hearings, with alarming consequences.

An alternative response for the field would be to accept our ambivalent position with respect to refugee families; we can take action but, given our complicity in their situation, will be unable to "do no harm." We would thus continue with wider report-writing, and disseminating it as an important advocacy skill, but would approach the clinical negotiation with families differently. We would have to attend to the risks outlined earlier in this chapter and try to mitigate the impact of diagnosis and medicalization on refugee children, youth, and families. This might involve being explicit with families about the fact that there are multiple ways of viewing their experience, including but not limited to medical pathology.[9]

The conversation with asylum-seeking families about what a psychiatric assessment is, and what it is not, is much more straightforward than many psychiatrists probably believe. Most refugee clients can instinctively grasp the idea that psychiatry is based on a Western worldview of medical pathology and individualism [37, 38]. Ideally, the physician acknowledges that they and the family are about to engage in a particular culturally based language of assessment, involving "symptoms" and "treatment." They are clear about their plans to write the report mostly in the language of medical symptoms and diagnosis. Refugee youth and families might benefit from knowing that these terms are well recognized in the host country as markers of many types of emotional reactions; this language is therefore useful in helping the immigration board to understand the family's story better [32]. In the encounter, however, the physician plans to explore the narratives and issues that the families feel are most important. Most importantly, the physician allies themselves with the family, using their status as a privileged insider to "translate" the mainstream system to them rather than simply and uncritically perpetuating the system's medicalized gaze and priorities.

While considering these "symptoms," however, the physician is careful to describe the child's or youth's experiences and feelings as fairly *normal* responses to *abnormal* conditions. They locate the true pathology in the external events leading to the family's flight from home as well as hardships in the new country as outlined above. The family may also have their own culturally based narratives that should be elicited and reflected upon in the assessment.

The child's or youth's story is thus reframed as one of survival, adaptation, and resilience, one that positions them not only as a "patient" but also as a political subject. Beyond outlining the signs and symptoms of suffering, the physician seeks out other aspects

---

[9] The following thoughts and ideas are not meant as a literal guide of items to discuss in detail during every assessment, which would be pedantic and alienating for a refugee family. They are simply thinking points to help practitioners reframe their assumptions and stance during their clinical negotiations and report-writing. It would be up to them as to which of these points are elaborated out loud, mentioned briefly, or simply processed internally and transmitted through their demeanor and language choice. The authors of this chapter cover these points in a myriad of ways and very quickly.

of the young person's identity, including their strengths and abilities to cope with highly difficult circumstances. Finally, the physician should consider treatment plans that are not simply aimed at individual symptoms (e.g., medication or traditional psychotherapy, which often emphasizes compensation or support without altering the status quo [39, 40]). There are many therapeutic approaches that promote empowering responses to oppression, not to mention the potential value of joining movements to enact broader change [41–46].

How would such an approach to the assessment affect the report produced afterward? Of course, the board will be interested in the psychiatrist's account of symptoms, diagnosis, and any relevant prognostication or treatment planning. A physician hoping to minimize the effects of medicalization on family dynamics could simply have the transparent discussion outlined above but still go on to write a fairly typical report based on their clinical findings. We submit, however, that the "tone" of these reports could also be altered to move away from purely pathologizing language. Indeed, the board would benefit from hearing a more nuanced discussion of the challenges faced by the family and the support needed moving forward.

A key area in which to alter this tone would be in the conclusion of the report. Instead of jumping automatically to diagnoses of Posttraumatic Stress Disorder or Major Depression, the physician could emphasize the primacy of parental safety and security on their caregiving capacity and the tangible risks to the child (beyond diagnosis) of disrupting these processes further. Comments about strengths will give the board a fuller sense of the child and family, as well as serving as "prognostic" considerations. The physician also names any factors that affect the child's or youth's narrative style – elements that might be culturally based, trauma-based, etc. – to contextualize the presentation to the board. They might include treatment plans that focus on basic resilience promotion, including addressing social determinants of health, supporting parenting capacity, working on problem-solving skills, etc., at least in a cursory manner. This would help to convey the reality that, in fact, most clinical work with this population does consist of relatively straightforward support without sophisticated medical interventions. Such a treatment approach is emphasized more in person with the family.

The authors are by no means suggesting that the cases of *Uppgivenhetssyndrom* in Sweden were simple enough that such a reorientation of approach would have avoided the level of serious pathology described in the article. It could be that this particular idiom of distress had already been firmly entrenched in the community of asylum seekers and their caregivers by this point or that the individual or family dynamics involved were more fraught to begin with; finally, the physician Dr. Hultcrantz may have had the sense (perhaps rightly) that their immigration cases were too precarious to experiment with less medically urgent language. There is risk inherent in using a less medically oriented approach; our suggestions could result in reports that are seen by immigration review boards as "too subjective," or less compelling, and we could thus be placing the immediate safety of families at risk.

That said, looking at the described zeal of Dr. Hultcrantz and her colleagues, we wonder about our urgent sense of these reports as a "make-or-break" factor in asylum claim hearings. This omnipotent attitude could simply be part of our professional culture as physicians; it involves us taking on globally oppressive processes over which we in fact have little control (and which are, as mentioned earlier, actually linked to our own social privilege). It is up to each individual physician to contemplate whether our image of ourselves as "saviors" of these families can tolerate the risk of doing things differently.

What we are suggesting is that there may, in fact, be a real reason to consider doing it differently, and that these well-meaning approaches are not without negative side effects.

Cases Revisited

Reflecting on the case in the light of the discussion above, D. S. realizes that she was caught in a very Hultcrantz-like scenario of high stakes, many symptoms, and a feeling of life-or-death urgency which had her "pull out all the stops" of medical language, going as far as to explicitly state in her report the extent to which the youth lacked resilience. It is situations like these that sometimes have us reflexively and unthinkingly don the psychiatrist's cap, discarding all that we know and believe about working interculturally.

D. S. has followed the youth for several years now. Alongside monitoring medication and symptoms and working to enhance the youth's surrounding supports at school and in her community, D. S. set out to repair this family's notion of her fragility; she began to focus on the youth's own understanding of her difficulties, her self-identified strengths of courage and persistence, and her goal of one day becoming a physician. It is humbling that to think that the "intervention" with clearly the most impact had little to do with D. S.'s attempts to reframe the youth's illness and dangerousness to herself: The change in the youth's thinking occurred after she became pregnant and gave birth to a baby girl. The discourse around suicide faded as this young mother now shifted her focus to nurturing and protecting her daughter.

In her assessment with the 11-year-old boy who had been kidnapped, P. R. did discuss with him the need to focus on "problems" to some degree, both for the sake of the report and also because – and here she shared her clinical suspicions frankly – it did seem that he was having some significant lingering reactions that were common and normal responses to his experience. She emphasized his relative good coping and likelihood of ongoing improvement, especially given his identity as a "helpful son" and his determination not to worry his parents. In line with this self-narrative, P. R. encouraged the youth to understand his symptoms while continuing to "protect his family" by pursuing ongoing good function. He initially resisted her suggestion of joining a school soccer team, citing lack of motivation, but when P. R. suggested that this might in fact reassure his mother, he immediately agreed to try it. At a second appointment he shared that he had begun to play again and tearfully related his happiness at seeing his parents' relief. He was feeling the stirrings of returning interest in the sport and was beginning to sleep better. In meeting with his parents, P. R. did not elaborate at length on the boy's level of distress; instead, she reassured them that he would get better so long as they took care of themselves (including continuing their own counselling supports) and showed themselves to be coping better around the house. She thus leveraged each family member's worry for the others and helped them to see themselves as a collective unit that could act as a resource for the individual members.

P. R. wrote a report for the Immigration Review Board emphasizing the boy's genuine posttraumatic symptomatology while noting that his symptoms did not meet criteria for a full diagnosis of PTSD and could be better described by the term Adjustment Disorder. In her formulation she included the self-narrative above, indicating that this contributed to the boy's masking of his own difficulties. She also emphasized that a sense of safety for the family – the parents in particular – would go a long way towards the clinical improvement of the youth. In her treatment plan, she mentioned extracurricular activities along with suggestions of a mild sleep aid and possibly family counselling. The in-person assessment process was thus heavily tilted towards discussions of the boy's resilience and measures to support this collectively, while the report focused more on individual pathology but attempted to reduce the medicalization of his experience to some degree.

Future Directions (Moving beyond the Clinic)

All of this said, physicians considering carefully how to approach these assessments and reports are still confining their actions to their individual work with families. In the end, these represent weak solutions to the problem. Indeed, a more structurally competent approach would have us move beyond the "microprocesses" of our clinical interactions to address the "macroprocesses of population-level inequalities" [20] on a larger scale:

> Nevertheless, the medical profession remains relatively weak in relationship to powerful government departments that control the fate of asylum seekers. Interagency coalitions with membership drawn from human rights groups, other nongovernment organizations, the legal profession, and health professionals may be more effective than individual health professionals in advocating for asylum seekers.
>
> (Silove et al., 2000, p. 609 [26])

An example relevant to current times would be physicians lending their voices to coalitions seeking changes to US immigration policy, emphasizing issues of rights and justice, rather than solely by predicting pathology in children. The difference may seem subtle, but it is important in not consistently painting refugees and migrants as victims, depoliticized bundles of symptoms or symptoms-in-waiting.

Silove describes how physicians can mobilize to promote the objectives of the 1951 Refugee Convention through larger-scale involvement, which could involve "contributing to the broad areas of education and awareness raising, undertaking further research, building constituencies for advocacy, and ensuring that the health needs of asylum seekers are given higher priority" (Silove et al., 2000, p. 608 [26]). We could begin by openly questioning the trend for rubber-stamping asylum claims with a psychiatric diagnosis and advocating for refugee rights without the use of medical language; this might involve engaging refugee lawyers and immigration review boards in a meaningful discussion about the role of the psychiatric report in substantiating asylum claims or disseminating these ideas further in scholarly, clinical, and lay media. Certainly, these discussions risk becoming an armchair exercise without broader action, but few physicians have the skills and knowledge to effect change at the level of local and global policy. This is where new developments in Structural Competency may be especially useful: Structural competency programs in psychiatry and in medicine more generally could "provide training and guidance on how to create coalitions, gain institutional support, and engage in a productive dialogue with stakeholder communities and policymakers" (Kirmayer et al., 2017, p. E2 [21]).[10] Equipped with hard skills in how to participate in these activities, we can operate effectively within our complex connection to the refugee predicament. We can use our positions of power as physicians to move the discourse *away* from the support and management of refugees as victims and medical patients to the recognition in word and deed of the rights of *all* refugees to safety and security.

---

[10] In Canada, we have already witnessed some ground-breaking changes which were the result of physicians mobilizing with other stakeholders to restore full medical insurance for asylum seekers [47] and to end the detention of asylum-seeking children [48].

References

1. J. Taylor, Confronting "culture" in medicine's "culture of no culture". *Academic Medicine*, 78(6) (2003), 555–559.

2. R. Aviv, (2017). *The Trauma of Facing Deportation*. New Yorker. www.newyorker.com/magazine/2017/04/03/the-trauma-of-facing-deportation (Accessed September 10, 2017.)

3. S. Brink, (2017). *In Sweden, Hundreds of Refugee Children Gave Up on Life*. NPR. ww.npr.org/sections/goatsandsoda/2017/03/30/521958505/only-in-sweden-hundreds-of-refugee-children-gave-up-on-life (Accessed September 10, 2017.)

4. B. Aronsson, C. Wiberg, P. Sandstedt and A. Hjern, Asylum-seeking children with severe loss of activities of daily living: Clinical signs and course during rehabilitation. *Acta Paediatrica*, 98(12) (2009), 1977–1981.

5. K. Sallin, H. Lagercrantz, K. Evers, I. Engström, A. Hjern and P. Petrovic, Resignation syndrome: Catatonia? Culture-bound? *Frontiers in Behavioral Neuroscience*, 10(7) (2016), 1–18.

6. Läkartidningen. http://lakartidningen.se/Sok-arkiv/?f=q:uppgivenhetssyndrom (Accessed January 25, 2018.)

7. A. Picard, Trump's Zero-Tolerance Policy Inflicts Anguish on Kids – With Toxic Health Impacts. *The Globe and Mail*. www.theglobeandmail.com/opinion/article-trumps-zero-tolerance-policy-inflicts-anguish-on-kids-with-toxic-health-impacts/ (Accessed July 12, 2018.)

8. C. Kraft, *AAP Statement Opposing the Border Security and Immigration Reform Act* (American Academy of Pediatrics, 2018). www.aap.org/en-us/about-the-aap/aap-press-room/Pages/AAPStatementOpposingBorderSecurityandImmigrationReformAct.aspx (Accessed July 12, 2018.)

9. V. Harrison, *Nauru Refugees: The Island Where Children Have Given up on Life*. www.bbc.com/news/world-asia-45327058 (Accessed September 23, 2018.)

10. D. Summerfield, Childhood, war, refugeedom and "trauma": Three core questions for mental health professionals. *Transcultural Psychiatry*, 37(3) (2000), 417–433.

11. A. Kleinman, V. Das and M. Lock, eds., *Social Suffering* (Berkeley, CA: University of California Press, 1997).

12. C. Pain, P. Kanagaratnam and D. Payne, The debate about trauma and psychosocial treatment for refugees. In L. Simich and L. Andermann, eds., *Refuge and Resilience: Promoting Resilience and Mental Health among Resettled Refugees and Forced Migrants* (New York: Springer, 2014), pp. 51–60.

13. T. Cross, B. Bazron, K. Dennis and M. Isaacs, *Towards a Culturally Competent System of Care (Vol I)* (Washington, DC: Georgetown University Child Development Center/CASSP Technical Assistance Center, 1989).

14. L. Kirmayer, K. Fung, C. Rousseau, H. T. Lo, P. Menzies, J. Guzder et al., Guidelines for training in cultural psychiatry. *The Canadian Journal of Psychiatry*, 57(3) (2012), S1.

15. K. Fung, H. T. Lo, R. Srivastava and L. Andermann, Organizational cultural competence consultation to a mental health institution. *Transcultural Psychiatry*, 49(2) (2012), 165–184.

16. L. Kirmayer, Rethinking cultural competence. *Transcultural Psychiatry*, 49(2) (2012), 149–164.

17. B. Agic, L. Andermann, K. McKenzie and A. Tuck, Refugees in host countries: Psychosocial aspects and mental health. In T. Wenzel and B. Drozdek, eds., *An Uncertain Safety: Integrative Health Care for the 21st Century Refugees* (Cham: Springer, 2019), pp. 187–211.

18. H. Hansen, J. Braslow and R. Rohrbaugh, From cultural to structural competency: Training psychiatry residents to act on social determinants of health and institutional racism. *JAMA Psychiatry*, 75(2) (2017), 117–118. DOI: http://10.1001/jamapsychiatry.2017.3894

19. H. Hansen and J. Metzl, Structural competency: Theorizing a new medical engagement with stigma and inequality.

Social Science and Medicine, 103 (2014), 126–133.

20. H. Hansen and J. Metzl, Structural competency and psychiatry. *JAMA Psychiatry*, 75(2) (2017), E2. DOI:http://10.1001/jamapsychiatry.2017.3894

21. L. Kirmayer, R. Kronick and C. Rousseau, Advocacy as key to structural competency in psychiatry. *JAMA Psychiatry*, 75(2) (2017), E1–E2. DOI:http://10.1001/jamapsychiatry.2017.3894

22. D. Silove, Z. Steel, I. Suslik, N. Frommer, C. Loneragan, T. Chey et al., The impact of the refugee decision on the trajectory of PTSD, anxiety, and depressive symptoms among asylum seekers: A longitudinal study. *American Journal of Disaster Medicine*, 2 (6) (2007), 321–329.

23. D. Ryan, F. Kelly and B. Kelly, Mental health among persons awaiting an asylum outcome in western countries. *International Journal of Mental Health*, 38 (3) (2009), 88–111.

24. D. Hocking, G. Kennedy and S. Sundram, Mental disorders in asylum seekers: The role of the refugee determination process and employment. *The Journal of Nervous and Mental Disease*, 203(1) (2015), 28–32.

25. R. Kronick, C. Rousseau and J. Cleveland, Mandatory detention of refugee children: A public health issue? *Paediatrics Child Health*, 16(8) (2011), e65–e67.

26. D. Silove, Z. Steel and C. Watters, Policies of deterrence and the mental health of asylum seekers. *JAMA*, 284(5) (2000), 604–611.

27. A. Kleinman, *Rethinking Psychiatry: From Cultural Category to Personal Experience* (New York: The Free Press, 1991).

28. C. Green-Pedersen and P. Odmalm, Going different ways? Right-wing parties and the immigrant issue in Denmark and Sweden. *Journal of European Public Policy*, 15(3) (2008), 367–381.

29. M. Eastmond, Egalitarian ambitions, constructions of difference: The paradoxes of refugee integration in Sweden. *Journal of Ethnic and Migration Studies*, 37(2) (2011), 277–295.

30. A. Ruth, The second new nation: The mythology of modern Sweden. In S. Grabaud, ed., *Norden: The Passion for Equality* (Oxford: Oxford University Press, 1986), pp. 240–282.

31. V. Pupuvac, Refugees in the "sick role": Stereotyping refugees and eroding refugee rights. *New Issues in Refugee Research (The UNHCR Policy Development and Evaluation Service)*, 128 (2006), 1–24.

32. J. Barrett, I. Baturalp, N. Gbikpi and K. Rehberg, An exploration and critique of the use of mental health information within refugee status determination proceedings in the United Kingdom. *Refugee Studies Centre*, 100 (2014), 1–15.

33. P. Raju, D. Stein and F. Dushimiyimana, Suffering as "symptom": Psychiatry and refugee youth. In S. Pashang, N. Khanlou and J. Clarke, eds., *Today's Youth and Mental Health: Hope, Power and Resilience* (Cham: Springer, 2018), pp. 341–358.

34. American Psychological Association, (2018). www.apa.org/advocacy/immigration/separating-families-letter.pdf (Accessed July 12, 2018.)

35. A. Frances, Robert Spitzer: The most influential psychiatrist of his time. *The Lancet*, 3(2) (2016), 110–111. www.thelancet.com/psychiatry (Accessed January 27, 2018.)

36. A. Frances, The past, present and future of psychiatric diagnosis. *World Psychiatry*, 12 (2) (2013), 111–112.

37. L. Kirmayer and D. Pedersen, Toward a new architecture for global mental health. *Transcultural Psychiatry*, 51(6) (2014), 759–776.

38. L. Kirmayer, Psychotherapy and the cultural concept of the person. *Transcultural Psychiatry*, 49(2) (2012), 232–257.

39. N. Phillips, G. Adams and P. Salter, Beyond adaptation: Decolonizing approaches to coping with oppression. *Journal of Social and Political Psychology*, 3(1) (2015), 365–387.

40. G. Adams, I. Doblesb, L. Gómezc, T. Kurtisd and L. Molina, Decolonizing

psychological science: Introduction to the special thematic section. *Journal of Social and Political Psychology*, 3(1) (2015), 213–238.

41. M. Schauer, F. Neuner and T. Ebert, *Narrative Exposure Therapy: A Short-Term Treatment for Traumatic Stress Disorders* (Cambridge, MA: Hogrefe, 2011).

42. J. Cienfuegos and C. Monelli, The testimony of political repression as a therapeutic instrument. *American Journal of Orthopsychiatry*, 53(1) (1983), 43–51.

43. S. Lustig, S. Weine, G. Saxe and W. Beardslee, Testimonial psychiatry for adolescent refugees: A case series. *Transcultural Psychiatry*, 41(1) (2004), 31–45.

44. C. Rousseau, M. Gauthier, L. Lacroix, N. Alain, M. Benoit, A. Moran et al., Playing with identities and transforming shared realities: Drama therapy workshops for adolescent immigrants and refugees. *The Arts in Psychotherapy*, 32(1) (2005), 13–27.

45. T. Tinkler, Transitory freedom: Political discourses of refugee youth in a photography-based after-school program. (PhD thesis.) (Santa Barbara, CA: University of California, 2006.)

46. S. Yohani, Creating an ecology of hope: Arts-based interventions with refugee children. *Child and Adolescent Social Work Journal*, 25(4) (2008), 309–323.

47. P. Berger, Physicians rise up against refugee health care cuts. *University of Toronto Medical Journal*, 93(1) (2015), 7–8.

48. R. Kronick, C. Rousseau, M. Beder and R. Goel, International solidarity to end immigration detention. *The Lancet*, 389 (10068) (2017), 501–502.

Reflexivity in the Everyday Lives and Work of Refugees and Therapists

Rukiya Jemmott and Inga-Britt Krause

> If we should start telling the truth that we are nothing but Jews, it would mean that we expose ourselves to the fate of human beings who, unprotected by any specific law or political convention, are nothing but human beings.
>
> *(Arendt, 1996, p. 118 [1])*

Introduction

The predicament of Jews referred to by Arendt above is shared by all refugees. Their journeys, while often characterised by extreme physical suffering, also involve the unbearable psychological and emotional contradiction associated with not belonging, that is to say, not receiving protection in their home country, not holding state membership in a new country and in this way being stripped down to 'mere' biological human beings, struggling to survive through everyday life activities and unable to participate in political action [2]. While Arendt's idea of 'humanity' has been contested particularly because of its negative view of the social (the everyday) as separate from and subsumed by the political and because she considers that rights can only be enjoyed from within the confines of political institutions such as the nation state [3], the contradiction to which she drew attention continues to define a refugee in current western ideologies [4]. The contradiction is further articulated in the 'discourses between compassion and repression' [5] which emerge in article 14 of the Universal Declaration of Human Rights, which states that 'everyone has the right to seek and to enjoy in other countries asylum from persecution' (Morsink, 1999, p. 332 [6]) and the way this principle is applied in practice. Refugees thus represent a failure of current political systems, because they are evidence that states and countries cannot protect their own citizens. They also represent a failure of a humanitarian ideal that being human ought to be enough to arouse compassion and protection. Both of these failures have far-reaching effects in the lives of refugees and asylum seekers and on what Watters has called the 'moral economy of care', referring to the caring services operating within 'a circumscribed context of societies' institutions and values' (2007, p. 395 [7]). Even after arriving in a new country and waiting for or having been granted asylum, these contradictions often remain palpable in the experiences of refugees, and political rights granted in the form of asylum do not by themselves necessarily translate into adequate social rights. Asylum seekers, refugees and especially refused asylum seekers experience much greater difficulties in accessing health services, housing, work and education than does the general population [8] and often have negative views and expectations of their own value as persons, of others as trustworthy and of the world as a safe place [9]. Such negative views may contribute to re-traumatisation, but may also contribute to other mental health difficulties and are of course a central concern of mental health professionals treating refugees or asylum seekers.

It is our argument here that as far as mental health services for refugees are concerned, it is our job as professionals to help restore trust [10] and the value of being human in our work with refugees and asylum seekers and also that this task implicates us in the contradictions outlined above and is far from straightforward. It cannot adequately be addressed through targeted cross-cultural mental health practice training or by applying treatment manuals, but in our view it requires a much more imaginative [11], cross-culturally intuitive and radical as well as tentative use of our own reflexivity. We consider that this is so for two reasons. First, as mental health practitioners we are ourselves members of institutions, which in our case are largely defined by the remit of government and the state on whose behalf we deliver our services. This predisposes and implicates us in political and institutional discriminatory practices, some of which we are not necessarily aware of, or not consistently aware. Second, we are ourselves persons with identities, languages and notions of specific cultural and professional meanings, some within and others outside our own awareness. We may feel that being human *is* having identities, passports, rituals and cultural memories. To connect to refugees' lived experience of 'humanity', either as an existential abstraction or as a biological condition, is impossible without imposing our own outlooks and assumptions, so working through and beyond these outlooks and assumptions *is* a central requirement. The field or the 'space' in which this work takes place is 'the everyday', and for refugees, ordinary routines and normality cannot be taken for granted partly because they very often point back to extraordinary events and ruptures in the past from which it is difficult to escape. We suggest that therapeutic work with refugees and asylum seekers presents a particular challenge to the reflexivity of professionals and therapists in working in and through this territory, precisely because extraordinary ruptures are concealed in and behind ordinary events.

In this chapter, we begin by describing our place of work, ourselves and our collaboration. We then sketch our notion of reflexivity in systemic psychotherapy, which will take us on to consider how to work with everyday meanings in order to foster trust and in order to move beyond these. We take this up in the final section, where, using examples, we show how we think about what we call the 'human condition' and how this notion helps us to go behind the immediate content of our therapy sessions to an awareness and understanding of our own relationship to our clients and the relationships both they and we ourselves have to our respective past histories. For us, 'past' includes both meanings in the lives of ourselves and our clients in the past and how this has been articulated in the structure of past relationships and events, often with the result of reproducing, restraining or rupturing those meanings. In this sense we see the past as embedded in contemporary[1] [12] everyday events, offering therapists and clients an opportunity for 'turning back' to the past as a necessary step in going forward [13]. In this move, the ordinary events, communications and interactions in the therapy room may come to stand out as extraordinary, pointing to what, following Das, we have called 'the everyday work of repair' (Das, 1998, p. 208 [13]), referring to finding a way in which the therapy and life itself can go on.

---

[1] Rabinow and Marcus define 'the contemporary' in the following way: 'if one no longer assumes that the new is what is dominant, [. . .] and that the old is somehow residual, then the question of how older and newer elements are given form and worked together, either well or poorly, becomes a significant site of inquiry. I call that site the contemporary' (p. 3 [12]).

The Setting and our Collaboration

We are systemic psychotherapists working in the same National Health Service Trust in the UK, although not in the same clinical team. Rukiya is also a social worker and Britt is also a social anthropologist. In fact, the separation of the services (Rukiya works in the Refugee Service, whereas Britt works in a general Child and Adolescent Mental Health Service) is typical of the organisation of specialist refugee services on the ground in the UK and perhaps reflects the contradictions referred to in the introduction, namely that refugees and asylum seekers suffer specific problems in the form of PTSD and accompanying symptoms and as such, being considered special cases, everyday issues encountered in the living of ordinary lives as well as access to specific cross-cultural expertise may receive less emphasis [14]. Apart from having different training backgrounds and working in different services, Rukiya and Britt are different in other ways. Rukiya is black of Caribbean descent, while Britt is white and from Denmark. We have both devoted much of our working lives and energy to working across culture, race and ethnicity in the context of mental health services in the UK, mostly with children and families [15], and Rukiya has also for many years worked in adult mental health services. These interests and commitments serve as points of connection but also of divergence, especially with respect to what in the UK are referred to as the 'Social Graces' [16], a dominant approach in this field. As a black woman, Rukiya has been and still is a fierce promoter of this approach [17], while Britt has been more sceptical [18]. However, neither of us takes a superficial and trivial view of politics, symbols or identity, and this is probably why we have been participating in the same peer supervision group for several years and why we trust each other. We are also both aware of the interest in and the influence of family relationships and the ways in which these have become ruptured in each of our own lives. We have come to frame this as 'kinship', referring not just to what systemic psychotherapists routinely associate with genograms, three-generational family relationships and family scripts, but also borrowing from social anthropology a wider field of structures, organisations and institutions and from psychoanalysis and psychoanalytic psychotherapy an emphasis on inter-subjectivity and unconscious processes. In particular, we see a common theme between us being a fascination with kinship relations and how to survive such relationships when they are ruptured, broken and betrayed, and it is this which we find resonates with the experience of our clients who have witnessed and been subjected to violence, criminality and torture. This may be captured in the work of Das, who referred to Wittgenstein's notion of the ideal [19] as something to which we must always turn back. Referring to events of communal violence (in Das's work about the Partition of India) and the ensuing rupture of trust and betrayal of the ideal of kinship solidarity, Das wrote: 'This image of turning back evokes not so much the idea of a return as a turning back to inhabit the same space now marked as a space of destruction in which you must live again' [1998, p. 208 [13]).

Although we might be seen to have fled our own families, neither of us has been a refugee or an asylum seeker, but we both believe that our own experiences of ruptures of trust have deeply influenced what we have become and that what we have become can be understood as a way of 'turning back'. Thus, Britt's preoccupation with kinship in her anthropological work and becoming a family therapist she understands as a 'turning back' from her experiences of a broken family, her father's suicide and a broken, acrimonious relationship with her mother. Rukiya, who, as a family therapist and social worker, has had a longstanding interest in genograms, understands this as a 'turning back' from being placed in foster care at the age of 18 months, returning to live with her mother and family at the age of 10 years with a strong sense of 'un-belonging'. Refugees and asylum seekers have experienced spaces of far more serious destruction and rupture in their relationships, but we consider that when it comes to repair, the processes may be similar and, as Das suggests, that 'you make such a space of destruction your own not through an ascent into transcendence but through a descent into the everyday' and with what she refers to as 'the everyday work of repair' (1997, p. 208 [13]). We do not wish to claim that this is all that refugees and asylum seekers need, but we do suggest that without this dimension of care, refugees and asylum seekers will have great difficulty in inhabiting the world again or in inhabiting a new world.

Reflexivity in Systemic Psychotherapy

In contemporary systemic psychotherapy, the therapeutic relationship – that is to say, the relationship between a therapist and their clients – tends to be conceptualised in terms of reflexivity. This is a complex term, which in one sense has been central to the discipline from its inception. Broadly, the notion of reflexivity refers to the interest in understanding how a system, be that a social system or a family system, operates as a collection of relationships in which one set of relationships is related to another set of relationships in such a way that there is feedback or constraint between them. This circularity was conceptualised as an almost mechanical process in the early development of systemic thinking, while contemporary notions about this are much more fluid and loose, indicating 'more-or-less' patterns. In this latter sense, systemic reflexivity is central to systemic thinking about the dynamic in family or indeed any relationships, interactions or communications [20–22]. When a therapist joins a family, they also join the relational dynamics of these relationships and communications, and the situation changes. This has been conceptualised in terms of dialogue [23, 24], reflecting teams [25], relational reflexivity [26] and attention to various aspects of identity [16, 17]. These recent conceptualisations have shifted the emphasis from patterns in relationships past and present to a focus on the social construction of the relationships between participants in the therapy encounter and on individual agency. In this way, continuity, history and past social patterns, as well as meanings and events which are wholly or partially outside the awareness of persons, have received much less attention in the discipline in recent years [27]. In short, in developing thinking about the therapeutic relationship, systemic psychotherapists have under-emphasised what we might call 'background understanding': the structure and organisation and meanings which constitute the background and history to the personal, social and political history of themselves and their clients. Even when the self-reflexivity of the therapist has been called forth, this has tended to be a somewhat solipsistic expression of liberal or neo-liberal western orientations. In our view, this will not do for refugee work, because the 'turning back' in refugee work requires particular attention to recognising, connecting and re-fashioning events in the past and how these are carried into the present. The past is articulated both in individual memories and in social and cultural institutions, which were the context for these memories, and it is our task to understand how as past events these have become incorporated into the present. This demands trust in the therapeutic relationship in order that these issues can be worked with. We therefore suggest that work with refugees and asylum seekers in particular calls for 'comprehensive reflexivity' [27], also referred to by others as 'radical reflexivity' [28, 29], 'operational perspectivity' [30] or methodological reflexivity [31]. This is a reflexivity which encompasses recursiveness between different aspects of meaning, interpretation and experience held or expressed by persons (either clients or therapists) *as well as* the reflexivity of both therapist and clients vis-à-vis their own history, development and background and the contexts in which they participate [27]. Citing Burke, Rabinow and Stavrianakis further note that 'experience is necessarily perspectival relative to the operational capabilities of an agent; but this is not to say that it is necessarily subjective' (2016, p. 417 [30]), and D'Arcangelis, referring to Ahmed, notes that this calls for a reflexive double turn, namely a 'turn towards and then away from the Self' (2017, p. 12 [29]). This implies an effort to understand the organisation and structures of social and political relations and events in the past and how these have impacted the contemporary ordinary everyday lives of our clients and of ourselves.

Comprehensive or radical reflexivity is an ongoing process and a struggle precisely because of the partial awareness which we hold of our own subjectivity and our inability to think outside the limits of categories and meanings. Our enquiries may reproduce the very relationships we are trying to help change, and at any time we may slip back into using reflexivity as a way of solving our own doubts as if this is a straightforward process. Pillow, writing about reflexivity in social science research, writes that our work 'would benefit from more "messy" examples . . . that do not seek a comfortable, transcendent end-point but leave us in the uncomfortable realities of doing engaged qualitative research' (2015, p. 193 [31]). We advocate a similar interrogation of discomfort and uncertainty in therapeutic work with refugees and asylum seekers, first, because such discomfort is likely to highlight the routines of everyday life for our clients that we may easily overlook, and second, because in work with refugees, in cross-cultural work – and indeed, we believe, in any therapeutic work – it is important to proceed as if the ordinary at any time can become extraordinary.

The following is such a 'messy example', which occurred during Britt's work with a Tigraian Muslim refugee, Radia. Radia had been coming for therapy for about three years and the therapy was progressing, albeit with many difficult turns and upsets. These processes had profound meaning for Radia's understanding of her existence and possibilities in the present, both as a displaced person but also as someone who in the midst of violent events had been denied compassion and protection from her own family in the past. At different times Britt felt that she needed to be a therapist, a mother or a friend to Radia, who sometimes asked for advice about cooking but who most of all struggled with not being able to conceive and become a mother [32]. The terrorist incident on 7 July 2005 in Central London in which Islamic terrorists detonated three bombs in the underground and on a bus, resulting in many casualties, became a significant event in their relationship. After this, Radia did not attend her weekly therapy session for many weeks. Britt tried to get in touch in different ways with no success at first. When she finally managed to contact Radia and she attended her next therapy session, the following conversation took place. As the session began, Britt said that she had been worried for Radia and also that she realised that something had happened in the social context, which might have some effect on, even be dangerous for, their relationship. Radia responded by telling Britt that in the days after the bombing incident she had been spat on by white youths in the street and that she had for the moment stopped wearing her headscarf in order to feel safer. A little later in the session, Britt wondered whether it was because of fear of going out that Radia had not attended her sessions, and Radia answered quietly,

'No, I did not want you to think that I thought you were one of them.' Britt remembers feeling bewildered and to this day struggles to understand fully what Radia meant. On the one hand, it seemed to convey that Radia was taking care of *her* rather than the other way around. Was she searching for a way of maintaining the bond in the face of increasing social tension? On the other hand, knowing Radia as Britt did, it also seemed that the atmosphere of hate which the bombing incidents incited in the general population played into Radia's feelings of shame and inadequacy. Perhaps more sobering, the trust which Britt felt they had built together was much more tenuous than she might have hoped, and a chasm had opened up. Britt remembers feeling grateful that the work did not stop, although subsequent therapeutic work had to be seen through the prism of these events.

The Human Condition: The Ordinary in Everyday Life

It seems reasonable to expect that unless the therapeutic relationship avoids reproducing a relationship of inequality and power it cannot optimise healing or hopes for clients who are refugees and asylum seekers in their new circumstances [32]. Aiming for comprehensive or radical reflexivity and encompassing messy, uncomfortable events may help the therapist to avoid becoming complacent and descending into more solipsistic forms of reflexivity. However, where, then, can the therapist start? How is reflexivity possible in the first place? We believe that therapeutic work with refugees in particular is best thought of as a process moving between the ordinary and the extraordinary in everyday life so that the ordinary may serve as a way into engagements, whereas the extraordinary poses the issue of how to live on from a space of destruction. Persons who have lost their place of belonging [33] and whose relationships have been ruptured may find comfort in new ordinary everyday patterns and routines, while the extraordinary events which brought the situation about still loom large. Similarly, ordinary past relational expectations such as rights and obligations based on kinship may have been ruptured, and returning to everyday life may necessitate living with 'turning back', as we suggested above. Here, we argue how, in order for it to be possible to make use of or have access to ordinary events and to connect or find resonance with our clients, it seems imperative to engage with an idea of 'humanness' and 'humanity', because not only does this idea haunt the treatment, services, thinking and politics in relation to refugees and asylum seekers as in the quote from Arendt above, the concept of 'humanity' can also all too easily serve as a type of self-reflexivity or self-awareness through which differences are ignored and which therefore offer solipsistic catharsis for the clinician. We prefer the term 'the human condition' to refer to the pre-discursive capabilities which we may relatively safely assume that persons in all societies and cultural contexts share. For us, 'the human condition' refers to capacities rather than to physical, mental or emotional states. All human beings have capacities for hunger, thirst, birth, death, ageing, suffering, communicating, symbol-making and some form of relationality or attachment, but this does not give information about how these capacities are expressed, experienced or articulated, whether they are hypo-cognised, hyper-cognised, over- or under-determined in any particular social, cultural or political context or situation. From this perspective, 'the human condition' is an assumption – we might even be tempted to say a fundamental assumption – about human beings, the articulation of which generally is only fleetingly experienced as a resonance and then through some symbolic formation in the therapeutic encounter. However, when it is felt, it can be put to good therapeutic and relational use in forging connections and in facilitating the emergence of significant events in the therapy. In what follows, we describe the emergence of three such significant events in our work with three different families. In this work, resonances between ourselves and our clients were picked up through a focus on the ordinary in everyday life, and this facilitated a turning back to extraordinary past experiences.

Falling Asleep

Rukiya worked with a 17-year-old adolescent boy, Mohsen, who is a Farsi speaker from Kabul in Afghanistan. Mohsen is about five feet tall, with dark curly hair; he has big bright eyes, which are a very dark brown. He felt sad rather than angry, and Rukiya became aware of a maternal instinct in her and that she wanted very much to help Mohsen. In this work they were joined by a male interpreter who spoke Farsi. Rukiya sensed a paternal warmth from the interpreter towards Mohsen, who had been self-harming. It was this which had alarmed the professionals, including the social workers who referred Mohsen to the refugee service. Mohsen spent quite some time telling Rukiya about his journey to England, having travelled through more than 12 countries and after that becoming separated from his family in Amsterdam. Mohsen described his father as aggressive, but he never said more when Rukiya tried to understand what this aggression looked and felt like or when she tried to find out more about the circumstances. Together they worked over this material during several sessions, and Rukiya felt that the slowness of the sessions had a mesmerising effect on her while she was working hard at keeping the conversation going. At the same time she had not been sleeping well at all and she met with Mohsen in the afternoon, which under these circumstances was the hardest time of day for her. On one particular day, she was aware that she was really tired and so she kept moving about in her chair, opened the window, etcetera so as not to fall asleep. This did not work, and for a second Rukiya nodded off. When she looked up, the interpreter and Mohsen were smirking at each other. Rukiya felt deep shame! She thought, 'This young man who is here with nobody has a therapist who cannot even keep awake for him.' Rukiya said nothing; she just reproached herself internally: 'You bad, bad therapist.' Later in the session, Mohsen asked if he had to keep coming to therapy here. Rukiya looked at him and said, 'Yes, you do need to keep coming. I am so tired at the moment because I did not sleep well; I am so tired I feel like my head could roll off and fall asleep right there on the floor. Even though I am that tired, I need you to know that you are really important. You, Mohsen, are here alone; your family is in Amsterdam and cannot look after you from there; I am here and it is important that I keep a check on you, as you know you have been cutting and therefore I do want to keep seeing you until I know you are safe and better.' After this, Rukiya asked Mohsen what he thought about what she had said. He looked at her, really looked at her, and said, 'Ok. I will come.' After that, Mohsen continued to attend regularly and the cutting stopped.

Rukiya had tried really hard to stay with Mohsen and shut out her sense of sleepiness. However, looking back at this moment, she was left wondering what else she may have been shutting out. Mohsen was meeting with her because he was in the UK alone; he did not know where his family was, as he had left them while en route to 'something better'. Rukiya, too, had spent many years in her childhood and adolescence separated from her family with a strong sense of being alone and not really belonging. She felt sure that there was something in Mohsen's silence and hard-to-reach suffering that was difficult for her to bear, while she wanted at the same time to be able to bear it. This sense, Rukiya believes, led her to keep her distance emotionally, and this was why she had drifted away into a kind of soporific state. The shame she had initially felt had also led her into silence, and at the same time she wanted to say something truthful and heartfelt to Mohsen. So she gave words to the sleep and in this way allowed space for her fallibility as a therapist to connect with Mohsen by showing something ordinary, human and transparent.

Disentangling

A 40-year-old Iranian woman, whom we shall refer to as Mahtab, was referred to CAMHS with her two children, Arash, who was 7 years old, and Yasmin, who was 15. All three were asylum-seeking refugees who had come to the UK two years previously in order to join Mahtab's husband, the children's father. The couple's own families came from different ethnic and religious backgrounds in Iran. After arriving in the UK, Mahtab's husband was extremely violent towards her and she escaped with Arash to a women's refuge. However, before she left, she had talked to Yasmin about all of them escaping. Yasmin was adamant that she wanted to stay with her father, and Mahtab and Arash moved to the refuge, the whereabouts of which the father did not know. During the next three months, the father was emotionally and physically abusive to Yasmin and she eventually joined her mother and brother. While there was no court order, there was a general agreement between refuge staff and social services that the children should not see their father. Arash begged her mother to be able to visit his father's brother and in this way meet up with his father. Mahtab, who knew how important the relationship between father and son is in Iranian ideas about kinship relationships and in the ideas which her family and her husband's family held about father/son relationships, as well as in her son's life, agreed. At the same time, the father had found out where Yasmin went to school and followed her home on a few occasions, in this way finding out the location of the refuge. Refuge workers were furious and adamant that Mahtab and her children would have to move, and social services considered that she was not able to keep her children safe and initiated Child Protection proceedings. At the same time, Mahtab and her children had been referred to the service in which Britt works but had not attended several appointments offered, and to social workers and refuge workers this further confirmed the negative view they had of Mahtab. Mahtab had turned up in CAMHS without an appointment, and Britt was able to follow this up. When Britt and Mahtab finally met with a Farsi-speaking interpreter, Mahtab was distraught, feeling triply persecuted and traumatised, first because of the persecution of her and her family in Iran, second because of the domestic violence which she had had to flee and third as a result of the bewildering and incomprehensible prospect of possibly having her children taken into care. Mahtab felt alienated, confused and overwhelmed, and Britt felt angry with her social work and refuge colleagues as well as worried about finding a way to work with Mahtab under these circumstances. An image of a ball of entangled wool with many colours all mixed up with no endings or beginnings occurred to her. She asked Mahtab whether there is a tradition of knitting in Iran and who knits – men or women, young or old? Mahtab said that, 'Yes, women knit in Iran and in my community.' Britt asked whether she 'knows how to knit'. Mahtab said yes, she used to knit back in Iran. Britt asked for the Farsi term which Mahtab and the interpreter had used for knitting. *Baftani* was the word they offered. Together they spoke about knitting and how easily wool becomes entangled so that one cannot find the beginning or the end. They both agreed that this task needs a great deal of *sabour*, patience. Britt thought further about this metaphor, about the present situation and about balls of wool, and she said that perhaps we also need hope, and Mahtab quickly translated this as *omidvar*. Britt speaks no Farsi, so each time she asked for the Farsi translation. All three women then spoke about *baftani* as a way of being productive and the challenges of both *sabour* and *omidvar* and how in difficult circumstances one might nurture these. At the end of the session, these three words were left on the whiteboard and they became a frame for the next few sessions, which have all been attended. During these sessions, Mahtab began to confront her bewilderment about social workers and refuge workers not understanding her actions as a good respectful Iranian mother vis-à-vis her children's relationships with their father and the betrayal she feels from her own family, who consider her a disrespectful wife both because she has left her husband but also because she is now instrumental in keeping her son from seeing his father.

In this example, the metaphor of knitting provided an image of the domestic space of family, while the ball of mixed-up thread pointed to something going wrong or being insoluble. Britt had been knitting herself, so this was an image which was alive for her. She could not, of course, assume that this image would be meaningful for Mahtab and therefore had to check it out. Once it was clear that this image was 'experience near' [34, 35] and reminiscent of Mahtab's ordinary everyday life in Iran, it could provide a metaphor both for 'turning back' to domestic life for Mahtab as a daughter and a wife and for the rupture in the past and the loose ends which she had been left to engage with in the present. For Britt, the knitting became 'a place to stand from where to begin', while the ideas of 'patience' and 'hope' are human capabilities, the meaning and process of which are still to be worked out in the specific case of Mahtab and her children.

Praying

Terrie and Amanda are sisters of 17 and 18 years of age. They came to the UK as asylum seekers from a war-torn country. They were referred to the refugee service and initially seen by two of Rukiya's colleagues. After some time, a decision was made for the sisters to be seen separately. When Amanda's individual worker left the service, Rukiya was asked to take over the work with her. This work started about a year after the sisters had joined the service, but Rukiya did not feel that she and Amanda were making progress. Amanda often did not attend, and when she did, she often spoke about her sister or wanted to know how Rukiya herself was keeping. After a conversation with the other worker, Lorraine, Rukiya suggested that they continue the work with the sisters together. After about seven months, due to work demands, it was decided that Lorraine would stop working with the sisters. At the beginning of one of the ending sessions, Rukiya, Lorraine and the interpreter were waiting for Terrie and Amanda to arrive. They were late. Rukiya felt that Lorraine was frustrated or anxious and asked her about this. Lorraine said that she was aware that they did not have enough time. At that moment, the phone rang, and at the same time there was a knock on the door. Amanda had gone to the reception, which was ringing to inform Rukiya and Lorraine that the clients had arrived, while Terrie had come straight to the room. There was a feeling that together the sisters had covered all possibilities through this division of labour.

During the session, Lorraine spoke to Terrie and Amanda, telling them what she had seen of them since their first meeting and how they had managed so many things. The older sister responded to Lorraine by saying that she too had watched Lorraine while Lorraine had spoken and while they had worked together. She said, 'I also know you.' Lorraine then spoke about her work with the sisters and about how the two sisters had managed so many new things. Amanda then described how she had been more open while Terrie had and still was wearing 'a bullet-proof vest'. Once Terrie opened this vest and let people come close, it would be much, much more painful for her to say goodbye. Rukiya and Lorraine had ideas as to why this might be so. They also knew that the sisters had struggled to talk about their family except to let their therapists know that they had a father, a stepmother and a younger sister with whom they had all lost contact. With the awareness of the ending of this phase of therapy in her mind as well as the idea that the bullet-proof vest protects the heart, an image occurred to Rukiya and she spoke about heart connections and how, while they had seen each other with their eyes and ears, as an outsider, Rukiya coming and meeting them here had seen how all three of them, Lorraine and the sisters, had also seen each other with their hearts, hearts that could also hear and see. She said, 'I feel that when you sisters met Lorraine, your hearts were broken, and you have sat together and slowly your hearts have started to heal. Now, you are at this place where you are going to say goodbye to Lorraine and your hearts may cry again.' Rukiya said that she saw this as a sign of progress, as both sisters had been able to trust Lorraine and that this was a sign for her that they were moving on in their lives. She finished by saying, 'As an outsider, I see that maybe your hearts have grown strong, strong enough to bear this ending, and will strengthen through the experience.' Terrie and Amanda sat still, really still, Amanda with her eyes closed, looking as though she had fallen asleep, and Terrie with her head down resting on her folded arms. Rukiya asked what they thought about what she had said – maybe it made no sense, maybe it was wrong or maybe they had a different view. Amanda and Terri were silent. Lorraine, who to Rukiya looked as if she was tearful and moved, said, 'Maybe you feel overwhelmed?' Terrie turned to her and said, 'No. When Rukiya said her sermon she said what is true.' Lorraine asked Amanda whether she was asleep, but Amanda said, 'No. I just needed to close my eyes to take it in.'

Rukiya had wondered about how the sisters had left their country, their home. Was it planned or sudden and unexpected? During the therapy, they had learnt that their departure from their homeland was unexpected, and they had talked about even planned endings being painful. As explained, Rukiya came to the work later than the other therapist, and the resounding message had been that the sisters did not want to talk about their family. Yet there was so much that Rukiya felt she needed to know. Later, she therefore asked the sisters whether they would allow her to ask them about their family. Terrie answered that it depended on what she wanted to know. Tentatively, Rukiya asked about the things they did together as a family, and specifically about praying, as earlier they had talked about their faith together and how this had helped them. Both sisters appeared to come to life as they told Rukiya that they all used to pray together on their father's bed, and it was clear from the looks on their faces that this was a good memory. At that point, Rukiya remembers feeling that she too knew something of the pain of endings unplanned and the pattern of pain such experiences can leave you with. So she said that they could pray right here in the session. Both girls and the interpreter turned to look at her with a look of surprise, and the session continued. At the end of the session, Rukiya said, 'Ok, so who will pray today?' The girls laughed, but Rukiya insisted that they should do this. With some to-ing and fro-ing between the girls, Amanda agreed to pray. She prayed in Lingala with the interpreter translating. Since then they have all, including the interpreter, taken turns to pray at the end of every session, and the tide has really turned, with a much lighter and more playful outlook as they both contest playfully that it is Rukiya's turn to pray.

How should we understand this act of praying together at the end of each session? We consider that this is an ordinary everyday act of turning back to something extraordinary, painful and ruptured for the sisters. They do not know if their father is alive or dead, but he lives on, as do they, in the moments of prayer at the end of every session.

The Ordinary and the Extraordinary in Everyday Life

How might one live? (May, 2005, pp. 1–25 [36].) This is perhaps a strange question to ask in relation to refugees and asylum seekers, who often do not seem to have much of a choice in the matter. However, in our work, this is a question which is always close to our thinking. It is a question both for us and for them. This is because it is a challenge in mental health work to avoid imposing one's own personal and professional ideas and theories to the exclusion of those held by our clients. The orientation with which we approach our own lives sets limitations or opens up possibilities as to how we approach this question of how to live for our personal and professional selves. This is an aspect of our 'comprehensive reflexivity' [27] or 'operational perspectivity' [30]. For us, this is articulated in three important ideas to which we consciously refer in our conversations with each other. The first of these is the idea that what we do in the world, in our work and amongst ourselves is in some sense discovering something new, but in this process we are also *creating* something new; something new emerges for which the possibility of existence was already present [36, 37]. The second is the idea of identity as being *encompassed by* difference rather than *preceding* it [36–38]. For our work with refugees, and actually for all our therapeutic work, this means that us coming together with our clients and co-workers creates the conditions for our own process of existence and work and that our own identities and the identities of our clients never are 'set in stone' but are always emergent and changing. Finally, the third idea refers to the background, experiences and relationships of all of us, but here specifically of refugees [18, 27]. When we first meet with clients, we do not know about these, their meaning or the weight these past contexts and events might have in the current situation. While we can have some general idea derived from the literature and previous work about trauma, rupture and loss, we do not know how this works for particular clients. Yet in order to facilitate a 'turning back', these past events are important for the present. For us, how we might live in the midst of these difficult issues is circumscribed by the capabilities we have referred to as 'the human condition', a capability of potentiality and possibilities for the future. We think that this can be captured well by the Deleuzian notion of 'becoming' [37, 39]. As May explains, 'becoming' is the expression of an ontology as 'the study of what is and of what unsettles it. It is a study that creates concepts that may open out onto new lands, onto terrains that have yet to be traveled' (2005, p. 56 [36]). We thus do not in any way consider these capabilities as determining. Rather, we suggest that in our work with refugees and asylum seekers, the relationships between them and us are fashioned in particular, contextual and emergent ways.

'Falling asleep', 'disentangling a ball of string' and 'praying' are all everyday activities and processes which originated in ourselves in the context of being with our clients. These processes and activities are thoroughly ordinary, even routine and repetitious. We find this a useful way of beginning and opening up our therapeutic work with refugees, which guards against, but does not entirely avoid, imposing our own conceptions and theories. Even when the symbol or metaphor derives entirely from the therapist, such as Britt's example of 'disentangling a ball of string', this image can – and did in this case – become appropriate and itself a symbol of the emerging relationship between Britt, the interpreter and Mahtab. In this way, we suggest that the everyday processes which became pivotal in initiating our work described here created a platform both for working with 'the turning back' to the place of destruction and loss experienced by our clients and for addressing this with us through a focus on the 'everyday work of repair' (Das, 1998, p. 208 [13]). Because all three processes involved a form of action and therefore embodiment, this helped the emergence of images and symbols which were 'experience-near'. This is important because refugees and asylum seekers have frequently arrived from societies in which language and texts are not privileged over action, interaction and experience. We also consider, and this is somewhat supported by the work of mirror neuron theorists, that in these examples the embodied aspects of the everyday processes and experiences in themselves helped convey a domain open to mutual recognition, a 'we-centric space' [40], even if the meaning of it may not have been immediately accessible. The examples are therefore presented here as an articulation of a useful place to begin the work [41, 42]. In this sense, the ordinariness of everyday life activities, which resonated with us, provided a bridge to extraordinary events to which we, through this process, eventually had the possibility of becoming secondary witnesses. We could not by ourselves, and have still not been able to, facilitate protection from 'specific law and political convention' [2] in the form of 'rights to citizenship' or 'leave to remain' in the UK for our clients, and, together with many of our colleagues referred to earlier in this chapter, we wonder about the contradictions in Human Rights Law referred to by Arendt and the ensuing conflict between the workings of political, legal and mental health service structures and organisations. However, we could help to provide a contemporary space in which to keep on living.

Conclusion

We began this chapter by talking about ourselves as white and black women with personal and professional stories who have shared areas of similarity and areas of difference. In this, our awareness of the need to turn back to our own past ruptures has enabled us to sit with refugee (and other) families in the present and reminds us to go beyond the content of the therapy session and find our way to a 'turning back' that can help find a journey forward. We have spoken of what we consider our task, namely to help restore trust in the value of being human and the importance of not losing sight of 'the human condition' as a way of finding resonance between ourselves and our clients. This we have stated overtly in order to address the much more obscure tension with which refugees always have to engage – the tension between being human and being a particular human such as a refugee from a certain background and country, to which Hannah Arendt referred in the quote with which we began this chapter. For our clients, the ordinary everyday of the present becomes mixed up with extraordinary traumatic physical and relational experiences and ruptures in the past, so that each time something routine or ordinary happens there is a germ of possible associations with these other devastating experiences. Mental health work with refugees and asylum seekers is work in which violent ruptures of relationships, betrayal, displacement and loss loom large, and where ordinary everyday relationships in the present may be rendered extraordinary precisely because these past events and relationships exist as shadows or reminders of the past. It is this which needs to be revisited so that people can go on living in it or with it, not in the past but in the present without erasing the past and at the same time keeping the potentiality of the future. This is what we think the 'turning back' helps families to do.

With respect for the differences between ourselves and the differences between ourselves and our refugee clients, we place great store on the idea of 'the human condition' rather than on the more general notion of humanity. The 'human condition' refers to the most fundamental aspects of life and experience which we share with others without directing us to the specific meanings of these, which we may not share. In this we insist on and aim to strive for a position of comprehensive or radical reflexivity, which connects us and our clients to myriads of ordinary daily events and contexts. So when Rukiya talks of the sisters and the praying in the sessions, it resonates with important connections and unspeakable losses in the past, but the resonance presents a potential to revisit this past in a new way within a different relationship and in a new context. Through this almost literal 'turning back', new possibilities may emerge. Likewise, when Britt enquires about knitting, this resonates with the domestic scene which Mahtab and her children have left behind and which was ruptured several times over, but it also points to possibilities and connections for what might emerge in the future. In this way, reflexivity, which is the bedrock of all therapy, reminds us that there can be no stark separation between the present and the past, between the ordinary, which is routine and expected, and the extraordinary, which is not expected, or between therapy, which articulates what is shared, and politics, which for refugees and asylum seekers in the contemporary context seems to set store by what is not.

References

1. A. Arendt, We refugees. In M. Robinson, ed., *Altogether Elsewhere: Writers on Exile* (London: Faber and Faber, 1996), pp. 110–19.

2. A. Arendt, *The Human Condition* (Chicago, IL: University of Chicago Press, 1958).

3. J. Lechte, Rethinking Arendt's theory of necessity: Humanness as 'way of life', or: The ordinary as extraordinary. *Theory, Culture & Society*, 35(1) (2018), 3–22.

4. UNHCR: The UN Refugee Convention, (1951).

5. D. Fassin, Compassion and repression: The moral economy of immigration policies in France. *Cultural Anthropology*, 22(3) (2005) 362–87.

6. J. Morsink, *The Universal Declaration of Human Rights: Origins, Drafting and Intent* (Philadelphia, PA: University of Pennsylvania Press, 1999).

7. C. Watters, Refugees at Europe's borders: The moral economy of care. *Transcultural Psychiatry*, 44(7) (2007), 394–418.

8. G. Morgan, S. Melluish and A. Welham, Exploring the relationship between postmigratory stressors and mental health for asylum seekers and refused asylum seekers in the UK. *Transcultural Psychiatry*, 54(5–6) (2017), 653–74.

9. F. J. ter Heide, M. Sleijpen and N. van der Aa, Posttraumatic world assumptions among treatment-seeking refugees.

Transcultural Pscyhiatry, 54(5–6) (2017), 824–39.

10. E. V. Daniel and J. C. Knudsen, eds., *Mistrusting Refugees* (Berkeley, CA: University of California Press, 1995).

11. L. L. Kirmayer, Failures of imagination: The refugee's narrative in psychiatry. *Anthropology & Medicine*, 10(2) (2003), 167–87.

12. P. Rabinow and G. E. Marcus, *Designs for an Anthropology of the Contemporary* (Durham: Duke University Press, 2008).

13. V. Das, The act of witnessing: Violence, poisonous knowledge, and subjectivity. In V. Das, A. Kleinman, M. Ramphele and P. Reynolds, eds., *Violence and Subjectivity* (Berkeley, CA: University of California Press, 1998), pp. 205–25.

14. C. Nakeyar, V. Esses and G. J. Reid, The psychosocial needs of refugee children and youth and best practices for filling these needs: A systematic review. *Clinical Child Psychology and Psychiatry*, 22(2) (2017), 1–23.

15. T. Afuape and I.-B. Krause, eds., *Urban Child and Adolescent Mental Health Services: A Responsive Approach to Communities* (London: Karnac Books, 2016).

16. J. Burnham, Development in social grrraaacceeess: Visible-invisible and voiced-unvoiced. In I.-B. Krause, ed., *Culture and Reflexivity in Systemic*

Psychotherapy: Mutual Perspectives (London: Karnac Books, 2012), pp. 139–62.

17. R. Jemmott, Gender-gender identity-geography-race-religion-age-ability-appearance- class -culture, -caste, -education, -ethnicity –economics-spirituality – sexuality –sexual orientation –writ large on the wall. *Context*, (2017), 3–4.

18. I.-B. Krause, Cross-cultural psychotherapy and neoliberalism. In R. Littlewood and B. Abadio, eds., *2nd Intercultural Psychotherapy Volume* (London: Routledge, 2019).

19. Wittgenstein, 1953, para. 103, quoted in V. Das, The act of witnessing: Violence, poisonous knowledge, and subjectivity. In V. Das, A. Kleinman, M. Ramphele and P. Reynolds, eds., *Violence and Subjectivity* (Berkeley, CA: University of California Press, 1998), pp. 205–25.

20. G. Bateson, *Steps to an Ecology of Mind: Collected Essays in Anthropology, Psychiatry, Evolution and, Epistemology* (London: Jason Anronson, 1972).

21. I.-B. Krause, *Culture and System in Family Therapy* (London: Karnac Books, 2002).

22. P. Watzlawick, J. B. Bavelas and D. D. Jackson, *Pragmatics of Human Communication: A Study of Interactional Patterns, Pathologies and Paradoxes* (New York: W. W. Norton & Company, 1967).

23. P. Rober, The therapist's self in dialogical family therapy: Some ideas about not-knowing and the therapist's inner conversation. *Family Process*, 44 (2005), 477–95.

24. J. Seikkula, Dialogue is the change: Understanding psychotherapy as a semiotic process of Bakhtin, Voloshinov and Vygotsky. *Human Systems: The Journal of Systemic Consultation and Management*, 14(2) (2003), 83–94.

25. T. Andersen, The reflecting team: Dialogue and meta-dialogue in clinical work. *Family Process*, 26(4) (1987), 415–28.

26. J. Burnham, Relational reflexivity: A tool for socially constructing therapeutic relationships. In C. Flaskas, B. Mason and A. Perlesz, eds., *The Space Between: Experience, Context, and Process in the Therapeutic Relationship* (London: Karnac Books, 2005), pp. 1–17.

27. I.-B. Krause, *Culture and Reflexivity in Systemic Psychotherapy: Mutual Perspectives* (London: Karnac Books, 2012).

28. S. Ahmed, Declaration of whiteness: The non-performativity of anti-racism. *Borderlands*, 3(2) (2004). http://www.borderlands.net.au/vol3no2_2004/ahmed_declarations.htm

29. C. L. D'Arcangelis, Revelations of a white settler woman scholar–activist: The fraught promise of self-reflexivity. *Cultural Studies: Critical Methodologies*, 18(5) (2017), 1–15.

30. P. Rabinow and A. Stavrianakis, Movement space: Putting anthropological theory, concepts and cases to the test. *Hau: Journal of Ethnographic Theory*, 6(1) (2016), 403–31.

31. W. S. Pillow, Reflexivity as interpretation and genealogy in research. *Cultural Studies: Critical Methodologies*, 15(6) (2015), 419–34.

32. I.-B. Krause, The complexity of cultural competence. In F. Lowe, ed., *Thinking Space: Promoting Thinking about Race, Culture and Diversity in Psychotherapy and Beyond* (London: Karnac Books, 2014), pp. 109–26.

33. R. Papadopoulos, ed., *Therapeutic Care for Refugees: No Place like Home* (London: Karnac Books, 2002).

34. H. Kohut, *The Analysis of Self: A Systematic Approach to the Psychoanalysis of Narcissistic Personality Disorder* (New York: International Universities Press, 1971).

35. C. Geertz, From the native's point of view: On the nature of anthropological knowledge. *Bulletin of the American Arts & Sciences*, 28(1) (1974), 26–45.

36. T. May, *Gilles Deleuze: An Introduction* (Cambridge, UK: Cambridge University Press, 2005).

37. G. Deleuze and F. Guattari, *A Thousand Plateaus* (London: Continuum, 1987).

38. M. Strathern, The nice thing about culture is that everyone has it. In M. Strathern, ed., *Shifting Contexts: Transformations in Anthropological Knowledge* (London: Routledge, 1995), pp. 153–76.

39. M. Nichterlein and J. R. Morss, *Deleuze and Psychology: Philosophical Provocations to Psychological Practices* (London: Routledge, 2017).

40. V. Gallese, Intentional attunement: A neurophysiological perspective on social cognition and its disruption in autism. *Cognitive Brain Research*, 1079 (2006), 15–24.

41. R. Malik and I.-B. Krause, Before and beyond words: Embodiment and intercultural therapeutic relationships in family therapy. In C. Flaskas, B. Mason and A. Perlesz, eds., *The Space Between: Experience, Context and Process in the Therapeutic Relationship* (London: Karnac Books, 2005), pp. 95–110.

42. T. J. Csordas, *Body/Meaning/Healing* (Basingstoke: Palgrave Macmillan, 2002).

Re-building Trust and Connectedness in Exile

16

The Role of Health and Social Institutions

Radhika Santhanam-Martin

Introduction: Humans as Co-operative Breeders

The evolutionary biologist Sarah Blaffer Hrdy [1] describes us as co-operative breeders shaped by our ancient heritage of communal care: groups that need to look after each other in order to survive. Many traditional societies, mythically and metaphysically, emphasize the interconnectedness that groups need in order to survive, adapt, and transform. For example, Ubuntu philosophy, according to Tutu, speaks particularly to human connectedness and the fact that you cannot exist as a human being in isolation: 'I am human because I belong, I participate, I share' (1999, p. 31 [2]). Given the critical need for connection to a group and belonging to a group for our species since the late Pleistocene period, people across all walks of human endeavour strive to fulfil this communal need in order to feel safe and to develop security. The evolutionary origin of the human species' unusual capacity for intuiting intentions, learning from others, sharing resources, and communicating ideas has been established robustly. Humans use their language and symbolic culture to co-operate with each other. After they understand others as intentional agents like themselves, a world of intersubjectively shared reality opens up [3]. Here, in this 'intersubjective space', is where help or harm is performed. We learn to love each other and in the same way we learn to harm each other. When our individual passions are reflected in the larger group, it consolidates our intentions and also our prejudices, biases, and assumptions.

As the explicit sharing of intentional states became a powerful force in human communities, this shifted our relational and attachment capabilities. Our capacity to bond, to form attachments, and to develop relationships became primarily an intersubjective process. The evolutionary need for human beings to (en)act as co-operative breeders radically shifted the centre of our attachments and relationships to a collective space, be it for communities or groups or societies [4].

As Bruner [5] noted, this intersubjectivity became the corner stone for shared meanings: our cultural view of life depended upon shared meanings. Shared meanings within a cultural universe foster a sense of belonging and bring a connection that is rooted in time and history. Such a sense of belonging and connection underlies human resilience and potential for growth.

With these theoretical notions as the backdrop, this chapter explores how this need for connection and belonging may be enhanced or disrupted by health care institutions and services that support individuals and families seeking refuge. The focus of the chapter is on the intersubjective or relational space between families seeking refuge and institutions providing support. That is, how do interactions occur in a host society between institutions (such as health and educational service providers) and families who have lost these relational spaces? This chapter builds on the evidence (research- and practice-based) that re-building trust and social connectedness by services and institutions are critical components for trauma reduction while working with refugee families who have suffered profound and complicated losses of human relatedness.

The Refugee Experience: Examining the Role of Institutions in the Resettlement Process

The published body of evidence in refugee research highlights a range of pre-migration, migration, and post-migration factors that affect the well-being and mental health of refugee adults and children [6–15].

Refugees are people who, as individuals or as families, are displaced, exiled, or coerced to move from their home country. As individuals and as families, they are displaced and separated from their homelands, their communal groups, their social environments, and their ecological roots. Typically, these families have lost all support that civic institutions and social/community services provided for them in their homelands. Most of these families have witnessed or experienced organized violence that has torn at the heart of communities, causing 'the destruction of human connectedness' [16] and disrupting the most primary communal ties within the family and social fabric [17–22].

This chapter is concerned with this particular experience of the destruction of human connectedness and with how connectedness may be either re-built or further weakened by the interactions that occur between refugees and institutions in host countries.

For refugee individuals and families, losses refer not only to safety, protection, and predictability but also to deep relational losses of extended families, communities, neigh-bourhoods, and networks. It is a web of interwoven connections that gets lost. And in some cases, the social and cultural fabric itself may have been the cause of violence, further complicating the process of building human connections. In this period of profound transition, families have to re-create, re-imagine, and re-connect with a new set of people, places, and spaces. It is during this transition time, where continuities have been disrupted in a tumultuous way, that refugee families and individuals come into contact with health care institutions and social and community organizations in host societies. How does the refugee experience impact upon the basic human capacities of intersubjectivity and belong-ing and influence the relational dynamics in exile? Particularly, how does the refugee experience and its destruction of human connectedness impact on interactive patterns with service providers?

Judith Herman [23] has cautioned that although traumatic experiences cannot be compared, in each event the salient characteristic that emerges is the traumatic predica-ment's power to inspire helplessness and terror. For refugee families who are fleeing brutal regimes or devastating catastrophe, this results not only in serious physical injury but also in failure to protect one's beloved family, friends, and community. Life histories of people who live in and with collective terror indicate that they use several strategies to cope with everyday collective violence that is impacting on their families' well-being. Although often seen as maladaptive or pathological (e.g., silence, denial, fragmentation, dis-association), some of these strategies may be highly adaptive and helpful in times of terror and intimidation, serving to protect or preserve the family's or individual's survival or the body's dignity [24]. These are valid and legitimate strategies even if they are seen as less relevant or pathogenic, or even pathological, by service providers in the host society context. These strategies validate the refugee's shattered worldview and world assumptions of what suffering humans are capable of inflicting on each other [25].

Another relational pattern in some refugee individuals and families is the loss of knowledge and memory of community engagement and practices of solidarity between community members. In some instances, transgenerational active engagements with community environs have been broken. The collective memory of community practices, when eroded, makes the family feel as if they don't have the capacity to engage with their community. This may be due to the fact that when a particular ethnicity gets targeted in a country, the collective memory and stories of community practices (be they rituals, rites, negotiations, mediation, etc.) gets obliterated and the community may get disempowered for generations (e.g., Hazaras from Afghanistan or Rohingyas from Myanmar). Or alternatively, as a group, members of a community in a new context may not be able to strengthen or build on available community resources as they still feel unable to trust each other and feel safe with each other. In these scenarios, it is critical for host society institutions to have a mature and moderating lens.

Sometimes, institutions and service providers that represent the host society perceive refugee communities in a dichotomy of 'all victims' or 'all survivors', generalizing their predicament into a 'one size fits all'. These kinds of assumptions do not do justice to the strengths that people bring and the resilience that they have but which they are unable to remember and re-connect with. This may lead to a context of learned helplessness or, worse, a form of self-affirming prophecy where communities and families become deeply dependent with no sense of agency or self-determination.

In the initial phase of resettlement, displaced communities that carry a history of collective violence (either as witnesses, forced participants, co-opted participants, or victims) come into direct contact with health care institutions (public, private, and community organizations) that shape and mould the host society experiences for the displaced refugee families. Indeed, two major sectors that are involved with these families are the health and welfare sectors (excluding the asylum-seeking process, where immigration policies and the legal sector play a dominant role). These places and spaces – that is, health and welfare institutions – are culture-bearing entities and they bring with them established rules, procedures, and protocols of relating and engagement. In the health and welfare system, the network of professionals – including, for example, medical professionals, counsellors, school and child welfare workers, and church/faith leaders – functions like a small community with its own set of rules and norms. When this network (a plethora of support workers) comes into contact with the family to offer supportive interventions, this interface mirrors the encounter between two networks of systems, each bringing their collective norms to bear upon the other.

From the perspective of such intersecting dynamics, we explore how health care systems connect or fail to connect with family systems. What processes help and hinder? How do these systems come to trust each other to give and to seek help? What could be the costs of distrust and disengagement for the families in a new country? And what would a sense of re-connection, trust, and belonging mean for the families in the host society? Here, we argue that systems that come to engage the refugee family can re-build social connectedness (and pathways that may lead to trust and safety) for the family. Alternately, systems can increase the sense of isolation and marginalization by not building social connections and not strengthening community networks, thus creating pathways that may lead to alienation, suspicion, and mistrust.

Health Care Services as Extended Networks of Support

Health care institutions and service providers quite often and quite naturally become extended networks of support for refugees in exile. For the individual who is seeking support, the services are an addition to the family or a substitute for the family. For the families seeking support, the services are in addition to or a replacement for close-knit community support. For example, a school teacher becomes a mentor, a swimming coach becomes the family's go-to for advice, the general practitioner becomes the 'trusted elder' for diverse issues, the counsellor becomes a 'big sister' in family functions, the youth worker is the first person to be called during any crisis, and so on. This process is also reflective of how families would have structured and mobilized their support networks and help-seeking pathways through extended family and close kinship ties in their home societies (from which they are now disconnected geographically and emotionally). The therapeutic players now become crucial anchor points for the refugee family in trying to navigate and negotiate the cultural references in the new country. This dynamic, with all its challenges, is the pathway that restores interconnectedness in the new social and cultural milieu. These therapeutic spaces act as an antidote to individuals' or families' sense of social isolation and alienation in the new country. Often, practitioners hear phrases such as 'You are like a family here, for us,' 'You are the only family we have here,' 'I wanted to share this good news with you, as you are like my family.' These statements are often balancing acts. That is, they are the individual's or the family's attempts to renew social bonds that have been lost from the old world and that need renewal in the new world. And when the connectedness occurs between service providers and families, it can function as a form of relational repair. The empathic failure that resulted from the destruction of human connectedness in the past has had an opportunity to restore and transform into faith in human encounters.

Alternately, the opportunity is also wide open for further disconnections. That is, these processes could also result in a reiteration of disrupted and displaced attachments. For example, it is equally common for practitioners to hear phrases like, 'Well, you are not any different to people back home. No one really wants to help,' 'Nothing really changes – things are the same where we are and where we came from,' 'God couldn't help me back then, why would he help me now?' and 'You will never be able to understand.' The human encounters are marred by entrenched patterns of disconnections and mistrust that result in utter hopelessness and deep despair.

At this juncture, it needs to be highlighted that these processes can become mirrored in intra-institutional and team dynamics, resulting in what has been called in the literature a 'parallel process' [26]. Of particular interest here are the political and social histories that are carried by service providers and practitioners working in mental health services. The service providers, just like refugee families, are not 'one size fits all'. They carry within them a diverse range of childhood and family experiences and, further, have wide-ranging political and historical influences. Thus, service providers can unwittingly or inadvertently repeat patterns of their own personal dynamics or professional histories in therapeutic relationships with refugee families. These parallel processes then become imbued with the risk of reiterating the rupture of relational stances or attachment bonds that has occurred in the past. Safety is a relational experience, be it for the displaced refugee or the distressed worker. Thus, service providers and institutions can come close to re-enacting the patterns of traumatic experiences that families have fled from. Systems that control and monitor their workers in punitive ways (e.g., excessive work hours demands, unreasonable expectations, inconsistent enforcement of trivial demands, micromanagement of workers, protocols and rules enforced without any flexibility, belittling workers and their practices, lacking in compassion, shutting down dialogical processes) give rise to a workforce that models similar punitive control of therapeutic spaces with families.

In addition, in the same societal space, refugees are under the authority of the institutions in charge of their migratory process, which first and foremost have the objective to control and securitize them. The families thus confront very different mandates in the host country institutions, some of which are trying to re-build trust while others are trying to reiterate suspicion and doubt. These distinct and contradictory mandates and agendas generate further confusion and distrust for the refugee. They may equally play a major role in punitive undercurrents of stereotyped or prejudiced institutional interpretations of refugee behaviours or actions. For example, in a recent consultation, a refugee mother was questioned by the government welfare agency that was providing some financial assistance with regard to their electricity bill. The agency staff questioned the mother about the use of electricity during the night, 'as this is paid by public money', while the mother accounted for this by stating her ongoing (quasi-paranoid) fear at night after a history of severe persecution. These dialogues that border on micro-oppressions echo broader social narratives that create suspicion, mistrust, and disconnection between marginalized communities and dominant systems. There is genuine concern under these circumstances that the bonding that may occur between these two sub-systems (a traumatized system and the traumatized family) carries the cluster of borderline traits across individuals and institutions. When this occurs, the patterns of splitting, triangulation, and disorganized communication become the norm.

First Vignette

K., a 42-year-old man of Kurdish background with a severe torture and trauma history, in detention camp for 2 years, develops a lung infection. He is flown to mainland Australia and becomes part of the cohort of community detention, the group of people detained in the community [27]. He is offered services by health and social care providers. The professional teams that get involved include clinical respiratory teams, a resettlement agency worker, a private counsellor, a torture and trauma service therapist, a clinical mental health nurse, a voluntary NGO worker, a support person from K.'s community, and an after-hours telephone crisis service worker. These workers, from the beginning, organize clear communication and role definition and discuss how best to add value to each other's functions. The workers rally around K.'s needs and inform each other regularly in writing of their individual efforts. The care team meets once every 6–8 weeks, exchanges updates, and plans the next steps.

At one point, as K.'s well-being significantly deteriorates (initially his lung functions, which then lead to psychosocial functions), the care team decides to have a weekly contact roster for K. That is, K. meets at least two workers each week, one at the beginning and one at the end of the week. This structure is different to the earlier structure, where K. had no contact from services some weeks but had three or four service contacts in another week. It is agreed at the care team meeting that, given the crisis, a regular, frequent, and predictable 'holding' space is needed for K. Consequently, the consensus is reached that K. will have contact with two workers each week who will gently monitor him and provide supportive spaces. This decision is considered by the care team to be better than emergency admission, crisis team referral, or an increase in anti-anxiety or anti-depressant medications. The reasoning by the care team is that K.'s fragility is due to external policy changes that have increased his vulnerability and thus he is in need of more support and safe holding. After eight months of sustaining this support structure, the situation gradually improves, and K. feels safer and relatively more secure in his well-being.

In this vignette, the way in which the care team created a circle of care around this vulnerable man is very similar to how extended families function, where people take on roles and organize each other's efforts to build up or care for a vulnerable member of the family. For this to work in a truly empowering way (both for the individual and for the system), a few critical elements are needed. From the above example, one can draw out a few of these: (a) to have clear communication, (b) to have regular, frequent communication, (c) to have clarity in roles and structures, (d) to not compete with each other in trying to 'outdo' one another; that is, to stay in the collective space, and (e) to keep the focus on the vulnerable individual and their needs rather than on the system's power (or the worker's pride/ego).

Second Vignette

A 30-year-old father and his 5-year-old son, who had fled persecution in their homeland, were seeking asylum. A range of services were providing support at different levels for social, psychological, and emotional needs: the housing service, the day care service, the torture and trauma counselling service, NGOs in the suburb, church pastors, a psychiatrist, community liaison officers, child protection officers, and a legal team.

The political history of this family was remarkably complex. There were many gaps in the narrative and the stories shifted often. There was never a linear, coherent account of what their past experiences were and what the sequence of events had been that led to their fleeing.

When services started working with the father-son dyad, there was a lot of trust and connection between services. There was also a fair amount of expectation for the family (father and son) and what changes the services could bring about. And in care team meetings there was a language of hope and empathy when the problems and difficulties faced by the dyad were discussed.

As time went by, the system started to grow perceptibly weary, largely due to an apparent lack of change in the dyad's presentation. There were a few plans that were implemented and some that fell by the wayside. The dyad was consistently engaged with the services, but no appreciable change occurred. For example, kindergarten attendance did not improve as expected; the father's weight, which was a concern for the medical team, did not improve with dietary interventions; the housing crisis continued as the dyad was unable to stay secure in one location; despite the dyad's co-operative engagement, finding community support was becoming harder; the pastor from the church felt that the dyad was shy and reserved and did not take up the community's offers of socialization and support.

As this continued, the service providers' narratives gradually started changing. Services started seeing the dyad as untrustworthy and un-co-operative. Even though there was no particular incident or evidence of untrustworthiness or lack of co-operation, service providers' frames of understanding gradually shifted towards less and less empathy and began leaning towards despair for themselves and anger towards the dyad. The very behaviour or actions (e.g., being reserved and not opening up, being less assertive) that had been seen in a generous, compassionate way early on were now scrutinized as evidencing secretiveness, defiance, and sabotage. The care team meetings took on a tone of resentment and contempt for the lack of drive shown by the dyad. Services slowly disconnected from the dyad, leaving the father and son with fewer and fewer networks and connections.

In this vignette, the service systems carried elements of both a re-building (repair) and a re-breaking (rupture) of connections. However, both the repair and rupture processes were underlined by the implicit assumption that help-seeking and help-giving are enacted around a polarized alliance which is perceived as either good or bad. That is, services either trust you or mistrust you. Services either hold hope for you or they don't. There is no process where both of these could co-exist: where services could hold hope for the client sometimes and despair at other times. Ambivalence, which requires that service providers accept being at times bad enough and at other times good enough, seems to have no place. And the awareness that violence is inherent in binaries of any sort is crucially missed. This 'all or nothing' view is not just the domain of professional teams. This dichotomous view of professionals 'all helping' or 'not helping at all' may be a lived and voiced reality for refugees as well, both in relation to service provision and in relation to broader societies. However, what was striking in this scenario as it played out was how the members of the dyad held and balanced multiple complex positionings in their everyday life. For example, the father would speak simply of how difficult housing is in suburban areas, without blaming any service; the dyad would compare an earlier life of trauma to current everyday struggles in an even manner without implicating any one country. When services are confronted with seemingly inconsistent narratives, the first attempt is to restore order or a certain 'truth' to the situation. For example, when the dyad went missing for a few weeks and, on return, did not give a 'convincing' story for the absence, the services found it impossible not to judge the veracity of the story provided and in fact came to doubt all the earlier stories. The naive assumption, or even yearning to see, that human suffering is linear, unambiguous, and not an experience full of contradictions, paradoxes, and absurdities is striking in service providers and in the systems they work in.

Service providers, understandably, are informed by reading patterns in vulnerable families with which they have come into contact in the past, or indeed by their own vulnerable family histories, and these inform their current understanding of experiences of displacement and suffering. In this context, a service provider or a service system can take on the role of the benevolent (or omnipotent) healer while exclusively locating trauma-related isolation or distress in the client space. To illustrate this point, in the second vignette, the institutional system positioned itself as the 'knowing' system. This kind of positioning or locating one knowledge against other forms of knowledge creates an ethical minefield. Is there 'one knowledge' for healing, or are there multiple ways of knowing? If we accommodate the view that there are multiple ways of 'knowing' and multiple ways of 'doing', then healing spaces also become multiple. Therapeutic impasses usually operate around the breakdown of trust between service providers who embody different knowledge paradigms and, consequently, differing belief systems on recovery and healing. This then resonates with the collective violence or harsh political oppressions that caused the original displacement (in the home context) for the refugee families. Further, it draws a parallel to the limits of understanding by the larger system that then brings about a breakdown in trust in interactions with any system/institution.

How, then, are practitioners to develop and reflect on 'balanced or nuanced relational stances [28] that embody divergent knowledge positions and complicated socio-political views in their everyday practice? How do practitioners balance the fine line between restoring or disrupting social connectedness in the post-trauma reconstruction without repeating the past patterns of tyranny? What therapeutic orientations support trauma reconstruction that restores balance in the system while creating a sense of connection and trust for the practitioner? In the next and final section, I will highlight a few principles that attempt to address these questions.

Restoring or Reiterating the Disruption of Social Bonds: Therapeutic Perspectives to Consider

I would like to consider some critical themes for reflection, for systems and service providers, when working with refugee families in post-trauma work. The goal of these reflections is to shift the responsibility of re-building or restoring trust and connectedness for refugee families to institutions and service systems. A space needs to be created for institutions and systems to develop practices that can enable relationship-building between professionals and families. Here, a trauma-informed framework is useful both for systems and for clients. Be it service providers or refugee individuals, experiences that invalidate and undermine people's sense of worth re-create traumatic impact [29]. Hence, having a trauma-informed lens while working with systems is a crucial first step, primarily operating from within the framework of 'safety, stability and structure' between service providers, in the way they co-operate, collaborate, and witness each other's strengths and struggles. The impact of this kind of approach or framework on the individual worker and/or the institution could be transformative.

I would like to highlight five practice frameworks that are trauma-informed while working with institutions and services that come together to provide care for a vulnerable family or an individual from a refugee background.

Holding Environment

This concept is borrowed from Winnicott [30] and his use of a 'facilitating environment'. An environment is facilitating when complex factors in that particular environment are made visible and 'held or contained'. Holding simultaneously dual or plural perspectives creates tension or fragility. Yet this kind of fragile holding is critical to containing spaces that are filled with uncertainty, instability, and sometimes fear. The process of holding becomes enabling rather than disabling, even if it is precarious. The goal of this process is not to fix or find solutions but to facilitate a relational containment. What I mean by relational containment is this: in a multi-system negotiation of care, practitioners with different power dynamics ought to embody and enact containment and not create more anxiety and despair. A holding environment is one that is not overwhelmed by an internal process that mimics the external process and that is cognizant of and able to separate the two – internal versus external. Illustrating a failure to create a holding environment is the despair or outrage that arises due to harsh governmental refugee policies and that gets projected as hopelessness and rage between and within teams providing services for the well-being of refugees.

Witnessing Struggles

Systems work best when they are compassionate and generous to each other. This does not mean that stakeholders agree on every aspect of intervention or supportive care. What this implies is that systems are able to witness each other's struggles: practitioners are able to acknowledge and honour the efforts of their peers or other service providers who are working with multiple constraints within their structures. Witnessing is a profound way of connecting where the practice of exclusion is not tolerated and the practice of inclusion is intentionally practised. For example, a young person in the refugee minor program, with the help of his trauma counsellor, wrote a therapeutic letter of thanks to the child protection team for giving their 'best shot' even though the outcome was not in his favour.

Imperfect Allies: Good Enough Peers

Winnicott's [31] legendary notion of 'good enough' and Reynolds's [32] concept of imperfect solidarity are vital perspectives for systemic work. We are all witnesses to each other's fragilities and vulnerabilities as much as we are to each other's triumphs. Reynolds highlights the need to make repair for our failures as allies or as constructive partners in creating cultures of critique and thereby resisting practices of attack, splitting, or triangulation. Building solidarity comes from knowing that our processes are flawed and our values are imperfect, which can then allow for 'good enough' connections and 'agreeable' alliances across time. For example, sitting in the room supporting the client who is being interviewed by the immigration detention officer makes all actors in the room culpable to varying degrees [27].

The Need for Critical Reflection to Address Rupture and Repair in Therapeutic Work

Bringing the dynamic of rupture and repair to the fore in therapeutic encounters is critical, as it informs the core dynamics of traumatic experiences and their aftermath. Exile stories are filled with ruptures, and families have escaped regimes that both protected and terrorized; governments that both helped and controlled. For clients to come into contact with systems that support and surveil may have a strong resonance with their past experiences. Practitioners in institutions need to create a dialogical space that brings forth this predicament: the quandary of systems that simultaneously control and care; of institutional routines that monitor and care, that provide agency and pose restrictions. These practices are best developed in reflective supervision, collectively or individually. In order to learn how to acknowledge and address ruptures (and repeated ruptures may well come to represent empathic failures), it is essential to develop a peer reflective intervision (supervision between peers) process. Without providing reflective dialogical spaces for workers, it is extremely difficult to acknowledge and/or address empathic failures in practice [33].

As defined by Fook and Askeland [34], critical reflection involves the identification of deep-seated assumptions, but with the primary purpose of bringing about some improvements in professional everyday practice. According to them, 'critical reflection must incorporate an understanding of personal experiences within social, cultural and structural contexts'. To illustrate an example, a therapist decides not to use an interpreter based on the client's request but fails to explore this further with the client, as it reminds her of her grandparents who similarly insisted on not using their language while talking about trauma. This resulted in very little progress in therapy for the client, as he was unable to use adequate English. Thus, reflective dialogue is one way to encourage or nurture collective accountability; to holdeach of us responsible for our actions and inactions.

Critical reflective sessions enable the creation of 'aspect-dawning' moments. According to Havercroft and Owen [35], aspect dawning – a concept first espoused by Wittgenstein – is forced from us: it arises from experience in the same way as a cry arises in response to pain (e.g., now I see! Aha, this is a new thing that I see!). This noticing or recognizing of the interconnection between experiences (be it by service providers or by families) and histories, between context and everyday reality, opens up a new space, a new perspective, and a new way of 'knowing more' of something that was hitherto familiar.

Here, it is important to acknowledge that these processes of collective accountability and ethical conversations are in direct opposition to the culture of individualism and work as a private activity, according to which our successes and failures are due to individual heroism or impotence.

A Sense of Humility

A sense of humility is interlinked with ethical reflections. Our professional cultures look down on self-doubt and self-disclosure. Workers who try to be critically reflective could easily become the targets of the mainstream culture of experts and competency. Humility brings with it an acknowledgement of 'not knowing'. It also brings with it the unknown and the unknowable in human experiences – what Rebecca Solnit calls 'the strange circuitous routes to what actually comes next' [36]. Valuing multiple perspectives leads us to appreciate diverse beliefs and a plurality of opinions in a way that opens our world to contradictions. And in valuing contradictions we are questioning the paradigm of knowledge that values certainty above all. Brookfield [37] speaks of this in critical reflection when he writes, 'an intellectual appreciation of the importance of contextuality and ambiguity comes to exist alongside the emotional craving for revealed truth'. He calls this phenomenon 'lost innocence'. I call it also 'discovering humility'. If we allow for this humility to be celebrated, might we then create the space for 'certain forms of perplexity' [38] to be embodied in our practices?

Conclusion

Reducing the impact of trauma is a key objective for services and institutions striving to provide resettlement support for refugees. If this objective is to be served to any degree, then it becomes an imperative for health and welfare services to be able to re-build trust and connectedness for and with refugee families. Without blaming or pathologizing families or institutional systems, we need frameworks and practices in institutions that can build trust and connectedness in exile. These are rarely straightforward. These are practices of kindness that are complicated and demanding. However, it is this delicate web of relational interdependence that has helped us to survive and thrive as a human community and as a species.

References

1. S. B. Hrdy, *Mothers and Others: The Evolutionary Origins of Mutual Understanding* (Cambridge, MA: Harvard University Press, 2009).

2. D. Tutu, *No Future without Forgiveness* (New York: Random House, 1999).

3. M. Tomasello, *The Cultural Origins of Human Cognition* (Cambridge, MA: Harvard University Press, 1999).

4. K. H. Hennighausen and K. Lyons-Ruth, Disorganisation of behavioural and attentional strategies toward primary attachment figures: From biologic to dialogic processes. In C. S. Carter, L. Ahnert, K. E. Grossmann, S. B. Hrdy, M. E. Lamb, S. W. Porges et al., eds., *Attachment and Bonding: The New Synthesis* (Cambridge, MA: MIT Press, 2005), pp. 269–99.

5. J. Bruner, *The Culture of Education* (Cambridge, MA: Harvard University Press, 1996).

6. K. E. Miller and L. M. Rasco, eds., *The Mental Health of Refugees: Ecological Approaches to Healing and Adaptation* (London: Laurence Erlbaum Associates, 2004).

7. M. Porter and N. Haslam, Predisplacement and postdisplacement factors associated with mental health of refugees and internally displaced persons: A meta-analysis. *Journal of the American Medical Association*, 294(5) (2005), 602–12.

8. R. Schweitzer, F. Melville, Z. Steel and P. Lacherez, Trauma, post-migration living difficulties, and social support as predictors of psychological adjustment in resettled Sudanese refugees. *Australian and New Zealand Journal of Psychiatry*, 40(2) (2006), 179–87.

9. T. Stompe, D. Holzer and A. Friedmann, Pre-migration and mental health of refugees. In D. Bhugra, T. Craig and K. Bhui, eds., *Mental Health of Refugees and Asylum Seekers* (Oxford: Oxford University Press, 2010), pp. 23–38.

10. H. Hermann, I. Kaplan and J. Szwarc, Post-migration and mental health in Australia. In D. Bhugra, T. Craig and K. Bhui, eds., *Mental Health of Refugees and Asylum Seekers* (Oxford: Oxford University Press, 2010), pp. 39–60.

11. D. Silove, The ADAPT model: A conceptual framework for mental health and psychosocial programming in post conflict settings. *Intervention*, 11(3) (2013), 237–48.

12. T. Measham, J. Guzder, C. Rousseau, L. Pacione, M. Blais-McPherson and L. Nadeau, Refugee children and their families: Supporting psychological well-being and positive adaptation following migration. *Current Problems in Pediatric & Adolescent Health Care*, 44(7) (2014), 208–15.

13. T. Puvimanasinghe, L. Denson, M. Augoustinos, and D. Somasundaram, Narrative and silence: How former refugees talk about loss and past trauma. *Journal of Refugee Studies*, 28(1) (2015), 69–92.

14. R. Kronick and C. Rousseau, Rights, compassion and invisible children: A critical discourse analysis of the parliamentary debates on the mandatory detention of migrant children in Canada. *Journal of Refugee Studies*, 28(4) (2015), 505–22.

15. M. Valibhoy, I. Kaplan and J. Szwarc, 'It comes down to just how human someone can be': A qualitative study with young people from refugee backgrounds about their experiences of Australian mental health services. *Transcultural Psychiatry*, 54(1) (2017), 23–45.

16. J. Herman, *Trauma and Recovery* (New York: Basic Books, 1997).

17. J. Garbarino, An ecological perspective on the effects of violence on children. *Journal of Community Psychology*, 29(3) (2001), 361–78.

18. D. Summerfield, Effects of war: Moral knowledge, revenge, reconciliation, and medicalised concepts of 'recovery'. *British Medical Journal*, 325 (2002), 1105–7.

19. R. J. Lifton, Destroying the world to save it. In B. Drozdek and J. P. Wilson, eds., *Voices of Trauma: Treating Psychological Trauma across Cultures* (New York: Springer, 2011), pp. 59–86.

20. M. H. Khalil, Access denied: Institutional barriers to justice for victims of torture in Egypt. *Torture*, 23(1) (2013), 28–46.

21. I. Agger, Calming the mind: Healing after mass atrocity in Cambodia. *Transcultural Psychiatry*, 52(4) (2015), 543–60.

22. P. Gobodo-Madikizela, *What Does It Mean To Be Human in the Aftermath of Historical Trauma? Re-envisioning 'The Sunflower' and Why Hannah Arendt was Wrong* (Uppsala: The Nordic Africa Institute and Uppsala University, 2016).

23. J. Herman, Complex PTSD: A syndrome in survivors of prolonged and repeated trauma. *Journal of Traumatic Stress*, 5(3) (1992), 377–91.

24. C. Rousseau and T. Measham, Posttraumatic suffering as a source of transformation: A clinical perspective. In L. Kirmayer and R. Lemelson, eds., *Understanding Trauma: Integrating Biological, Clinical and Cultural Perspectives* (New York: Cambridge University Press, 2007), pp. 275–91.

25. F. J. ter Heide, M. Sleijpen and N. van der Aa, Posttraumatic world assumptions among treatment-seeking refugees. *Transcultural Psychiatry*, 54(5–6) (2017), 824–29.

26. L. S. Bloom, Trauma-organized systems and parallel process. In N. Tehrani, ed., *Managing Trauma in the Workplace: Supporting Workers and Organizations* (London: Routledge, 2010), pp. 139–53.

27. Refugee Council of Australia, (2016), *Australia's Detention Policies*. Accessed on September 30, 2019. www .refugeecouncil.org.au/getfacts/seekingsaf ety/asylum/detention/key-facts/

28. C. Rousseau, J. Guzder, R. Santhanam-Martin and E. de la Aldea, Trauma, culture, and clinical work: The 'House of Stories' as a pedagogical approach to transcultural training. *Traumatology*, 20 (3) (2014), 191–8.

29. J. Herman, Justice from the victim's perspective. *Violence Against Women*, 11 (5) (2005), 571–2.

30. D. W. Winnicott, The maturational processes and the facilitating environment: Studies in the theory of emotional development. *The International Psycho-Analytical Library*, 64 (1965), 1–276.

31. D. W. Winnicott, The theory of the parent-infant relationship. *International Journal of Psychoanalysis*, 41 (1960), 585–95.

32. V. Reynolds, Fluid and imperfect ally positioning: Some gifts of queer theory. *Context*, 111 (2010), 13–17.

33. T. Ghaye, A. Melander-Wikman and M. Kisare, Participatory and appreciative action and reflection (PAAR): Democratizing reflective practices. *Reflective Practice: International and Multidisciplinary Perspectives*, 9(4) (2008), 361–97.

34. J. Fook and A. Askeland, Challenges of critical reflection: 'Nothing ventured, nothing gained'. *Social Work Education: The International Journal*, 26(5) (2007), 520–33.

35. J. Havercroft and D. Owen, Soul-blindness, police orders and Black Lives Matter: Wittgenstein, Cavell, and Rancière. *Political Theory*, 44(6) (2016), 739–63.

36. R. Solnit, *Hope in the Dark: Untold Histories and Wild Possibilities* (Edinburgh: Canongate Books, 2016).

37. S. Brookfield, Tales from the dark side: A phenomenography of adult critical reflection. *International Journal of Lifelong Education*, 13(3) (1994), 203–16.

38. T. Nagel, *The View from Nowhere* (Oxford: Oxford University Press, 1986).

Family-School Relationships in Supporting Refugee Children's School Trajectories

Mina Fazel and Aoife O'Higgins

Refugee Families and Schools

Schools play an important role in supporting a positive post-migration experience for refugee children and their families [1–4]. Across the world, schools provide a system of instruction and care for children and families, although with great variation in how schools function and where they are located [5, 6]. The differences across schools can include how large the class sizes are, the staff-to-pupil ratio and mix, the opportunities for staff to receive additional support and training, the curricula and extra-curricular activities that are offered, the extra learning support that might be available, the school's theoretical and organisational philosophies, the populations they serve and their approach to broader family and community engagement.

In considering the needs of refugee families entering the context of resettlement, schools are often one of the first institutions that they, as a family, might have contact with. Children can sometimes be placed relatively quickly into schools in order to try to provide some structure and a system of support around them and their learning. How this is done, however, is important, especially when considering the potential vulnerability of some of the forcibly displaced families, especially those that have been exposed to trauma. The first section of this chapter discusses the barriers to accessing education. Second, we focus on the importance and complexity of comprehensive assessments of the learning needs of children. Third, we review specific educational interventions and highlight some mental health approaches that have been tried in schools to support refugee children and families. Indeed, alongside potentially poor educational literacy amongst refugee families, there is often equally poor mental health literacy in refugee populations, exacerbated by different health care and belief systems, as mental illness is highly stigmatised in many cultures across the globe [7]. In each section, we consider the perspective of the school, the family and the child. This multidimensional approach is represented in Figure 17.1. In high-income countries, schools can provide a bridge to psychosocial and mental health provision, further amplifying the role of the school as a space for social support and integration and thus highlighting the importance of facilitating for refugee children better engagement with school.

Barriers to Accessing Education and Quality of Provision of Education

Enrolling children in schools is one of the first tasks that newly arrived families will carry out on arrival in a host country. However, accessing schools and ensuring that their children

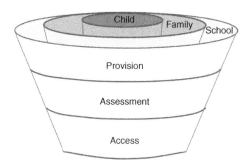

17.1 Key responsibilities of schools for refugee families

benefit from the appropriate educational provision may, for refugee parents, be fraught with difficulties from the outset. Characteristics or circumstances of the children or their families may make accessing school challenging, but schools also play an important role in facilitating, as well as impeding, access to their provision and programmes. This section draws on findings from recent research to describe these barriers from the perspective of the school, the family and the child [8–11].

Schools are key to facilitating access to their provision and programmes. In the first instance, schools and their administrations should be easy to locate and contact, whether in person, over the phone or online. In some areas, however, admissions are managed centrally by local or regional administrative bodies. Some schools also have strict admission criteria, which may not be immediately available or comprehensible to newly arrived refugee families. How and where this information is obtained and how the admission process is managed are likely to vary by locality within and across host countries. Refugee families often lack access to this information and may encounter additional barriers if they do not speak the host language, use current technology and lack support to engage with the admissions process [8, 11, 12]. While many schools and local authorities aim to provide simple and clear information, this is rarely offered in other languages. Many refugee families also arrive in the host country in the middle of a school cycle, so schools may be full or refuse access to newly arrived children [8, 11]. The majority of refugee families arriving in high-income countries also have limited financial means and are more likely to live in areas of high deprivation. These neighbourhoods also tend to have lower-resourced and therefore lower-performing schools, which as a result are more likely to be less popular by local standards and hence might not be at capacity [13]. If refugees happen to live in higher socio-economic status neighbourhoods, schools may well be full and less experienced at catering for newly arrived children arriving at non-traditional points of entry. Families can appeal schools' decisions to refuse access to children, but this can be cumbersome and often requires resources and knowledge of the administrative system. Finally, a school's culture and ethos are important to facilitating access to refugee families [10]. The role that schools play in the lives of children and families, and in the community, varies widely across cultures; when schools are sensitive to this and have practices in place to support the transition into the new context, smoother access can be facilitated.

While refugee families will be impacted by the barriers some schools put up to accessing education, their unique circumstances and experiences may also make finding suitable provision for their children a challenge. Language and cultural barriers make communication with schools and local administration difficult. Some families may also choose not to disclose their immigration status for fear of discrimination and stigma, meaning that schools are unable to provide appropriate support [14]. Parents may also suffer from mental health problems, including post-traumatic stress disorder (PTSD), which may impinge on their ability and confidence to carry out important tasks such as communicating effectively to advocate for their needs with the school and local authorities, attending appointments or providing information about the family's past and present circumstances [12].

Children's individual circumstances may make access to school and quality provision more or less of a challenge. First, a child's age has been shown to affect the ease with which they assimilate into the host culture and school context. Younger children may find the integration task easier than adolescents, who might face a raft of other social, emotional and educational difficulties [15]. Second, children may acquire the host language relatively fast, and in some cases sooner than their parents, meaning that they effectively play the role of a linguistic and cultural interpreter, and in some cases that of a proxy carer for other family members [9]. This may contribute to their resilience but might place children in a complex position which can affect their subsequent relationships and interactions with schools, teachers and other social services as well as their peers.

Finally, refugee children may experience significant mental health difficulties as a result of their exposure to organised violence and conflict or because they have witnessed acts of violence against family members. While school may play a role in stabilising and normalising through increasing structure, significant mental health difficulties, and trauma in particular, can impede language acquisition and learning [16]. Peers play an important role in the lives of children, and past research has shown that children's social adjustment is influenced by the quality of their peer relationships [4, 17]. As school is often the main locus of children's social worlds, refugee children must be provided with sufficient support and opportunity to develop those important relationships. Finally, as with their families, children's cultural backgrounds and values will impact on their interactions with schools and teachers. For example, where children in the USA are expected to be collaborative and independent learners, children from Asian countries, like Cambodia, are likely to be unaccustomed to this, leading to reports of increased misunderstandings or being misunderstood by their teachers and peers [9]. This can have important negative consequences for learning, socialising and acclimatising to the school context.

A Broad-Based Assessment of Refugee Children in School Settings

In order to determine what the learning needs of refugee children are and to identify high-quality educational provision, a broad-based assessment is required. However, there is a dearth of research on assessment of refugee children [16, 18], in particular cognitive assessment, despite evidence that comprehensive educational assessments of refugee children are associated with better educational outcomes [18]. Indeed, research indicates that many children are not correctly assessed and either inappropriately placed in special educational needs settings or denied the support they require in order to learn [19–21]. Other studies point to refugee children being placed in classrooms which are unsuitable for them, either because these are too advanced or not challenging enough [22, 23]. Therefore, placing children in the wrong grade can have short- and long-term consequences for children's educational outcomes as well as their well-being [10, 23]. High-quality assessments are therefore essential to comprehensively support refugee children's school trajectories, understand their educational and psychosocial needs and identify high-quality provision.

Assessment of refugee children is a complex process: it requires knowledge of stress-related disorders and how these affect learning, skills to identify learning disorders in refugee populations, and sensitivity to the changing dynamics of refugee families which will impact parents' ability to support children and engage with schools. These challenges are compounded by language and cultural barriers to engagement, limited resources available to schools and other professionals and a lack of evidence-based guidance on carrying out such assessments. We discuss the challenges of assessments below.

Many refugee children have experienced multiple stressful life events, especially those who arrive in host countries at an older age. They may have witnessed conflict or war, been subject to persecution and had to flee their countries of origin, with or without their families. Stressful life events can continue to occur in transit to a safe country and can, furthermore, be exacerbated by post-migration experiences if they are subject to discrimination and have uncertain futures due to immigration determination processes. Such events, and in particular cumulative stressful life events, are likely to give rise to mental health problems, including anxiety disorders, depression and PTSD [24–27]. Children are also more likely to suffer from mental health problems if their parents have PTSD [28]. These mental health difficulties may impact on refugee children's cognitive functioning as well as on their ability to engage in learning activities in school [29]. For example, research with children who are not refugees has shown that trauma affects children's cognitive development [30]. Indeed, different types of traumatic experiences and accompanying symptoms (e.g., anxiety and depression) can affect various aspects of functioning and cause problems such as difficulty sustaining attention, listening, completing tasks or memory problems and irritability [16, 17, 28, 30]. These tasks are all central to school readiness and functioning in a classroom setting and are critical to learning and school progress [29]. Symptoms of PTSD also include impaired sleep, intrusive thoughts and disassociation, which will also have an impact on children's ability to engage in school and learning activities [29, 31]. In some cases, the impact of traumatic events can also interfere with language development in young children, with reports of resultant selective mutism [32]. Understanding how PTSD interacts with cognitive functioning is therefore critical for schools carrying out assessments of refugee children's learning needs.

Research also indicates that children and adults with low IQ are at greater risk of developing PTSD and that high IQ may be a protective factor [15, 28, 33]. Many refugee children have lived in dangerous and precarious conditions for several years prior to their re settlement, either in conflict zones, refugee camps in third countries or in transit to the host country. This hardship may impede parents' abilities to provide adequate nutrition, stimulation and warmth to their children, resulting in sub-optimal physical and emotional growth and ultimately stunted cognitive development and low IQ. Such adversity may mean that children are more vulnerable to PTSD, while impaired cognitive function has implications for engaging in school tasks and acquiring academic skills and knowledge. Assessments therefore require gathering a comprehensive history of the family and the child's past experiences.

Research has also found that ADHD (attention deficit hyperactive disorder) is common in refugee children and that it often presents alongside PTSD [28, 31]. However, it is not clear from the current available evidence whether there is high co-morbidity or whether ADHD and PTSD symptoms simply overlap. Overlapping symptoms include inattention, difficulties listening or completing tasks, poor organisation and avoidance of mental tasks, memory problems, hyperactivity and irritability [31]. Such behaviours constitute a barrier to learning and may present as challenging to teachers responsible for large pupil groups [29, 31]. Refugee children with either PTSD or ADHD or both therefore run the risk of being misdiagnosed and offered the wrong, if any, treatment. In addition, there is a dearth of evidence about the prevalence of other learning difficulties or special educational needs among refugee children in high-income countries, suggesting that many children are either wrongly diagnosed or undiagnosed [10, 21]. This poses further challenges for assessment, as it requires that school professionals have a good knowledge of the manifestations of learning difficulties in culturally diverse populations and how these are distinguished from mental health problems in refugee populations.

Further complexities of adequately assessing refugee children in schools include cultural differences, language barriers and, for some children, illiteracy and no prior schooling. Families may also be unaware of their child's learning needs or learning difficulties. Available assessment tools, including non-verbal tests, are not culturally validated for children coming from different contexts, as most have been developed in and are specific to the 'Western' context [16, 34]. While some have shown validity across cultures [35], these have not been tested for the countries that most refugees originate from. Research has documented different cultural behaviours of migrant children in schools (including, for example, body language or expression), which can be misinterpreted in Western contexts [9, 23, 34]. Moreover, assessment tools are not standardised when used with an interpreter or validated for assessments of children who are illiterate or who have no basic schooling experience [34]. As a consequence, the cognitive functioning of children may be misunderstood or misdiagnosed, precluding the provision of effective educational interventions and support.

Supporting children's cultural needs is a critical component of school assessments. Cultural stereotyping or a general lack of awareness or understanding of children's cultural backgrounds and experiences can make assessments inaccurate, which in turn can lead to misdiagnoses and subsequent poor relationships between schools and children and their families. Different cultural assumptions held by schools or families may also result in a lack of communication or miscommunication and lead to fraught relationships between the school and the family [22, 23]. These complexities highlight the importance of involving families in the assessment process as early as possible. Parents can provide critical information about their children's circumstances and needs as well as their cultural background, so involving parents and families ensures as broad a picture of the children's needs as possible. Immigrant and refugee parents commonly have high educational aspirations for their children, as educational success is seen as the key to greater economic and employment opportunities [36–41]. These aspirations are often a vehicle of hope, and parents' sacrifices are made worthwhile when their children thrive in education and beyond. Schools should be sensitive to these family dynamics and seek to engage with parents to support their children's development throughout assessment processes.

In addition, schools may seek cultural brokers, internally or externally, to support children's school trajectories. These may be teachers, teaching assistants or community members who share the same cultural backgrounds as the children. Examples of their involvement include participating in or reviewing assessments to ensure that children are not wrongly placed in or denied access to special educational provision, working with schools to create environments which welcome and promote diversity and organising activities to promote the value of education for success in host countries [10]. In addition, some research has shown that children whose teachers were interested and engaged with their cultural heritage performed better than those whose teachers were not [10, 23, 42].

Assessing the learning needs of refugee children is therefore a complex task which requires an appreciation of how mental health difficulties and cognitive and learning difficulties manifest in children. Given the scarcity of resources to help in these assessments, in practice, refugee children are likely to require repeated multi-disciplinary assessments, ideally with families, community members and education and mental health professionals collaborating.

We acknowledge the structural limitations that many schools will have in conducting such an assessment, with many experiencing poor access to the resources of time, support and expertise when first accepting refugee families into their schools. However, a commitment to a comprehensive assessment, over time, will be beneficial for all involved; children's developmental histories might be gleaned and parents will have a chance to meet and appreciate the staff in the school and build bridges from which their children will probably benefit. This can also give an opportunity to introduce the host country's educational system and assumptions, which, given the number of novel and different components of post-migration life that families have to deal with, might be overwhelming.

Emerging research has suggested different strategies and priorities to assess the learning needs of refugee children [16, 18]. These suggest a holistic assessment framework which goes beyond the use of standardised tools to determine cognitive functioning. Kaplan et al. (2016) advocate for a broad-based assessment of the children which considers the cultural background of the child, charts their experiences in their country of origin and includes a comprehensive developmental and medical history [16]. Within this assessment, practitioners should determine the number of languages the child can speak and write and the degree of proficiency. This information should then be used to decide what language(s) further assessments should be conducted in, or whether the support of a bilingual aide or qualified interpreter is appropriate. To differentiate language abilities from cognitive deficiencies, specific strategies have been suggested, such as 'dynamic assessments'; here, children are given feedback on their performance and tested again with similar items and any changes in performance evaluated. This allows children to familiarise themselves with test structures, and some evidence suggests that these approaches can distinguish learning difficulties from other, language or cultural, barriers to test performance. Given the impact of family functioning and parental mental health on child well-being, a family history is also recommended. Similarly, Minhas et al. [18] provide a mnemonic checklist, EMPOWER, to guide the assessment of the developmental needs of refugee children. This checklist covers Education, Migration history, Parents and family (including well-being and educational background), Outlook (the child's aspirations for the future), Words (for language proficiency), Experiences of trauma (pre- and post-migration) and Resources (including housing, finance, etc.). We suggest incorporating cultural background into the checklist, given its critical importance.

Whether the assessment is conducted in school, in the home or in a clinical setting might best be determined by where the child and the family are most comfortable. This can often be in the school or other community setting, which can be perceived as carrying a low risk of stigmatisation [22, 23].

Given the assessment challenges, an important question is its timing. Most schools will seek early assessment of children: for orientation purposes before grade placement, or in the early weeks of entry into school, or as soon as difficulties are identified. Such an approach, if successful, aims to place children in the appropriate grade and provide early intervention to avoid children falling further behind. However, there are a number of reasons why this may not be in the child's best interests. First, newly arrived children may be extremely vulnerable and traumatised to the extent that they are unable to engage in any meaningful assessment. Allowing children to settle and establish emotional safety over a period of time may be necessary; indeed, in some contexts practitioners wait two years before administering any standardised assessments [16, 23]. However, assessments should only be delayed if this is in the best interests of the child, as a failure to assess may have significant consequences, including being placed in the wrong grade or being denied special educational provision. Second, the lack of validated assessment tools means that qualitative assessments are needed, including observations from children's teachers and other school professionals, and these often require time to obtain. Moreover, children's mental health and cognitive development are dynamic and fluctuate over time. Overall, this highlights the benefit of ongoing assessments and flexible planning to best meet the learning needs of refugee children.

Different Approaches to Working with Refugee Families in Schools and the Importance of Maintaining Relationships

It is essential to note that with refugee families there might be an increased likelihood that relationships between families and schools might suffer, and this fragility needs to be considered and anticipated [43]. Refugee families might have the experience of numerous relationships breaking down, exacerbated by how exposure to previous traumatic events might compromise the ability to build relationships, especially with authority figures or those who might be perceived as threatening (possibly informed by their own childhood relationships with teachers).

There are a number of challenges that might be faced by families who have experienced trauma and displacement. These are worthy of note here, as school can play a role in helping to redress them. Parental roles can be undermined by experiences in countries of origin, especially if parents feel that they were unable to protect their children from the disruption and desecration often accompanying mass violence. Many feel a sense of shame and humiliation which can impact on their parenting capacity [44]. On arrival in a host country, there are often changes in intrafamiliar dynamics and relationships which can be made worse if family members are suffering from mental health problems such as PTSD. An ongoing fear and instability on arrival in the host country, often exacerbated by numerous house moves and possible immigration/asylum uncertainty, can make things even harder for a family trying to settle and find new stability; in the interim, often until parents have found meaningful ways to sustain their livelihoods, their lives can be difficult to manage. For some refugees, this downward mobility will be temporary; others may suffer from it all their lives and even pass the disadvantage on to their children [45]. In the context of this, parents need to find ways to continue their parenting role, despite the many changes taking place around them [46, 47]. There have been some reports of higher rates of parent-to-child aggression in refugee families, with other evidence that family relationships and parent-adolescent conflict is the strongest post-migration risk factor for aggressive behaviour in migrant families, further highlighting the importance of trying to support the family unit [48].

Many of the experiences of migration and resettlement for refugee families can challenge family norms, and it is not uncommon for these complex changes and struggles to be observed by the staff in schools, who are well-placed to act and support the family in a timely manner. Furthermore, if there are any emerging concerns about the well-being of the child and if they are experiencing any abusive situations, then often schools are the first places where these are observed or raised and can facilitate support, if needed, for any changes (this often includes consultation and/or working with statutory services). Therefore, refugee children and their families need to navigate the choppy waters of resettlement in their relationships with each other as well as with educational and other external agencies. Supporting them with a focus on maintaining relationships is an important component of many interventions.

Educational Interventions

There is a paucity of evidence available generally about the learning outcomes and needs of refugee children [10]. In one systematic review of learning problems in refugee children, only 8 studies reported on educational outcomes and 14 included some prevalence data on developmental or learning needs. The authors did not identify any which reported on autism spectrum disorders, specific language impairments or dyslexia; however, one has subsequently been published [21]. This limits our knowledge and understanding of what educational provision and interventions should be offered to refugee children.

Usually, younger children are placed in mainstream school and offered additional support through one-to-one tutoring or group interventions [49]. These may be specific to refugee children or migrant children or offered to all children needing additional support in schools. The availability and type of educational provision will vary by country, locality and school. It may also be different for primary and secondary school children and will depend on the available resources.

Educational provision for adolescents may be more complex, as the demands of the curriculum for older children and particularly during exam years might be too ambitious for newly arrived young people with limited host language skills. This is particularly the case when young people arrive in the host country in the middle of the school year and, critically, in years when young people sit examinations. Some young people may be denied a place in mainstream education and instead offered bespoke educational programmes. These are usually intended to provide information about living and settling in their host country, support the development of language skills and teach them additional life and vocational skills. Few such programmes have been evaluated [10], and it is not clear that delaying young people's access to mainstream education is always in their best interests. The question of whether the educational needs of young refugees are better served in mainstream education, which may include additional support, or by placing them in alternative provision before they enter mainstream school remains unresolved in research.

Psychosocial Interventions for Families in Schools

The opportunity and challenge of conducting mental health interventions for refugee children and their families in the school context is substantial. As described above, many refugee families make early contact with schools, and these are often the places that know the family and children best. Many perceive the school to be a relatively 'safe' environment, so finding ways to enhance what is offered in the school context is important to consider. Schools can therefore be a place where schools, health services and other allied professionals work closely together to find a way to deliver mental health services that are potentially more acceptable and accessible than in more traditional settings [50], especially as there is good evidence that engagement by refugee families with mental health care is otherwise poor when compared to the host population. This is because of differences in the cultural expressions of mental distress and illness, causal explanations and beliefs about mental illness and beliefs and experiences of seeking help [51]. The evidence shows that refuges under-utilise mental health services, with little known about barriers and facilitators to accessing care [52, 53]. Refugee children are dependent on carers to access services, and their carers might have poor knowledge of such services and poor mental health literacy, distrust as a result of stigma, and poor language services to assist in interpretation, in conjunction with limited financial means if services need to be purchased [7]. The low priority placed on mental health by adult refugees, as shown in some studies, highlights the need for practical solutions to social, legal and economic difficulties and the hierarchy of such needs in relation to mental health. Therefore, mental health needs are often considered as part of the broader psychosocial needs of a traumatised refugee family.

A number of systematic reviews have been conducted exploring the role of school-based interventions in the mental health of refugee children and their families [2, 3] and also of treatments for children exposed to violence and armed conflict [51]. The school setting provides a number of different ways that mental health interventions can be delivered by either mental health professionals or trained school staff or other professionals depending on the intervention and its evidence base [54–56]. A systematic review of family interventions for traumatised refugees, although identifying only six studies, highlights the importance of family-level processes in the treatment of traumatised refugees, such as building family relationships, communication and resilience, which can also potentially be successfully delivered within the school context [57].

Broadly, the types of mental health interventions of relevance for refugee children and their families fall into three areas, although the overall state of the evidence base is limited [2].

First, interventions that support the verbal processing of past traumatic events, for which there is the strongest evidence base [58]. These are mainly to treat the sequelae of past traumatic events and include the treatment of PTSD. Cognitive behavioural therapy and narrative exposure therapy have both been studied in schools for refugee children. The Cognitive Behavioral Intervention for Trauma in Schools (CBITS) is a group intervention that has been studied for traumatised migrant and local populations in the USA, with evidence of reductions in PTSD in children and increases in the levels of functioning of children [59]. Interestingly, CBITS has been used with families, although not refugee families, and has demonstrated how adding a family component to CBITS has enhanced treatment outcomes in school-based PTSD treatment for Latinx families [60]. Families that do best seem to engage more with schools and have less 'inconsistency'. Given the prominent intergenerational impact of PTSD, few studies have been designed to influence multiple domains, with little involving refugee families in PTSD treatments within schools, although this would be important to study [61].

Second, schools can be a locus for parenting interventions, although most available studies have involved migrant families, some of which have been refugees. A randomized controlled trial (RCT) of the Oregon model of Parent-Management Training (PMTO) for two migrant groups (Somali and Pakistani) showed that PMTO was effective in enhancing parent practices, with a decrease in harsh discipline and an increase in positive parenting, but these did not translate into teacher-identifiable effects on the children's conduct and social competence [62]. A support programme for Somali-born parents showed improvements in children's behaviour problems [63] and another, Families And Schools Together (FAST), for Mexican immigrants showed reductions in children's aggressive behaviours [64]. Given the acculturation stressors that can impact on refugee families through each stage of child development, it has been suggested that parenting support might be beneficial throughout the child's time at school [65].

The final broad area where interventions have been developed is to assist with managing the change in living circumstances on arrival in a host country [2]. These interventions include broad psychoeducation interventions, enhancing coping skills and adjustment difficulties. The evidence base supporting these remains limited, although many interesting innovations have been tried in schools, including cultural brokers and home support workers and a commitment to fostering diversity in the school community by celebrating different religious and cultural festivals. Involvement in the school and developing a sense of belonging are crucial components, especially as supporting peer relationships, often helped by participation in extra-curricular activities, have been identified as useful [4, 10]. Family involvement and finding ways to help them contribute to and feel part of the school community can be important key components to health settlement.

Conclusion

In conclusion, schools can play a key role in helping traumatised families to manage the transition into the host society. When considering how best to support refugee children, schools should first consider how accessible they are to refugee families in the community and what tools and skills they may need to ensure a broad approach is taken and to carry out a holistic assessment. In turn, this means that schools can provide appropriate and high-quality provision to these children. Throughout, they should maintain a family lens. Indeed, schools are likely to be best placed to facilitate these families feeling a sense of belonging in their host country as well as signposting them to other services as any additional needs become apparent. The importance of a family perspective is vital given how traumatised families have often experienced some trauma together, with PTSD clustering in families [66]. Moreover, PTSD has negative effects on attachment and parenting [67].

The importance of building a sense of belonging was highlighted in the Good Starts Study investigating 97 refugees in Australia where the key factors strongly associated with well-being outcomes were those most closely related to belonging: subjective social status in the broader community, perceived discrimination and bullying [43]. The study authors concluded that our perspective needs to change to embrace refugee families within a broader socially inclusive society, one that offers real opportunities for those with refugee backgrounds to flourish. Schools can exert significant influences on facilitating acculturation in young people [68], and studies of immigrant populations and peer violence show the important influence of classroom environments and levels of support – thus the question remains about how best to foster this in classrooms [69].

Finally, a broader focus on resilience can help us to inform any interventions for refugee families in schools. A systematic review identified social support (from friends and community), a sense of belonging, valuing education, having a positive outlook, family connectedness and connections to their home culture as factors promoting resilience in refugee children [70]. Another study on resilience in refugee children identified factors that appeared to promote psychosocial well-being in adolescent refugees, and these additionally included finances for necessities, host language proficiency, cultural guidance, educational support, and faith and religious involvement [71]. The authors conclude that because resilience works through protective mechanisms, greater attention should be paid in research and practice to enhancing these components [57, 71]. Successful educational adaptation includes language acquisition opportunities, institutional supports, instructional practices and teacher-student engagement strategies [72].

In the context of violence and displacement, efforts to improve the mental health of refugee children and their families require thoughtful consideration of the mental health cascade across generations and the cluster of adversities that impact family well-being. The school can potentially play an important role in supporting families and providing a significant contribution to the mental health of refugee children and their families [73, 74].

References

1. M. Fazel, R. V. Reed, C. Panter-Brick and A. Stein, Mental health of displaced and refugee children resettled in high-income countries: Risk and protective factors. *The Lancet*, 379(9812) (2012), 266–82.

2. R. A. Tyrer and M. Fazel, School and community-based interventions for refugee and asylum seeking children: A systematic review. *PLoS One*, 9(2) (2014), e89359.

3. A. L. Sullivan and G. R. Simonson, A systematic review of school-based social-emotional interventions for refugee and war-traumatized youth. *Review of Educational Research*, 86(2) (2016), 503–30.

4. M. Fazel, A moment of change: Facilitating refugee children's mental health in UK schools. *International Journal of Educational Development*, 41 (2015), 255–61.

5. M. Fazel, K. Hoagwood, S. Stephan and T. Ford, Mental health interventions in schools in high-income countries. *The Lancet Psychiatry*, 1(5) (2014), 377–87.

6. M. Fazel, V. Patel, S. Thomas and W. Tol, Mental health interventions in schools in low-income and middle-income countries. *The Lancet Psychiatry*, 1(5) (2014), 388–98.

7. S. May, R. M. Rapee, M. Coello, S. Momartin and J. Aroche, Mental health literacy among refugee communities: Differences between the Australian lay public and the Iraqi and Sudanese refugee communities. *Social Psychiatry and Psychiatric Epidemiology*, 49 (5) (2014), 757–69.

8. C. Gladwell and G. Chetwynd, *Education for Refugee and Asylum Seeking Children: Access and Equality in England, Scotland and Wales* (London: UNICEF, 2018). www .unicef.org.uk/wp-content/uploads/2018/0 9/Access-to-Education-report-PDF.pdf

9. J. L. McBrien, Educational needs and barriers for refugee students in the United States: A review of the literature. *Review of Educational Research*, 75(3) (2005), 329–64.

10. H. R. Graham, R. S. Minhas and G. Paxton, Learning problems in children of refugee background: A systematic review. *Pediatrics*, 137(6) (2016), e20153994–e20153994.

11. M. Arnot and H. Pinson, *The Education of Asylum-Seeker and Refugee Children* (Cambridge, UK: Faculty of Education, University of Cambridge, 2005). www .educ.cam.ac.uk/people/staff/arnot/Asylu mReportFinal.pdf

12. J. Stevenson and J. Willott, The aspiration and access to higher education of teenage refugees in the UK. *Compare: A Journal of Comparative and International Education*, 37(5) (2007), 671–87.

13. L. Sanbonmatsu, J. R. Kling, G. J. Duncan and J. Brooks-Gunn, Neighborhoods and academic achievement results from the Moving to Opportunity experiment. *Journal of Human Resources*, 41(4) (2006), 649–91.

14. N. Sigona and V. Hughes, *No Way out, No Way in: Irregular Migrant Children and Families in the UK: Executive Summary* (Oxford: ESRC Centre on Migration, Policy and Society, 2012).

15. M. Porter and N. Haslam, Predisplacement and postdisplacement factors associated with mental health of refugees and internally displaced persons: A meta-analysis. *Journal of the American Medical Association*, 294(5) (2005), 602–12.

16. I. Kaplan, Y. Stolk, M. Valibhoy, A. Tucker and J. Baker, Cognitive assessment of refugee children: Effects of trauma and new language acquisition. *Transcultural Psychiatry*, 53(1) (2016), 81–109.

17. K. Almqvist and A. G. Broberg, Mental health and social adjustment in young refugee children 3½ years after their arrival in Sweden. *Journal of the American Academy of Child and Adolescent Psychiatry*, 38(6) (1999), 723–30.

18. R. S. Minhas, H. Graham, T. Jegathesan, J. Huber, E. Young and T. Barozzino, Supporting the developmental health of refugee children and youth. *Paediatrics and Child Health*, 22(2) (2017), 68–71.

19. D. Vega, J. Lasser and A. F. M. Afifi, School psychologists and the assessment of culturally and linguistically diverse students. *Contemporary School Psychology*, 20(3) (2016), 218–29.

20. B. Nykiel-Herbert, Iraqi refugee students: From a collection of aliens to a community of learners –the role of cultural factors in the acquisition of literacy by Iraqi refugee students with interrupted formal education. *Multicultural Education*, 17(3) (2010), 2–14.

21. A. O'Higgins, Analysis of care and education pathways of refugee and asylum-seeking children in care in England: Implications for social work. *International Journal of Social Welfare*, 28(1) (2018), 53–62. DOI: http://10.1111/ijsw.12324

22. C. Rousseau, A. Drapeau and E. Corin, School performance and emotional problems in refugee children. *American Journal of Orthopsychiatry*, 66(2) (1996), 239–51.

23. L. M. Usman, Communication disorders and the inclusion of newcomer African refugees in rural primary schools of British Columbia, Canada. *International Journal of Progressive Education*, 8(2) (2012).

24. I. Bronstein and P. Montgomery, Psychological distress in refugee children: A systematic review. *Clinical Child Family Psychology Review*, 14(1) (2011), 44–56.

25. J. Huemer, N. S. Karnik, S. Voelkl-Kernstock, E. Granditsch, K. Dervic, M. H. Friedrich et al., Mental health issues in unaccompanied refugee minors. *Child Adolescent Psychiatry & Mental Health*, 3 (1) (2009), 13.

26. S. L. Lustig, M. Kia-Keating, W. G. Knight, P. Geltman, H. Ellis, J. D. Kinzie et al., Review of child and adolescent refugee mental health. *Journal of American Academy of Child Adolescent Psychiatry*, 43(1) (2004), 24–36.

27. M. Fazel and A. Stein, The mental health of refugee children. *Archive of Disease in Childhood*, 87(5) (2002), 366–70.

28. A. Daud and P.-A. Rydelius, Comorbidity/ overlapping between ADHD and PTSD in relation to IQ among children of traumatized/non-traumatized parents. *Journal of Attention Disorder*, 13(2) (2009), 188–96.

29. M. M. Perfect, M. R. Turley, J. S. Carlson, J. Yohanna and M. P. Saint Gilles, School-related outcomes of traumatic event exposure and traumatic stress symptoms in students: A systematic review of research from 1990 to 2015. *School Mental Health*, 8(1) (2016), 7–43.

30. M. Rutter, C. Beckett, J. Castle, E. Colvert, J. Kreppner and M. Mehta, Effects of

profound early institutional deprivation: An overview of findings from a UK longitudinal study of Romanian adoptees. *European Journal of Development Psychology*, 4(3) (2007), 332–50.

31. K. Szymanski, L. Sapanski and F. Conway, Trauma and ADHD – association or diagnostic confusion? A clinical perspective. *Journal of Infant, Child, Adolescent Psychotherapy*, 10(1) (2011), 51–9.

32. P. Wong, Selective mutism: A review of etiology, comorbidities, and treatment. *Psychiatry (Edgmont)*, 7(3) (2010), 23.

33. I. Kira, L. Lewandowski, J. Yoon, C. Somers and L. Chiodo, The linear and nonlinear associations between multiple types of trauma and IQ discrepancy indexes in African American and Iraqi refugee adolescents. *Journal of Child and Adolescent Trauma*, 5(1) (2012), 47–62.

34. I. Kaplan, Effects of trauma and the refugee experience on psychological assessment processes and interpretation. *Australia Psychology*, 44(1) (2009), 6–15.

35. J. Georgas, L. G. Weiss, F. J. Van de Vijver and D. H. Saklofske, eds., *Culture and Children's Intelligence: Cross-Cultural Analysis of the WISC-III* (Elsevier, 2003).

36. S. Gorard, B. H. See and P. Davies, *The Impact of Attitudes and Aspirations on Educational Attainment and Participation* (York: Joseph Rowntree Foundation, 2012).

37. N. E. Hill, D. R. Castellino, J. E. Lansford, P. Nowlin, K. A. Dodge and J. E. Bates, Parent academic involvement as related to school behavior, achievement, and aspirations: Demographic variations across adolescence. *Child Development*, 75 (5) (2004), 1491–509.

38. N. E. Hill and D. F. Tyson, Parental involvement in middle school: A meta-analytic assessment of the strategies that promote achievement. *Developmental Psychology*, 45(3) (2009), 740–63.

39. C. Goldenberg, R. Gallimore, L. Reese and H. Garnier, Cause or effect? A longitudinal study of immigrant Latino parents' aspirations and expectations, and their children's school performance. *American Educational Research Journal*, 38(3) (2001), 547–82.

40. G. Kao and J. S. Thompson, Racial and ethnic stratification in educational achievement and attainment. *Annual Review of Sociology*, 29 (2003), 417–42.

41. S. Roubeni, L. De Haene, E. Keatley, N. Shah and A. Rasmussen, 'If we can't do it, our children will do it one day': A qualitative study of West African immigrant parents' losses and educational aspirations for their children. *American Educational Research Journal*, 52(2) (2015), 275–305.

42. G. Bitew, P. Ferguson and M. Dixon, Ethiopian-Australian students' experience of secondary schooling in the Australian education system in the state of Victoria. *Australasian Review of African Studies*, 29 (1–2) (2008), 78–91.

43. I. Correa-Velez, S. M. Gifford and A. G. Barnett, Longing to belong: Social inclusion and wellbeing among youth with refugee backgrounds in the first three years in Melbourne, Australia. *Social Science & Medicine*, 71(8) (2010), 1399–408.

44. B. K. Barber, C. A. McNeely, E. El Sarraj, M. Daher, R. Giacaman, C. Arafat et al., Mental suffering in protracted political conflict: Feeling broken or destroyed. *PLoS One*, 11(5) (2016), e0156216.

45. H. J. Gans, First generation decline: Downward mobility among refugees and immigrants. *Ethnic and Racial Studies*, 32 (9) (2009), 1658–70.

46. R. Raffaetà, Migration and parenting: Reviewing the debate and calling for future research. *International Journal of Migrant Health and Social Care*, 12(1) (2016), 38–50.

47. E. Riggs, J. Yelland, J. Szwarc, S. Wahidi, S. Casey and D. Chesters, Fatherhood in a new country: A qualitative study exploring the experiences of Afghan men and implications for health services. *Birth*, 43(1) (2016), 86–92.

48. P. R. Smokowski and M. L. Bacallao, Acculturation and aggression in Latino adolescents: A structural model focusing

on cultural risk factors and assets. *Journal of Abnormal Child Psychology*, 34(5) (2006), 657–71.

49. C. Rousseau, C. Beauregard, K. Daignault, H. Petrakos, B. D. Thombs and R. Steele, A cluster randomized-controlled trial of a classroom-based drama workshop program to improve mental health outcomes among immigrant and refugee youth in special classes. *PLoS One*, 9(8) (2014), e104704.

50. M. Fazel, J. Garcia and A. Stein, The right location? Experiences of refugee adolescents seen by school-based mental health services. *Clinical Child Psychology and Psychiatry*, 21(3) (2016), 368–80.

51. F. L. Brown, A. M. de Graaff, J. Annan and T. S. Betancourt, Annual research review: Breaking cycles of violence – a systematic review and common practice elements analysis of psychosocial interventions for children and youth affected by armed conflict. *Journal of Child Psychology and Psychiatry*, 58(4) (2017), 507–24.

52. E. Colucci, J. Szwarc, H. Minas, G. Paxton and C. Guerra, The utilisation of mental health services by children and young people from a refugee background: A systematic literature review. *International Journal of Culture and Mental Health*, 7(1) (2014), 86–108.

53. H. Fenta, I. Hyman and S. Noh, Mental health service utilization by Ethiopian immigrants and refugees in Toronto. *Journal of Nervous and Mental Disease*, 194(12) (2006), 925–34.

54. K. Pottie, G. Dahal, K. Georgiades, K. Premji and G. Hassan, Do first generation immigrant adolescents face higher rates of bullying, violence and suicidal behaviours than do third generation and native born? *Journal of Immigrant and Minority Health*, 17(5) (2015), 1557–66.

55. S. J. J. Lim and J. L. Hoot, Bullying in an increasingly diverse school population: A socio-ecological model analysis. *School Psychology International*, 36(3) (2015), 268–82.

56. A. Hjern, L. Rajmil, M. Bergström, M. Berlin, P. A. Gustafsson and B. Modin, Migrant density and well-being: A national school survey of 15-year-olds in Sweden. *European Journal of Public Health*, 23 (2013), 823–8.

57. O. Slobodin and J. T. V. M. de Jong, Family interventions in traumatized immigrants and refugees: A systematic review. *Transcultural Psychiatry*, 52(5) (2015), 723–42.

58. S. M. Chafouleas, T. A. Koriakin, K. D. Roundfield and S. Overstreet, Addressing childhood trauma in school settings: A framework for evidence-based practice. *School Mental Health*, 6(1) (2018), 1–14.

59. S. A. Hoover, H. Sapere, J. M. Lang, E. Nadeem, K. L. Dean and P. Vona, Statewide implementation of an evidence-based trauma intervention in schools. *School Psychology Quarterly*, 33(1) (2018), 44.

60. C. D. Santiago, J. M. Lennon, A. K. Fuller, S. K. Brewer and S. H. Kataoka, Examining the impact of a family treatment component for CBITS: When and for whom is it helpful? *Journal of Family Psychology*, 28(4) (2014), 560.

61. K. Peltonen and R. Punamäki, Preventive interventions among children exposed to trauma of armed conflict: A literature review. *Aggressive Behaviour: Official Journal of the International Society for Research on Aggression*, 36(2) (2010), 95–116.

62. R. Bjørknes and T. Manger, Can parent training alter parent practice and reduce conduct problems in ethnic minority children? A randomized controlled trial. *Prevention Science*, 14(1) (2013), 52–63.

63. F. Osman, R. Flacking, U.-K. Schön and M. Klingberg-Allvin, A support program for Somali-born parents on children's behavioral problems. *Pediatrics*, 139(3) (2017), e20162764.

64. L. Knox, N. G. Guerra, K. R. Williams and R. Toro, Preventing children's aggression in immigrant Latino families: A mixed methods evaluation of the Families and

Schools Together program. *American Journal of Community Psychology*, 48(1–2) (2011), 65–76.

65. F. Osman, M. Klingberg-Allvin, R. Flacking and U.-K. Schön, Parenthood in transition: Somali-born parents' experiences of and needs for parenting support programmes. *BMC International Health and Human Rights*, 16(1) (2016), 7.

66. W. H. Sack, G. N. Clarke and J. Seeley, Posttraumatic stress disorder across two generations of Cambodian refugees. *Journal of the American Academy of Child and Adolescent Psychiatry*, 34(9) (1995), 1160–6.

67. E. van Ee, R. J. Kleber, M. J. Jongmans, T. T. M. Mooren and D. Out, Parental PTSD, adverse parenting and child attachment in a refugee sample. *Attachment and Human Development*, 18 (3) (2016), 273–91.

68. C. Ward and N. Geeraert, Advancing acculturation theory and research: The acculturation process in its ecological context. *Current Opinion in Psychology*, 8 (2016), 98–104.

69. S. D. Walsh, B. De Clercq, M. Molcho, Y. Harel-Fisch, C. M. Davison, K. R. Madsen et al., The relationship between immigrant school composition, classmate support and involvement in physical fighting and bullying among adolescent immigrants and non-immigrants in 11 countries. *Journal of Youth and Adolescence*, 45(1) (2016), 1–16.

70. K. A. Pieloch, M. B. McCullough and A. K. Marks, Resilience of children with refugee statuses: A research review. *Canadian Psychology*, 57(4) (2016), 330.

71. S. Merrill Weine, N. Ware, L. Hakizimana, T. Tugenberg, M. Currie, G. Dahnweih et al., Fostering resilience: Protective agents, resources, and mechanisms for adolescent refugees' psychosocial well-being. *Adolescent Psychiatry (Hilversum)*, 4(4) (2014), 164–76.

72. L. Stermac, A. K. Clarke and L. Brown, Pathways to resilience: The role of education in war-zone immigrant and refugee student success. In C. Fernando and M. Ferrari, eds., *Handbook of Resilience in Children of War* (New York: Springer, 2013), pp. 211–20.

73. C. J. Trentacosta, C. M. McLear, M. S. Ziadni, M. A. Lumley and C. L. Arfken, Potentially traumatic events and mental health problems among children of Iraqi refugees: The roles of relationships with parents and feelings about school. *American Journal of Orthopsychiatry*, 86(4) (2016), 384–92.

74. C. Panter-Brick, M.-P. Grimon and M. Eggerman, Caregiver-child mental health: A prospective study in conflict and refugee settings. *Journal of Child Psychology and Psychiatry*, 55(4) (2014), 313–27.

Chapter 18

Collaborative Mental Health Care for Refugee Families in a School Context

Garine Papazian-Zohrabian, Caterina Mamprin, Alyssa Turpin-Samson, and Vanessa Lemire

Introduction

School- and community-based collaborative services, inspired by systemic intervention approaches, aim to respond to refugee children's various needs in the face of the multiple challenges facing refugee youth and their families in ways that avoid stigmatizing or pathologizing their psychological and psychosocial vulnerabilities. In this chapter, the first section defines collaborative care, presenting various models of community-based collaborative services. Second, we discuss collaborative care models in school contexts, with a particular focus on the model developed in the course of an action research project we conducted in Quebec. Lastly, we exemplify school-based collaborative care through reflecting on two case studies.

Community-Based Collaborative Services for Refugees

According to the American Psychiatric Association [1], collaborative care has to be team-driven by a multidisciplinary group, considering the professional training of each individual involved in the process. In this medical approach, the team is responsible for the patient's care and the outcomes of decisions taken on the basis of clinical data (e.g., characteristics of the targeted population, symptoms). It is expected that the care-providing professionals adapt evidence-based treatments to the individual and their life context. Yet this model enhances the interprofessional collaboration without involving the community at stake.

Concerning refugees, the American Psychological Association (APA) proposes that treatment of this population must use evidence-based, comprehensive and community-based services that are culturally adapted [2]. As described by Rousseau et al. [3], the frontline or primary care team which provides mental health care can work in association with community organizations or schools to create a support network for the families. In this context, collaborative care can facilitate the comprehension of needs from a social and cultural perspective [3]. Furthermore, the association between primary care clinics and other organizations frequented by the individual (e.g., community centers, schools) may also create a context of help that is less stigmatizing than specialized mental health care.

Adopting this perspective and following the Inter-Agency Standing Committee Mental Health and Psychosocial Support Guidelines [4], Measham et al. elaborated a collaborative care model based on a stepwise community approach [5]. Schematized as a pyramid, this four-step model describes the progression from general psychosocial services to specialized psychiatric services. At the bottom level, the authors represent the support provided by local community-based health and social service providers. Those services are dispensed in a clinic, at home or at school and are offered to refugee children and families. At the second level, in order to support children and adolescents who need more assistance, the community-based youth mental health services are represented. Those services can be provided in community-based clinics. The service providers are mainly social workers, psychologists, educators, therapists and mental health nurses. At the third level, professionals in community-based services collaborate with psychiatric consultants. This collaborative team provides culturally sensitive mental health intervention: Youths can receive culturally adapted mental health interventions provided by community-based mental health providers in association with child psychiatric consultants. Further, for those children and adolescents who are experiencing significant mental health difficulties, community-based services may refer them for psychiatric consultation if they are overwhelmed. Finally, children and adolescents can be referred to specialized trauma child mental health services. The use of a stepwise collaborative care model is an asset in needs comprehension. It also provides a wider network support for children and families.

Various initiatives targeting the mental health care needs of refugee families within a collaborative approach are documented throughout the world, including in Canada and Quebec. The following section provides an exemplary overview.

In London, Durà-Vilà et al. [12] conducted action research among refugee youth in school and community institutions. The aims of the intervention were to provide direct therapeutic intervention to refugee children and their families, to develop consultations with teachers about vulnerable students, to train school staff members to recognize and manage children's psychological distress, and to enhance appropriate referrals to mental health services. When a teacher, a social worker or a volunteer referred a student, the child and their family could benefit from several psychological consultations, with an interpreter if needed. Among the various types of therapy proposed, individual narrative psychotherapy, support therapies, family therapy and cognitive approach on loss issues were the most popular. According to the teachers' and parents' assessment, behavioral problems, hyperactivity, attention difficulties and relational problems with peers improved significantly.

In 2013, Ellis et al. developed a multi-tiered intervention program for refugee youth in New England [9]. Following a public health approach, this program offers personalized mental health care to refugee youths and their families. Four different service levels are provided. The first layer involves community resilience-building through engagement, education and outreach. Second-layer services take place in schools. Therefore, refugee students learning English benefit from a nonstigmatizing intervention that consists of building preventive skills to manage acculturative stress and emotions. It also allows teachers, parents and group leaders to identify children in greater need. Finally, layers three and four are individual services based on trauma systems therapy. The third level is school-based advanced care for young refugees. As for the fourth level, it consists of intensive home-based care for highly distressed children. The advantage of this program was its broad outreach as well as the fact that it addressed social and environmental stressors.

Community-based sociotherapy was initially developed in postgenocide Rwanda and aimed at reducing distress among genocide survivors by enhancing relationship-building in a group. Later, this therapy has been implemented in the Netherlands with refugees [16]. This therapeutic approach takes place in a community setting, and group facilitators are recruited from within the community and trained. Groups can share everything, from daily life problems to exposure to traumatic events. Facilitators must be open-minded observers and listeners. Sociotherapy sessions are ruled by five main guidelines: a nonjudgmental attitude, two-way communication, decision-making at all levels (which promotes sympathy), shared leadership, consensus in decision-making and social learning by social interaction. Progressively, these guidelines are integrated within the group. Concretely, facilitators establish and maintain a safe atmosphere, trust in others, care and respect towards others.

In Canada, Yohani [17] conducted community-based action research. The Hope Project is a preventive intervention in school settings after classes. Social workers, counselors and educational professionals lead the action. Using arts (e.g., collages, drawings, paintings and photography), children aged between 6 and 18 define what the word 'hope' represents for them. After attending several workshops, they write or tell their conception to the group, assisted by interpreters if needed. Then, children create a 'hope quilt' which consists of drawing their own hope story. Here, the children's creation becomes a medium to share their personal experiences. Meanwhile, a group interview with parents and cultural brokers is conducted to discuss their own hope for their child, how to enhance it and what might impede it. Following this interview, children present their hope quilt to their parents and to cultural brokers. This project aims to create and develop intergenerational connections through art.

Marsh [18] conducted a piece of research in Sydney, Australia, developing a creative therapeutic intervention within a collaborative setting. Youths, parents, caregivers, community leaders, teachers, multicultural teaching assistants and community workers were offered the opportunity to participate in a seven-month musical activity program in order to promote social connections and cohesion. Activities were elective music and dance groups, public performances and community celebrations within school and community organizations. The objectives were to develop different forms of communication, a sense of belonging and empowerment. It also contributed to cultural maintenance, identity construction, emotional release and integration into the host culture.

Based on the results of their research, Stewart and Martin produced a guide about the best supportive practices for professionals working with newcomer and refugee families in Canada [15]. In this summary, we present some of the recommendations, as formulated by the authors. First, they suggest that partnership between school, family and community is a key factor. More precisely, the school can be a point of reference for these families, supporting refugee families to settle and understand the functioning of the Canadian society (e.g., citizenship, the school and work system) and introducing them to available community services. In addition to academic goals, schools can offer diverse programs to facilitate the social integration of students. These programs can be oriented toward professional knowledge such as work skills and employees' rights, arts or psychosocial challenges. These actions can be implemented according to the needs of the students. In order to help the school community to have a better cultural knowledge, schools can complete their team with a cultural broker to support the workers. In addition, teachers can receive cultural competency training. Moreover, students with low literacy levels can receive financial support to attend after-school classes. In this way, the school can become a community hub, offering different programs to newcomers in after-class hours. Second, and in support of students with greater needs, family therapists, grief counselors, resource teachers, community support workers and social workers can complete the school team. By applying these recommendations, the developmental needs of young refugees and their families should be better addressed [19].

According to Persson and Rousseau [20] and Kirk [21], schools can have a nodal place in the development of the psychological wellbeing of children traumatized by war. Hamilton and Moore conducted research aiming for the promotion of the psychological wellbeing and the academic success of these children through an intervention affecting the various systems in which they evolve [21]. Working in the same field, Rousseau et al. highlight the importance of schools promoting refugee youth mental health by developing various strategies such as creativity and socialization [22, 23].

From the perspective of a collaborative mental health care model, the school context may operate as a primary care context where different professionals cooperate in providing mental health care. As a natural and positive environment, trusted and highly accessible [6] to refugee families and youth, schools can be an excellent location for mental health services [7]. Here, different studies show the benefits associated with actions taking place in a school setting [8, 9], showing a reduction of PTSD symptoms, a lower rate of depression, a decrease in hyperactivity and less mental distress. Several studies emphasize the relevance of collaborative health care as mental health provision in school settings [8–12].

Refugee children, who may be unable to access mental health care because of fear of stigma and lack of resources, are often more likely to receive services when those are delivered in school settings [13]. Indeed, school represents a key component of everyday life for both refugee youths who establish a social network within the host community and for their families, who often invest very positively in the education of their children [8, 14, 15]. Indeed, considering the potential stigma related to mental health problems, children and parents are often worried that teachers or peers will perceive them differently if they are considered as having a mental illness [24]. Some studies have shown, however, that school-based intervention is less stigmatizing than specialized services [25], and that schools are perceived as a safe and convenient place [24] in which premigratory trauma may be worked through. School-based interventions can thus be seen as a powerful approach to decreasing stigma [7]. Furthermore, school- and community-based collaborative services address the diverse needs of refugee youth and families without pathologizing their psychosocial difficulties. Rather, although acknowledging their vulnerabilities, they emphasize the resources and strengths of youth and families and aim to empower refugee families through including their voices on migration histories, the challenges of cultural belonging and the postmigration social predicament.

Moreover, school may also provide refugee families with a space where they can establish contact with the community [26]. For instance, some studies have described the importance of the community leaders' involvement within the school [27]. Equally, schools can host some extracurricular activities supported by community leaders or help families in need of services by directing them to the corresponding resources, like the medical center [27]. In sum, collaborative health care can promote access to services for refugee families and, simultaneously, support primary care professionals in increasing their expertise in working with refugee communities

However, to bridge the gap between families and appropriate services, it is important for school staff to be aware of the reality of refugee families. Moreover, in order to support traumatized refugee children it is important that school staff and teachers propose a caring and understanding attitude [28].

Understanding the Reality of Refugee Families: A Necessity for School Actors

As described above, schools can be depicted in the literature as one of the best entry points for psychosocial interventions [28]. However, schools can also be the scene of power dynamics between minorities and ethnic groups, racism and discrimination [29–31]. With that in mind, it is important for school actors to welcome refugees with an inclusive attitude [32] and consider the social, political and economic structures in which the school is embedded [33].

Research highlights the importance of teachers and other school professionals who are delivering interventions to refugee youth having some generic information about participants' culture and the variety of challenges that children and their families face and have faced [8]. For instance, teachers can be sensitized to some manifestations related to trauma and grief that may have an influence on the academic achievement of refugee youth (e.g., social withdrawal, regressive behavior, hyperarousal, dissociation, memory difficulties, sleep disturbance, feelings of guilt, depression, posttraumatic stress disorder and anxiety disorder [34]). Equally, teachers and professionals have to be interested in the history of the family because, despite the similarities among certain refugees, there are some differences related to their experiences and their cultural norms that have to be addressed [35]. The family has to be considered as a partner for the teachers and other school professionals [35].

Addressing the individual particularities implies the comprehension of teachers and school professionals of the past scholarly experiences of the refugee youth as well as their parents, which may provide an understanding of parental practices of involvement in their children's school trajectories [46]. For example, in some cultures parents aren't involved in school because they consider the teachers experts and they have complete trust in them [36]. In North America, those behaviors may be interpreted as disinvestment or lack of interest. By the same token, the school actors should clarify the values conveyed by the schools and the foundations of certain practices that can be misunderstood by parents [37]. With refugee youth, another element should be particularly considered: school delay. Depending on the pre- and perimigratory context, children may have experienced limited or disrupted access to school [38, 39]. Even if reintegration into a new school system requires adjustments from the students, it is relevant for teachers and school staff to understand the past academic histories of the refugee youth.

Assessing and Addressing Refugee Youth's Psychosocial and Educational Needs

Even though school staff are aware of the particularities related to working with refugee children and families, it is also important for them to be able to assess their psychosocial and educational needs. As mentioned before, some basic information can be known prior to their arrival at school (e.g., general challenges related to immigration, general information related to the culture, information about the school system). Nonetheless, contact with the families is essential to establish their individual needs and address them. It is important to mention that sometimes the lack of knowledge about the experiences of refugee youth and the possible psychological problems provoked by them can induce misdiagnosis [40]. Language barriers and diagnosis tools that are not culturally appropriate [24, 41] may further reinforce this phenomenon. One of the cases we present in this chapter is an illustration of such a situation in a school setting.

Schools can be a point of reference for information and assistance, and yet communication between schools and refugee families can be difficult due to linguistic or cultural barriers, exacerbated by thresholds in finding access to resources for translation [42]. Several texts mention the advantages of having access to an interpreter [43, 44] or cultural broker [45] to facilitate the communication between family and school. Nonetheless, even in the face of cultural and linguistic barriers complicating communication with refugee families, it is important to consider them as partners in their child's education.

This documentation regarding various mental health care services based in community and school settings reveals the complexity related to the welcoming of refugee populations in general, and youth in particular. Premigratory as well as postmigratory psychological, social and environmental stressors and their negative influence on the refugees' mental health makes it essential to address the complexity of their life context and the influence it has on all welcoming initiatives. The approach that makes comprehension of the situation possible and authorizes the conception of appropriate actions capable of addressing this complexity is the systemic approach. Our approach is shared by several authors who emphasize that working with refugee youth and families requires a holistic approach [34, 46] as well as an ecological or systemic one [7, 34, 47]. The action research we conducted in several schools with refugee youth is based on this approach.

Promoting the Psychological Wellbeing of Young Refugee Students in Schools: Action Research in Quebec Schools

As a response to the international context, the Canadian government decided in 2015–17 to welcome a large number of refugees, of which 46,700 were Syrian refugees, 47% of them being minors [48]. The province of Quebec welcomed 7,583 of these refugees [49].

According to Hassan [50] and Sirin and Roger-Sirin [38], many of these young Syrian refugees had experienced different traumatic events: violations of their rights to security and protection, including danger of death and injuries; exposure to violent scenes, including killings, corpses and injuries, as well as grief relating to separation and human and material losses. Various psychosocial needs have been documented, in particular the chronic lack of care, food, and health and education services.

In this context, our team proposed an action research project in one of the schools which was welcoming those refugee children. A school-based psychosocial and collaborative intervention was developed. The school would provide protection and safety as well as healing opportunities and intercultural encounters in order to promote the psychological wellbeing of the young refugee students as well as their sense of belonging to the school and to the wider society.

The main objective of this research action, *"Promoting the social and educational integration of Syrian refugee students by developing their sense of belonging to the school, their psychological well-being and that of their families"*, was to evaluate a short systemic school action aiming to support wellbeing in refugee children. Families and community organizations, as well as primary care providers in their neighborhood, were invited to participate in the promotion of the psychological wellbeing and the sense of belonging of newly arrived young Syrian refugee students. Discussion groups and psychosocial support for refugee students showing signs of distress were organized. The participants were reception class students from three schools (one elementary school and two high schools welcoming Syrian refugees). A qualitative evaluation of the implementation of the project was conducted.

The Action

Discussion groups were held in one primary school (two classes) and two high schools (three classes) in Montreal and Laval, addressing sensitive topics of traveling, migration, perceived differences (social, cultural, racial), death and loss, faith, violence, identity, family, life and the experiences of the discussion groups. A translation service from Arabic was offered when children had difficulty expressing themselves in French. The teacher was always present and took part in the activity. Specific space and time were framed by opening and closing rituals. These groups proposed a context that aimed to enhance human and intercultural encounters and the necessary free symbolic expression for the promotion of mental health. The basic principles of this activity were free expression, a nonjudgmental attitude, mutual respect and the confidentiality of shared information. A detailed guide was produced by our team in order to spread this approach and equip the school actors with a new classroom psychosocial intervention tool [51].

The psychosocial support for refugee students and for their families consisted of a school-based collaborative service, aiming at the promotion of their mental health and enhancing the relation between the school workers and the families, as well as families and community and health services. The first step of the intervention consisted of teachers' referral of refugee students in psychological distress or presenting signs of ill-health to our team. The referral was followed by several meetings and clinical interviews with parents and sometimes the student as well as the teachers. The main objective of these interviews consisted of the evaluation of the students' psychosocial, developmental and educational needs, based on a detailed anamnesis of the child's development as well as the detailed pre- and postmigratory family history. After these interviews, we observed the students in different contexts: the classroom, the playground, etc. Once the evaluation was complete, the research team analyzed each case and proposed an individualized multimodal intervention: advice and counseling for the teacher, advice and counseling for the parents, educational adaptations or adjustments, psychosocial intervention with community workers and sometimes referral to local primary health care services.

Figure 18.1 represents the collaborative care model we developed in order to provide psychosocial support to refugee youth and to their families as well as to promote their mental health.

Research Method

Data collection was based on pre- and post-intervention semi-structured interviews with reception class teachers, community and school workers and the school principals. All of these interviews, as well as the group discussions, were recorded. Regarding the psychosocial support for the targeted students, the interviews with their parents and teachers were also recorded. All research assistants or facilitators (animators, observers and psychosocial workers) kept field notes regarding the details (e.g., modalities, conditions) of the implementation of the project. These qualitative data, the field notes and the verbatim transcriptions of these audio recordings were analyzed with QDA-Miner.

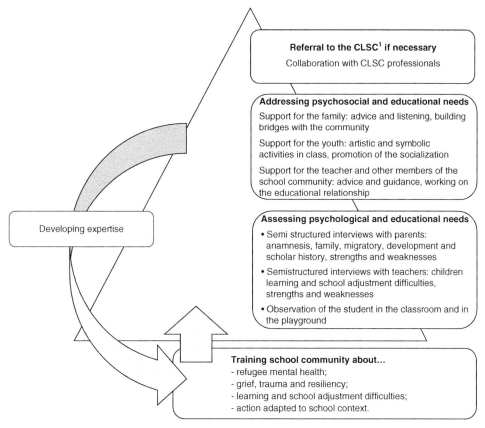

Referral to the CLSC[1] if necessary
Collaboration with CLSC professionals

Addressing psychosocial and educational needs
Support for the family: advice and listening, building bridges with the community

Support for the youth: artistic and symbolic activities in class, promotion of the socialization

Support for the teacher and other members of the school community: advice and guidance, working on the educational relationship

Assessing psychological and educational needs
• Semi structured interviews with parents: anamnesis, family, migratory, development and scholar history, strengths and weaknesses

• Semistructured interviews with teachers: children learning and school adjustment difficulties, strengths and weaknesses

• Observation of the student in the classroom and in the playground

Developing expertise

Training school community about...
- refugee mental health;
- grief, trauma and resiliency;
- learning and school adjustment difficulties;
- action adapted to school context.

18.1 School-based collaborative care model promoting youth mental health[1]

Results

The analysis of our data showed that the discussion groups, participated in the development of the reception class students' psychological wellbeing. They enabled the expression of grief, enhanced the mourning process and the symbolic expression of trauma and supported the healing process. They also provided a space and a time to construct a new meaning of life and to express emotions and thoughts.

> It was like something was on our shoulders and now it has fallen. We could give our . . . like take out our feelings.

The discussion groups also promoted the psychological wellbeing of the students by developing a good relationship between them and their teachers as well as improving ties among them. We noticed an increase in their empathy towards each other.

---

[1] CLSC refers to local community service center (Centre Local de Services Communautaires).

We concentrate on each person. The person who is crying, she has feelings. Everybody has the same feelings.

Regarding the development of the sense of belonging, the results were positive concerning their sense of belonging to the class but negative concerning their sense of belonging to the school. The research highlighted a sense of exclusion and 'ill-being' among the refugee students in the school. The participants, students and school actors described the use of violent and discriminatory gestures and words against young Syrian refugees in the school by Quebecers of various origins, including other Arabs. The students also testified that they and their families were victims of verbal abuse outside the school. All the participants emphasized the fact that the reception classes and their students are marginalized in the school. These results corroborate the results of several studies [29] underlining the fact that postmigratory adverse conditions and negative experiences deteriorate the refugees' mental health, making the presence of various care services in school settings a necessity.

In what follows, we further explore in more depth the second part of our action research, focusing on the proposed provision of psychosocial support to refugee students in distress as well as their families.

The following case studies will illustrate, although briefly, the model of the school-based collaborative care service we proposed in the context of this research. It is important to underline that with these two students the psychologist/researcher involved had a good knowledge of Arabic and we didn't ask for the services of an interpreter. In a different situation we would have done so.

In the Name of the Father: From Distress and Nonsense to a Construction of Meaning with and Through the School and the Community

S. and R. are two Syrian refugee brothers. They are, respectively, 12 and 9 years old. Their parents being of different religious affiliations, when the war in Syria intensified, their father, an academic working in a university in Syria, found a way to send his wife and their two children to Montreal. As usual, like other newcomers, they were registered in reception classes in order to learn French and to be able to join their age group classes.

At the beginning, both children were very motivated and engaged in their learning. After a while, they began having difficulties, and their knowledge of French remained elementary. After two years in the reception classes, following regulations, the school administrators transferred them to the regular classes. The oldest boy was incapable of any progress and the school professionals were thinking about evaluating his cognitive and linguistic abilities. As he was in the sixth grade, they were in the urgency of evaluating him in order to prescribe the orientation he should take in high school.

That was the situation when our research began and when we proposed training on trauma and grief and their influence on the students' school adjustment and learning difficulties to all the teachers in the participant school, pointing out the signs of distress and the symptoms that should be detected in order to refer a student to our team.

Detecting the refugee student's distress - S.'s teacher referred him to us, highlighting the signs and symptoms she noticed after the training: distraction and the impression of being disconnected, irritability, restlessness, difficulties related to memorization, general fatigue and lack of cognitive availability for tasks.

The collaborative care proposed within the school - With the mother's consent, our research team (represented by an Arabic-speaking psychologist/researcher) organized a meeting with her. The objective of this first meeting was to understand the family's situation and its history and to assess the psychosocial needs of the family and the children. What we learned, combined with the school's urgency to evaluate S's abilities, accelerated the process of the intervention.

We learned that the children were born in a loving and educated family. Their development was normal. Before the war, they used to go to a well-known private school in Damascus. Their school performance and achievements were good. That information was verified by the former school's report cards. At the beginning of the war, the family was in Syria, but when the conflicts intensified, the father, a Shiite, sent his wife, a Sunnite, and their children to Montreal in order to protect them from the civil war. At first, he was in regular contact with them by a videoconference platform. He was very attached to his sons and he talked with them every day, encouraging them in their studies, giving them hope regarding the reunion of their family. Then one day he was not online. They were worried. The mother tried to explain his absence by telling them that he had work to do. But the days passed and their father was never online. The anguish of the family intensified. The mother was very worried, but she always found a plausible explanation to give to her children. She contacted her family in Syria and was informed that her husband had been kidnapped. She kept the information to herself, trying to protect her sons. S. and R. were alternately sad, worried and angry with their father. Their mother continued covering for him, trying not to show her anguish, simultaneously trying to get some information regarding his whereabouts. Then one day she received an email from a family friend saying that her husband had been tortured in prison and declared dead. At first she didn't believe it and tried to find some proof. After a while, a photo was sent to her. It was a photo of her husband's body. She broke down and cried a lot but couldn't say anything to her children.

Meanwhile, the children, anxious and destabilized, imprisoned behind a wall of silence, became more and more restless and unable to study. The mother thought that if she told them the truth, they would be devastated and she would lose them completely. So she kept up the lie until our meeting.

Our research team, represented by the psychologist/researcher, supported them in the mourning process, proposing to their mother a space to talk and professional advice regarding her children's grief. We listened to her, knowing that talking about the people or the things that are lost is key to the mourning process. We supported her grief by helping her to accept her husband's violent death, knowing that the circumstances of his death and her incapacity to bury him were aggravating factors in her mourning process. We gave her advice concerning her children and the way to tell them the truth about their father. We supported her in the process. We explained to her that the uncertainty and the unknown reinforce the anxiety and that her sons needed to know the truth in order to be able to mourn their father – that the three of them needed to be real, to cry and to live their grief.

During this rather long but crucial meeting (three hours), we also realized that she was very isolated; she didn't have any friends, she didn't know the neighborhood and she had a lot of questions regarding the school system in Quebec.

A second meeting was then organized with the mother, the vice-principal of the school, the community school worker and an interpreter. The objective of this meeting was to form the basis for a school-family collaboration as well as to organize the necessary services for the children.

The community school worker ensured the link between the mother and several neighboring community organizations and took the time to explain to her the educational system in Quebec.

The vice-principal ensured and supervised all the necessary adaptations and adjustments the students needed in order to improve their academic performances and results: encouragement, understanding, help with homework, more time and less stimulation during tests and evaluations.

We also met S.'s teacher, thanked her for her awareness and gave her advice regarding the attitude she should have with S. (patient, encouraging, soothing) and the extra time she could take with him in order to catch up on certain concepts.

Two weeks after these meetings, after the March break, the teacher called us saying that S. was better; he was working better, concentrating and his academic results were improving. She told us that after he had learned the truth from his mother, he had come to her and said:

I learned that my father is dead. He saved us. He sent us to Canada and he wanted us to succeed. He was a professor at the university. I am able to study now. I will do it for him.

In this case study, we recognize how silence can be broken and primary care can be provided within the school, how school administrators, professionals and community workers can support refugee children in their psychological difficulties, grief and trauma by proposing an adequate setting, intervening differently and assessing the psychosocial and educational needs before doing any other psychological or language evaluation. The case also illustrates how school staff and teachers can misunderstand a student's difficulties and increase the possibility of misdiagnosis.

Ghosts from the Past: When Cumulative Grief and Amplified Distress Pour into School. School-Based Collaborative Care as an Answer to a Paralyzing Situation

K. is a young female refugee student in one of the reception classes participating in our research. She is 11 years old and she arrived in Canada at the end of 2015 with her family: her parents and a little brother.

Detecting the refugee student's distress - K. was referred to our research team by her teacher, who noted that she lacked motivation and curiosity toward school activities and learning; she frequently forgot her school material. The teacher said that although K. had skills, she lacked cognitive availability and was failing in the majority of the academic subjects. K. also had a tendency to have conflicts with some teachers and some classmates. According to her teacher, when she arrived she used to pull out her own hair (trichotillomania).

The collaborative care proposed within the school - The first two meetings with K.'s mother were dedicated to the anamnesis and the family pre- and postmigratory history. These are the most important elements that were released: The symptoms that were described by the teacher appeared or developed after the family's resettlement in Canada. We also noted the presence of depressive symptoms masked by a resistant/aversive attitude. The family, as well as K., have lived through potentially traumatic events and several losses.

This table summarizes the family's migratory path:

18.2 K.'s family history

Pre-migration

– Many events had an influence on K's pre-migratory life:

- sudden death of her older brother at three days old;
- medical complications at the birth of the student;
- sudden death of maternal grandfather;
- beginning of the war in Syria and first attack in Aleppo – car bomb near the family home;
- besieged neighborhood and food shortage;
- the mother escapes a terrorist attack;
- the father loses his job;
- the father suffers from a heart discomfort.

Migration

– Long journey to Turkey (Istanbul) by land.

Post-migration

– Difficulties related to their resettlement in Montreal:

- precarious health of the father;
- communication problems;
- inability to have the equivalence of their diplomas;
- difficulties finding a job.

The analysis of K.'s and her family's history leads us to understand that the death of her elder brother as well as the medical problems she had at birth had profoundly traumatized her mother. Therefore the attachment that she proposed to K. was influenced by the grief of losing her first child as well as the anxiety of potentially losing K. The loss of her own father, as well as the traumatic events linked to the war, exacerbated her anxiety and reinforced her overprotectiveness towards K. In addition to all this, her father's health issues as well as all the socioeconomic difficulties related to their resettlement in Montreal had amplified K.'s distress. K. and her mother were in a paralyzing anxiety dynamic and it was affecting both her academic and her social life at school. K. was transferring her attachment patterns to school, and the educational relationship she was developing with her teacher, as well as her social relations with her classmates, were echoing her psychological problems.

The proposed intervention was multimodal. We had several consultations with K.'s mother. We proposed to her a space within the school where she was able to express herself and distance herself from the potential traumatic events she had lived through. The first two sessions aimed to instill a climate of trust and security between the psychologist/researcher and the mother. As a result of these two interviews, the mother was able to relate K.'s symptoms to the family experience and to give a meaning to certain behaviors that she had considered confusing at first. Thus, enabling speech allowed the emergence of a certain psychological flexibility. The mother was therefore more open to the advice that we offered in the following sessions. The following three meetings aimed to increase the mother's awareness regarding the cumulative traumas experienced by the family and how they had influenced the family dynamics as well as the need to break the wall of silence regarding these issues. We encouraged her to talk about these events with the various members of her family, to encourage them to verbalize the emotions related to these events. This was a perspective that the mother initially dreaded but was eager to follow in the end, understanding the importance of symbolization and expression. These meetings made her also realize the way she had transmitted her grief and her anxiety to her daughter. Another suggestion that was given to the mother was to avoid having a reproachful attitude over K.'s academic delay and to adopt a more understanding approach to the problem without giving her a sense of guilt. We also encouraged her to initiate direct and regular contact with K.'s teacher.

We had four consultations with the teacher in order to help her understand K.'s difficulties and the particularities of the relationships that she had developed at school. We also gave her some advice regarding her symptoms and the way to deal with them in class without stigmatizing her. Some clues were also proposed as to how to deal with her social problems and the conflicts she often created with her peers.

At first, we developed the teacher's awareness regarding K.'s pre- and postmigratory history and emphasized the importance of making K. feel welcome and accepted, understood and not judged despite her negative behavior and her tendency to have conflicts with others. We suggested to the teacher to work on her educational relationship with K., to help her put words to and give a meaning to her attitude and behavior. We encouraged the teacher to keep in close contact with K.'s parents and by her positive attitude to try to decrease K.'s and her parents' anxiety regarding homework and school achievement.

A meeting was also organized between K.'s teacher, K. and her mother. The main purpose of the meeting was to lay the foundation for a future collaboration between them. Our role was mainly to facilitate the exchange but also to provide K. with a support system.

After three months, K.'s situation had improved. Although no longer critical, K.'s difficulties were persistent. At the end of our research project, we referred the family to the youth mental health care team at the CLSC, knowing that there would be a period of waiting before the first appointment. But primary care had already been given and the situation was less urgent. Unfortunately, our partnership with the CLSC, as well as its involvement in primary schools, was very limited. Despite that, we were able to transfer K.'s file to the relevant specific services.

In this case study, we identify the importance of a school-based primary care service as well as the necessity of understanding as quickly as possible how family dynamics and parent-child relationships can influence school dynamics and teacher-student relationships. We also underline the paralyzing effect of trauma and anxiety on refugees and point out how it can be relived in a school context, as well as underlining the importance of early intervention and family-school collaboration. The need for a stronger collaboration between schools and social and health services is also revealed.

Conclusion

The discussion groups, as well as the collaborative care we proposed through this action research, revealed the diversity of life contexts, paths, stories, war- and violence-related experiences, cultures and beliefs among refugees sharing the same country of origin and sometimes even the same language. That is why the same activities did not have a similar impact on all the participants. The same collaborative care model did not lead to the same type of collaboration between school workers, teachers and refugee students and their families.

The collaborative primary health care model that we proposed in the context of our action research gave us the opportunity to address refugee youth psychological needs differently, by taking into account their preferences (collective or individual intervention), their culture (translation facilities) and their needs. With the adopted systemic approach, we were able to answer the individual psychological needs by offering different spaces and opportunities to break paralyzing traumatic silences and to elaborate losses and progress in grief. Our actions in the school setting with the parents, the school and community actors enabled us to bring modifications to the refugee youth psychosocial context and cause changes in family and school dynamics as well as students' psychological well-being. Their pre- and postmigratory history was addressed, highlighting the positive and negative moments lived by the refugee youth and their families – moments of rupture, moments of bonding, and constructive and destructive moments sustaining trauma and resiliency.

Several initiatives around the world, in Canada and in Quebec have attempted to meet the psychosocial needs of refugee youth and their families. Many of these initiatives use a systemic approach. A partnership between the community and the school is a good way to address these needs. Whether through a hierarchical organization of the services offered, the establishment of focus groups or the use of visual arts or music, these initiatives work preventively, thereby reducing the stigma that is generally associated with mental health care. The school-based collaborative care model promoting youth mental health described in this chapter illustrates an initiative aiming at the psychological rehabilitation of the one of the most vulnerable populations in the world today: refugee youth, who cannot be considered independently from their families. Proposing community- and school-based primary care programs makes it possible to overcome obstacles like stigma and difficulty accessing services and helps to promote the mental health of refugee families within a broader approach.

References

1. American Psychiatric Association, (2018). *What is the Collaborative Care Model?* www.psychiatry.org/psychiatrists/practice/professional-interests/integrated-care/get-trained/about-collaborative-care (accessed September 1, 2018).

2. American Psychological Association (APA). *Resilience and Recovery after War: Refugee Children and Families in the United States.* www.apa.org/pi/families/refugees.aspx (accessed February 1, 2018).

3. C. Rousseau, T. Measham and L. Nadeau, Addressing trauma in collaborative mental health care for refugee children. *Clinical Child Psychology and Psychiatry*, 18 (2013), 121–36.

4. Inter-Agency Standing Committee, *IASC Guidelines on Mental Health and Psychosocial Support in Emergency Settings* (Switzerland: IASC, 2006).

5. T. Measham, J. Guzder, C. Rousseau, L. Pacione, M. Blais-McPherson and L. Nadeau, Refugee children and their families: Supporting psychological well-being and positive adaptation following migration. *Current Problems in Pediatric and Adolescent Health Care*, 44 (2014), 208–15.

6. R. Quinlan, R. D. Schweitzer, N. Khawaja and J. Griffin, Evaluation of a school-based creative arts therapy program for adolescents from refugee backgrounds. *The Arts in Psychotherapy*, 47 (2016), 72–8.

7. C. Rousseau and J. Guzder, School-based prevention programs for refugee children. *Child and Adolescent Psychiatric Clinics*, 17 (2008), 533–49.

8. A. Sullivan and G. Simonson, A systematic review of school-based social-emotional interventions for refugee and war-traumatized youth. *Review of Educational Research*, 86 (2016), 503–30.

9. B. H. Ellis, A. B. Miller, S. Abdi, C. Barrett, E. A. Blood and T. S. Betancourt, Multi-tier mental health program for refugee youth. *Journal of Consulting and Clinical Psychology*, 81 (2013), 129–40.

10. R. Berger, R. Pat-Horenczyk and M. Gelkopf, School-based intervention for prevention

and treatment of elementary-students' terror-related distress in Israel: A quasi-randomized controlled trial. *Journal of Traumatic Stress*, 4 (2007), 541–51.

11. K. A. Ehntholt, P. Smith and W. Yule, School-based CBT group intervention for refugee children who have experienced war-related trauma. *Clinical Child Psychology and Psychiatry*, 10 (2005), 235–50.

12. G. Durà-Vilà, H. Klasen, Z. Makatini, Z. Rahimi and M. Hodes, Mental health problems of young refugees: Duration of settlement, risk factors and community-based interventions. *Clinical Child Psychology and Psychiatry*, 18 (2013), 604–23.

13. M. Hodes, D. Jagdev, N. Chandra and A. Cunniff, Risk and resilience for psychological distress amongst unaccompanied asylum seeking adolescents. *Journal of Child Psychology and Psychiatry*, 49 (2008), 723–32.

14. Refugee Trauma Task Force, (2005). *Mental Health Interventions for Refugee Children in Resettlement*. www.nctsnet.org/nctsn_assets/pdfs/materials_for_applicants/MH_Interventions_for_Refugee_Children.pdf (accessed February 1, 2018).

15. J. Stewart and L. Martin, *Bridging Two Worlds: Supporting Newcomer and Refugee Youth* (Toronto: CERIC, 2018).

16. A. Richters, C. Dekker and W. F. Scholte, Community based sociotherapy in Byumba, Rwanda. *Intervention*, 6 (2008), 100–16.

17. S. C. Yohani, Creating an ecology of hope: Arts-based interventions with refugee children. *Child and Adolescent Social Work Journal*, 25 (2008), 309–23.

18. K. Marsh, The beat will make you be courage: The role of a secondary school music program in supporting young refugees and newly arrived immigrants in Australia. *Research Studies in Music Education*, 34 (2012), 93–111.

19. M. Fazel, J. Garcia and A. Stein, The right location? Experiences of refugee adolescents seen by school-based mental health services. *Clinical Child Psychology and Psychiatry*, 21 (2016), 368–80.

20. T. Persson and C. Rousseau, School-based interventions for minors in war-exposed countries: A review of targeted and general programmes. *Torture: Quarterly Journal on Rehabilitation of Torture Victims and Prevention of Torture*, 19 (2009), 88–101.

21. J. Kirk, (2002). Les enfants touchés par la guerre dans les écoles de Montréal. www.cgtsim.qc.ca/images/documents/enfants_guerre.pdf (accessed February 1, 2018).

22. R. J. Hamilton and D. Moore, Education of refugee children: Documenting and implementing change. In R. Hamilton and D. Moore, eds., *Educational Interventions for Refugee Children* (New York: RoutledgeFalmer, 2004), pp. 106–16.

23. C. Rousseau, G. Ammara, L. Baillargeon, A. Lenoir and D. Roy, *Repenser les services en santé mentale des jeunes: La créativité nécessaire* (Quebec: Les Publications du Québec Montréal, 2007).

24. M. Fazel, J. Garcia and A. Stein, The right location? Experiences of refugee adolescents seen by school-based mental health services. *Clinical Child Psychology and Psychiatry*, 21 (2016), 368–80.

25. G. Hughes, Finding a voice through 'The Tree of Life': A strength-based approach to mental health for refugee children and families in schools. *Clinical Child Psychology and Psychiatry*, 19 (2014), 139–53.

26. H. B. Ellis, A. B. Miller, H. Baldwin and S. Abdi, New directions in refugee youth mental health services: Overcoming barriers to engagement. *Journal of Child & Adolescent Trauma*, 4 (2011), 69–85.

27. S. J. Lee and M. R. Hawkins, 'Family is here': Learning in community-based after-school programs. *Theory into Practice*, 47 (2008), 51–8.

28. T. Idsoe, A. Dyregrov and K. Dyregrov, School based interventions. In M. A. Landolt, M. Marylène Cloitre and U. Schnyder, eds., *Evidence-Based Treatments for Trauma Related Disorders in Children and Adolescents* (Switzerland: Springer, 2017), pp. 465–82.

29. C. Suárez-Orozco, M. Onaga and C. de Lardemelle, Promoting academic engagement among immigrant adolescents through school-family-community collaboration. *Professional School Counseling*, 14 (2010), 15–26.

30. C. Baker, M. Varma and C. Tanaka, Sticks and stones: Racism as experienced by adolescents in New Brunswick. *Canadian Journal of Nursing Research Archive*, 33 (2016), 87–105.

31. J. Stewart, *Supporting Refugee Children: Strategies for Educators* (Toronto: University of Toronto Press, 2011).

32. S. Taylor and R. K. Sidhu, Supporting refugee students in schools: What constitutes inclusive education? *International Journal of Inclusive Education*, 16 (2012), 39–56.

33. M. Bajaj, A. Argenal and M. Canlas, Socio-politically relevant pedagogy for immigrant and refugee youth. *Equity & Excellence in Education*, 50 (2017), 258–74.

34. K. Block, S. Cross, E. Riggs and L. Gibbs, Supporting schools to create an inclusive environment for refugee students. *International Journal of Inclusive Education*, 18 (2014), 1337–55.

35. E. G. Kugler, (2009). *Partnering with Parents and Families to Support Immigrant and Refugee Children at School*. www.lacgc.org/pdf/PartneringSupportImmigrantChildren.pdf (accessed February 1, 2018).

36. D. A. Stegelin, (2017). *Strategies for Supporting Immigrant Students and Families: Guidelines for School Personnel*. http://dropoutprevention.org/wp-content/uploads/2017/10/supporting-immigrant-students-and-families-2017-10.pdf (accessed February 1, 2018).

37. J. Charrette and J.-C. Kalubi, Collaborations école-famille-communauté : L'apport de l'intervenant interculturel dans l'accompagnement à l'école de parents récemment immigrés au Québec. *Education, Sciences & Society*, 2 (2016), 127–49.

38. S. R. Sirin and L. Roger-Sirin, (2015). *The Educational and Mental Health Needs of Syrian Refugee Children*. www.researchgate.net/profile/Selcuk_Sirin/publication/287998909_The_Educational_and_Mental_Health_Needs_of_Syrian_Refugee_Children/links/567ccd6c08ae19758384e4bf.pdf (accessed February 1, 2018).

39. A. O. Mace, S. Mulheron, C. Jones and S. Cherian, Educational, developmental and psychological outcomes of resettled refugee children in Western Australia: A review of School of Special Educational Needs: Medical and Mental Health input. *Journal of Paediatrics and Child Health*, 50 (2014), 985–92.

40. M. E. Williams and S. C. Thompson, The use of community-based interventions in reducing morbidity from the psychological impact of conflict-related trauma among refugee populations: A systematic review of the literature. *Journal of Immigrant and Minority Health*, 13(4) (2011), 780–94.

41. R. A. Tyrer and M. Fazel, School and community-based interventions for refugee and asylum seeking children: A systematic review. *PLoS One*, 9 (2014), e89359.

42. S. S. Kupzyk, B. M. Banks and M. R. Chadwell, Collaborating with refugee families to increase early literacy opportunities: A pilot investigation. *Contemporary School Psychology*, 20 (2016), 205–17.

43. Y. Pang, Barriers and solutions in involving culturally linguistically diverse families in the IFSP/IEP process. *Making Connections: Interdisciplinary Approaches to Cultural Diversity*, 12 (2011), 42–51.

44. R. Georgis, R. J. Gokiert, D. M. Ford and M. Ali, Creating inclusive parent engagement practices: Lessons learned from a school community collaborative supporting newcomer refugee families. *Multicultural Education*, 21 (2014), 23–7.

45. S. Yohani, Educational cultural brokers and the school adaptation of refugee children and families: Challenges and opportunities. *Journal of International Migration and Integration*, 14 (2013), 61–79.

46. M. Arnot and H. Pinson, *The Education of Asylum-Seeker and Refugee Children: A Study of LEA and School Values, Policies and Practices* (Cambridge, UK: University of Cambridge, 2005).

47. B. Soller, J. R. Goodkind, R. N. Greene et al., Ecological networks and community attachment and support among recently resettled refugees. *American Journal of Community Psychology*, 61 (2018), 332–43.

48. United Nations High Commissioner for Refugees, (2017). *Refugee Resettlement Facts.* www.unhcr.ca/wp-content/uploads/2017/04 /Canadian-Resettlement-Fact-Sheet-ENG-April-2017.pdf (accessed February 1, 2018).

49. Ministry of Immigration, Diversity and Inclusion, (2017). *Bienvenue aux réfugiés syriens.* www.immigration-quebec.gouv.qc .ca/fr/informations/accueil-refugies-syriens/ (accessed February 1, 2018).

50. G. Hassan, L. Kirmayer and A. Mekki-Berrada, (2015). *Culture, Context and the Mental Health and Psychosocial Wellbeing of Syrians: A Review for Mental Health and Psychosocial Support Staff Working with Syrians Affected by Armed Conflict.* www.unhcr.org/55f6b90f9.pdf (accessed February 1, 2018).

51. G. Papazian-Zohrabian, V. Lemire, C. Mamprin, A. Turpin-Samson and R. Aoun, (2017). *Mener des groupes de parole en contexte scolaire.* www.sherpa-recherche.com/wp-content/uploads/2017/ 12/Mener-des-groupes-de-parole-en-contexte-scolaire.pdf (accessed February 1, 2018).

Chapter 19

Interrogating Legality and Legitimacy in the Post-migratory Context

Working around Traumatic Repetition and Reenactment with Refugee Families

Cécile Rousseau

War, armed conflicts and other forms of organized violence shatter the protective nature of society. In these violent contexts, institutional power becomes at best inefficient, when governments are unable to protect their citizens, at worst oppressive, when it participates directly in abuse. In both cases, the state and its institutions lose their legitimacy. Organized violence contexts often also transform and undermine the judicial power, which may then, in many ways, support or even encourage persecution, human rights violations and discrimination toward citizens or noncitizens. In the official international organizations' discourse about refugees, it is this incapacity of the state to defend and protect their citizens which justifies the right of asylum. In their narrative, refugee families seeking protection are expected to resettle in host countries with laws which defend human rights, institutions which are legitimate and in a society which is, overall, protective.

Beyond this official narrative, what is meant by "protection," "family" and "legitimacy" may be quite different for the host country agencies and for the refugees themselves. Furthermore, the significance of the concept of protection is rapidly evolving with the emergence of the antirefugee rhetoric associated with globalization [1]. As discrimination against refugees increases, the host country social context sometimes becomes a more important risk factor for mental health than premigration trauma [2]. This challenges the myth about the protectiveness and benevolence of European and North American host societies and changes specifically the trauma repetition experiences and the reenactment dynamics of refugee families.

In this chapter, I will argue that the notions of protection and family are negotiated in complex and often conflictual ways among refugee families and host country institutions, sometimes becoming pivotal parts of reenactment scenarios in which the apprehended repetition of trauma transforms the potential protective nature of the host society into a space perceived as violent. These common inversion processes may sometimes be associated with host country policies or practices, which act as triggers of retraumatization. They may also be related to refugee family members acting out and risk-taking, which may provoke retaliation on the part of institutions when they are perceived as transgressive. Very often, however, the perceived loss of the protective nature of the host country is the product of a complex interplay between discrimination and exclusion experienced by the refugee families in the host society and reenactment dynamics on the part of refugee family members. These dynamics encroach in different ways upon clinical encounters with the refugee families. They first put forward the diversity of pathways reflecting the internalization of trauma and the coping strategies to address it. They may also reflect both the cultural differences which are present in the clinical encounter and the structural discrimination processes which structure the place of the refugees in the wider community.

After briefly situating this topic in the field of legal consciousness studies, I will first examine the plurality of meanings evoked by the concepts of family and protection and illustrate some of the ways in which the present refugee resettlement context transforms the perceptions of family members' obligations and rights in a specific social space. I will then present clinical situations to show how what clinicians consider as legal obligations and boundaries need to be constantly interrogated from a legitimacy point of view and how this raises challenging ethical and clinical dilemmas for mental health and social professionals.

Legality, Legitimacy and Legal Consciousness

The term *legality* is used to refer to the meanings, sources of authority and cultural practices which, together, operate to define, regulate and pattern social life. Silbey [3] proposes that legality is constituted through everyday actions and practices and that most of the time it is just this "Invisible constraint, suffusing and saturating our everyday life. Most of the time, legal authority, forms and decisions go uncontested or are challenged only with the legally provided channels of context" [3]. This legal world order is, however, not neutral and has been described as ideological by the critical legal studies movement, which has highlighted repeatedly that law serves to buttress the established power rather than to protect the rights of the vulnerable [4]. The concept of hegemony is put forward to represent the ways in which meaning is produced, challenged and perpetuated in social structures. These meanings are so embedded in daily life that representational and institutional struggles are no longer visible and, in general, subjects do not question the hegemony, which is accepted as shared evidence [3].

This analysis of the hidden nature of structures favoring the perpetuation of the majority privileges can be seen in parallel with the growing awareness of the importance of structural determinants in public health [5]. In structural discrimination situations, the organization of relations and resources blurs the mechanisms that systematically allocate status and privileges. "Social actors are thus constrained without knowing from where or whom the constraint derives" [3].

In the situation of refugees, the host country law is considered by health and social professionals and by educators as the norm. Religious and traditional laws are either disqualified or presented as alternative or counter-hegemonic legalities [6]. In situations of pluralism, claims of legitimacy of the majority norm or of alternative norms are usually supported by invoking higher morality and are, according to Benda-Beckman et al. [7], indissociable from political struggles for hegemony. These processes can, for example, simultaneously confer acceptability on illegal acts like suspending civil rights in the name of national security and banish a pluralist interpretation of the law regarding family matters, which may be presented and perceived as an unacceptable attack on the majority core values. Legal pluralism mirrors the great complexity of cognitive and normative conceptions in contemporary societies. These complex systems provide standards to evaluate actions as well as ideas for dealing with delicate situations, for example, the management of family conflicts [7]. Thus, presently, globalization may simultaneously promote the legitimate coexistence of a diversity of norms and representations of families and, because of increasing hegemony, impose more than ever international norms and standards forged by and for the powerful.

What are some of the consequences of this situation for social and clinical intervention with refugee families? A first level of impact for families seeking care may be the shift in the professional interpretation framework of what is legal and legitimate. The ways in which people invoke and enact legality is called *legal consciousness*. These interpretations, which may be highly individualized, may also be influenced by collective representations circulating widely through the media. This process may influence the professional evaluation of the level of danger or the compromisation of a particular conflictual couple or parent-child relationship and may subsequently alter the tendency of these professionals to signal youth protection or to call the police. A second level of impact may be associated with a decrease in the relative trust that the refugee families may have in health and social services professionals and institutions. When their communities are portrayed publicly in a negative light, refugees may fear that the professional that they will meet will be prejudiced [8, 9]. They may as a result refuse to disclose any information which they feel could be misinterpreted or be an indication of family difficulties. Simultaneously, they may turn toward community resources or toward transnational networks to find what they consider legitimate advice and appropriate support. On the part of the host country institution, the distrust of the families is often perceived as a sign of resistance, which further confirms the belief that they have something to hide and should be the object of suspicion.

In summary, although clinicians are trained to recognize their own emotional bias in therapeutic encounters, their perceptions of the law and of their legal obligations often remain unquestioned. In working with refugee families, clinicians need to become aware of the hegemonic dimension of the law in the host country and of the diverse ways in which the social context surrounding them will allow or prohibit a pluralist interpretation of the legal frame. Clinicians also need to elicit the eventual alternate norms to which the family may adhere in order to establish a dialogue and negotiation between different levels of legitimacy.

Hegemonic Discourses around Legality and Clinical Intervention with Families

Hegemonic discourses impose mainstream representations of family relations, gender roles and what constitutes violence both directly, through laws, and indirectly, through clinicians' interpretative frames. Uncovering the blind spots and becoming aware of the majority biases is a necessary first step to establishing relationships with refugee families.

When Law Defines and Prescribes Family Relations

Although the concept of family is universal, the definition of what is meant by a family and of the obligations and rights of family members vary not only across settings and cultures but also over time within societies. Legally, family relations are enshrined within a complex set of codes and roles which define couple and gender relations and parent-child relations, among others. Gender equity, autonomy of the subject and protection against abuse and violence are at the forefront of the laws which regulate family life in European and North American countries. Applied mechanically to refugee families, with goodwill but without cultural sensitivity, protection-oriented measures meant to guarantee the preservation of these rights can often cause distress and destabilize the families [10]. For example, in Canada, youth autonomy is valued, and adolescents are guaranteed confidentiality at the age of 14 years old, which means that from that age they can consult a health professional without their parents' knowledge. This measure ensures that adolescents can have confidential access to family planning, sexual counseling and abortion, among other things. For migrant families, this confidentiality clause is often understood as a way of telling adolescents that the state and the professionals of the host country are considered more trustworthy than their parents, as an invitation to transgress cultural and religious codes of conduct and as directly undermining parental authority. In the case of refugee families who have endured organized violence, there is often an additional layer of meaning. Because persecution is almost always founded on complex networks of denunciation, this legal provision is a reminder of the dangers of family betrayal, which evokes a conflict of loyalty. When, in addition, the families are dysfunctional, the youth are often caught in a double bind. Disclosing family conflicts, interpersonal violence and abusive physical discipline may reenact denunciation scenarios which have been harmful or deadly to the family. Keeping silent, on the other hand, may be a way of condoning ongoing intrafamily violence and becoming an accomplice of traumatic repetition, thus endorsing the aggressor role.

Defining who is a family member and who can be a legal caretaker is another situation in which there is frequently a gap between the law in the host country and what the family may consider legitimate. During flight, children are often entrusted to adult caretakers who are not their biological parents but who may be legitimate authorities for the children. This is frequently the case in polygamous marriages, with children and youth fleeing with one of their father's wives, but also with unaccompanied refugee minors, who may consider as an invested relative someone they have never met.

> Hassan is a 13-year-old unaccompanied minor from Somalia. At the Canadian border, he explains to the migration officers that he has an uncle in Canada whose name he ignores. The Somali interpreter asks him a few questions about his lineage and suggests that Mr. B., who lives in Montreal, may be related to the child. Hassan becomes happy and overexcited and declares, "Mr. B. is my uncle; bring me there." When realizing that this will not be the case immediately, he becomes furious.

Although precautions are, of course, warranted before giving a child into the care of any adult, identity verification (identity papers and DNA testing) has often resulted in significant harm and disruption to refugee families, sometimes even revealing painful family secrets which are associated with subsequent exclusion and rejection processes. The European and North American representation of families as essentially nuclear further interacts with the legal premises about parental authority. In a qualitative study of Vietnamese refugee families, Tingvold et al. [11] showed how aunts, uncles and cousins were significant figures in the lives of many adolescents. This extended kin network proved to be particularly important at critical stages and in crisis situations in family life. Most of the time, however, grandparents, aunts and uncles are not consulted when psychological help or counseling is required by refugee families in health and social institutions, because they are often automatically assumed to have a secondary or negligible role.

Although child protection agencies increasingly take into account the significance of the child's or youth's multiple attachments in the assessment of who can be an acceptable caretaker or who are the significant caretakers, the legal dimension continues to predominate over cultural definitions of families' obligations and relations, interfering with a more emic understanding of what the family is and often hindering interventions.

Refugee families may also experience the host society discourse as paradoxical. On one hand, our societies over-rely on biological proof of family relations, delegitimizing the authority of other parental figures. On the other hand, the state has the power to decide that these biological caretakers are not protective enough and that the children can be entrusted to strangers. As some refugee parents told us, one of the first things they learned before they landed in Canada was: "Be careful, here they can take away your children."

Growing Xenophobia Expressed in the Gender and Age Profile of Prejudices

The representation of the "other," the member of a minority group or the migrant or refugee, as the "barbaric other" can be found throughout human history. In modern times, with the adoption of the International Charter of Human Rights and of the Charter for the Rights of Children, these representations have progressively attributed to the "others" the nonrespect of child protection and of gender equity. (Interestingly, although the northern countries tend to believe that this is their predicament, the same arguments are used by groups like ISIS, among others.)

Although both gender equity and child protection are essential values, the ways in which they are interpreted in a situation of cultural gaps often tends to mirror minority–majority power relations and may become more harmful than protective for women and children and for families in general. As part of the Canadian Medical Association Guidelines for Immigrant and Refugee Health, two systematic reviews of the literature discussed the available evidence for intimate partner violence and for child maltreatment [12, 13]. With regard to conjugal violence, they conclude that immigrant and refugee women are particularly vulnerable to the consequences of false positives and that screening does not reduce the recurrence of violence. With regard to child maltreatment, screening instruments were shown to result in unacceptably high false positive rates, which are associated with significant harm because of the disruption created within the family and its network by the often erroneous suspicions of parents.

Studies in black American communities, but also in Arabic Muslim communities, have repeatedly demonstrated how men and youth are particularly targeted by the prejudices portraying them as violent [14]. Women, on the other hand, are most often portrayed as submissive and helpless, a situation which has led female scholars in postcolonial studies to critique this instrumentalization of the gender position to consolidate the hegemony of the west [15]. Similarly, Kleinman and Kleinman [16] have argued that the portrayal of low-income-country children as helpless and isolated could be a way to confirm the domination and the image of benevolence of the European and North American countries. Far from being erased by globalization, these representations have been fueled by polarization processes and by the increase in social hostility around ethnic, religious and racial differences [17]. The "war on terror" discourse, which has been justified largely by the hypothesis of the clash of civilizations [18], has also instrumentalized women and children and described southern refugee families as patriarchal and oppressive, often portraying European and North American countries as representing a higher standard of morality and an example of social progress.

The growing xenophobia which is structured explicitly or implicitly in these discourses is internalized in diverse ways by health and education professionals in the receiving country and influences their gaze on refugee families and their understanding of family dynamics as well as their preference in terms of therapeutic avenues.

Protection as a Double-Edged Sword for Refugee Families

In this landscape of relative confusion and divergence around the family concept and the attached semantic networks, the notion of protection, although advocated by all and central to the refugee predicament, is embodied and negotiated through complex and often contradictory processes. The idea of risk, of danger, of threat is indissociable from the idea of protection. In clinical encounters, what is perceived as a threat and as a danger may evoke trauma repetition, be interpreted as traumatic reenactment and/or represent an entanglement of both. When the refugee family suffers from particular forms of organized violence within the host country (most commonly structural discrimination and exclusion) which are characterized by De Certeau [19] as "clean violence," these experiences may evoke past trauma and shatter the idealized vision of the new society. At the same time, family members may act out and stage in diverse ways scenarios evoking more or less explicitly the violence that they have endured in the past and that they expect to happen again. This is particularly the case for adolescents, for whom reenactment and risk-taking behaviors are at the forefront of post-traumatic stress disorder (PTSD) symptomatology [20]. Family members' expectations are often partially confirmed by their experiences in the host country, and, because recognizing the violence of our own society is not easy, clinicians may have a hard time disentangling what belongs to the family and what is the responsibility of the receiving society. The following clinical accounts illustrate the diverse forms in which these dynamics may emerge during clinical encounters.

Meriem: You Are Free and Equal, but We Will Decide What Is Good for You

Meriem is a 15-year-old adolescent living with a large extended family headed by her mother. She has slight cognitive limitations, is struggling to learn the host country language and is teased within the family and at school because of her analphabetism. The youth protection agency has been involved because of her school's concerns about Meriem's behavior with boys and men. She hangs out late with them and accepts money and food from them in exchange for sexual interactions. Social workers have done some unsuccessful psychoeducation interventions in which they have explained to Meriem that she is putting herself at risk of abuse. They have also met with her mother to ask her to better control her daughter, but they felt that her mother was avoiding talking about her daughter's issues and was minimizing the significance of her behavior. Because the family was Muslim, this seemed awkward to the social worker, who concluded that the mother was not protective and that the girl should be placed in an institution under the care of Youth Protection. In placement, Meriem became severely depressed, made a risky suicide attempt and ran away from the emergency department.

In a subsequent family assessment with a transcultural team, some of Meriem's older sisters revealed privately to the clinicians that Meriem had been a major provider for the family in the refugee camp. In the gaps of the story, the clinician understood that Meriem had been "sacrificed" or "sold" to older men in the camp and that this had enabled this large, female-headed family to survive. On one hand, Meriem suffered from this sexual exploitation, while on the other, she was proud to be able to help her family significantly. In exile, she was both reenacting the trauma and asserting her agency through her promiscuous behavior. The placement, which shamed both her mother and herself, shifted the meaning of their history in the camps, deprived her of a certain control over her life and led her to make a desperate gesture.

In this situation, the decision of youth protection services to protect Meriem from a real risk of abuse had invalidated both her understanding that she was able to protect her family and her mother's painful (and questionable) decision to expose Meriem to such risks in order to feed and protect the whole family. Because of the sexual freedom of youth in Canada, Meriem had naively imagined that her dating behavior with men (which was not approved by her brothers) would not be problematic in Canada. She felt disoriented: "They tell me I can have a boyfriend. They tell me here you can have sexual relations. Then they tell me it's bad." The mother's authority was shattered by the youth protection intervention, and the family (which was already dysfunctional) became much more disorganized.

Meriem's story illustrates how different representations of protection may be antagonistic in situations of traumatic reenactment and how a justified concern for a youth's safety, if it does not take into account the family's strengths and system of meaning, may further disempower the family.

Juana: I Cannot Do What You Are Asking Me to Do

Juana, a 35-year-old Salvadoran refugee, presented at the community health center with multiple bruises. During the assessment, she disclosed a chronic situation of conjugal violence. She told the nurse that her husband had been hitting her from time to time in El Salvador but that it had become much worse recently. The family had two young children who sometimes witnessed the outbursts of violence. The nurse explained that Canadian law prohibited conjugal violence and told Juana that she had to call the police and youth protection services in order to protect her and the children, who were witnessing the abuse. Juana began to cry loudly. She admitted that she had thought about it but could not do it because her husband had suffered from torture in jail and that if she called the police she would feel as though she was torturing him again, like in the nightmares he always had.

In Juana's situation, the legal protection available for battered women in Canada represented some hope, but it also evoked the repetition of the political trauma perpetuated by the army in El Salvador. We helped the nurse to talk with Juana about what would be eventual acceptable alternatives which could protect the whole family. When asked why things were better before exile, Juana mentioned first the pride of her husband, who was engaged with the guerillas, then his present irritability and sadness, which she attributed to the sequelae of the torture he had endured. Finally, she explained that in El Salvador, the presence of her brothers, who lived nearby and whom he respected, was also an important moderating factor and concluded: "Help me bring my brothers here." While this was not possible, we searched for other masculine figures who could have the same form of legitimacy for her husband and who would be in a position to address with him both the violence and his need for help.

For Juana, the Canadian protocol criminalizing conjugal violence was absolutely unacceptable because it identified her husband, whom she also considered a victim, as being only an aggressor. The engagement of her husband with treatment to buffer some of his reenactment behaviors was delicate and required the identification of legitimate figures who could question his behavior while supporting his pride and agency.

Hamid: Stabbing a Mother

Hamid is an 11-year-old Afghan refugee boy, recently arrived in Canada with his mother. He was referred to a youth mental health clinic because he hit his mother and insulted her, accusing her of being a prostitute. The assessment revealed a trajectory of disrupted attachment in a mixed marriage context. As a baby, Hamid had been in the care of his maternal grandmother for about two years. Subsequently, he endured hunger and poverty with his mother until the age of six. After being transferred to his father's family, he was severely neglected and suffered from repeated physical abuse for about two years. When he moved back to his mother, he had more or less learned to live on the street in a high-intensity armed conflict area. He repeatedly witnessed war atrocities, saw mutilated and beheaded corpses and was exposed to combat violence. In Canada, soon after their arrival, Hamid's mother established a relationship with a young man. For Hamid, this confirmed what his father's family had always said about his mother being a bad woman. The clinical team tried to address the ambivalent attachment and the war traumas and to reestablish some forms of legitimate cultural markers that would signify acceptance of his mother's desire to find a companion while reassuring her son that he did not have to defend the family's honor.

A few weeks after the beginning of the intervention, Hamid stabbed his mother and was placed as an emergency in a closed center for delinquent youth. Obviously, we had under-evaluated the risk of violence, even if our understanding of its relation to both the attachment disruption and the cumulative traumas was probably valid. In spite of this, as expected, the placement was deemed unfair and highly traumatic by both the mother and the son, who united against a common aggressor – the host country institutions. During the following two years, there were complex negotiations to preserve the invested and detested mother-son relationship. Through this process, both mother and son were able to partially mend the split between victim and aggressor positions and to use the host country professionals and institutions as a "bad enough" holding space which could provide a relative distance from threatening community interpretations and constitute an intrusive yet comforting third party which, by decreasing the fusion between mother and son, was also decreasing the risk of violence.

For Hamid and his mother, the violence within the family was repeatedly minimized while the relational disruption caused by the placement became a source of cohesion for mother and son, who united against an external agency identified as a common enemy. It was difficult for the clinical team to navigate between a realistic evaluation of the risk of violence and a recognition that the placement constituted a violent repetition of the multiple ruptures of attachment previously endured.

Abdi: When You Will Understand, You Will Agree with Us

Abdi is a 16-year-old Somali refugee. He was placed by youth protection services in a closed facility because he was potentially dangerous, connected with a Tourette syndrome diagnosis. A transcultural psychiatry team consultation was requested to create an alliance with the family, which was depicted as resistant to the intervention. The assessment revealed that

Abdi was the second child of a family of eight siblings. Easily distracted and bit impulsive, he often adopted a clown role at school, which irritated his teachers. On one occasion, an argument with some of his peers led to physical escalation in which nobody was hurt. Although he had been teased because of facial tics, Abdi was identified as the main problem after this incident and brought to an emergency department to evaluate the risk of violence. A diagnosis of Tourette syndrome with impulsivity was given to Abdi, who, in agreement with his mother, who was the head of the family, refused to take the prescribed medication. The subsequent decision to place Abdi in a Youth Protection Center seemed to rely on the idea that the mother was refusing treatment and that Abdi could constitute a risk for the other youth at school.

The family had been resettled in Canada for five years. The father was reported to have disappeared and the older siblings, including Abdi, were helping their mother with chores but also with paperwork and relationships with schools and health institutions.

His mother described Abdi as a good son, caring and respectful. Although she acknowledged that he could be impulsive, she explained that he had been bullied repeatedly by his peers and that the school staff did not intervene to protect him. He felt that it was because he was black. In Abdi's and his mother's minds, the diagnosis and the proposed medication were means to confirm that Abdi was crazy by treating him as such. During the assessment, the mother acknowledged experiences of discrimination since their arrival. She attributed them to the fact that they were black, but also to their Muslim identity. She interpreted the placement as a sign of distrust toward her, a sign that she had failed as a mother. Trying to mediate between youth protection services and the family, we emphasized how the placement was perceived and proposed ambulatory services and a reintegration of Abdi into his family. Our intervention was perceived as disqualifying by the social worker in charge of the case. She turned to the mother, telling her, "We know you want what is best for your son; when you understand what is really going on, you will agree with us." The placement continued.

In this situation, our alliance with Abdi's mother led us to feel viscerally how violent the placement was for the family. In our understanding, the prejudices against black Muslim youth had coalesced with the prejudices and fears about Tourette syndrome to create a perception of heightened risk in the absence of objective indications of danger. The social worker from the youth protection services had probably felt our irritation and the associated unspoken questioning of the intervention plan and resented it as a form of blame. Far from helping the family, our intervention had rigidified the system and deepened the split between the family and the youth protection institution. This sad story illustrates how a culturally sensitive understanding of the family's perspective may sometimes be harmful if the alliance process neglects to support all the parties involved and to take into account the vulnerability of host country professionals.

Omar: Asking Too Effectively for Help?

Omar is a nine-year-old boy born in Canada in a resettled refugee family from the Middle East. Quiet and relatively withdrawn, he is an average student who did not attract the school's attention. One day he disclosed to the school counsellor that his father had just come back from an armed conflict zone where he was fighting. He said that his father had weapons at home and confided that he was afraid for his family's safety, because his father had plans to go on fighting. There was a crisis intervention involving the police and youth protection services among others. The involved professionals discovered that the story was false. The father had a regular job, had not been traveling, had no involvement with armed or ideological groups and no weapons at home.

The family had been going through some relational turmoil. The parents' relationship was increasingly conflictual, with frequent shouting spells and some psychological violence but no physical violence. When asked about his "lie," Omar stated that he wanted help for the family and wanted the fights between his parents to stop. He added, "I did not invent everything; there are some decorative swords hanging on the wall of my house dining room."

Omar had used the polarized social context and the prejudices of the host society to call attention to his family's difficulties. At the fantasy level he had maybe also reconstructed the heroic position of warrior for a father who had fled the armed conflict and, in a situation of social status loss, was struggling to earn a living in the host country. By transforming the family story, Omar was portraying his father as potentially dangerous but also as very powerful and courageous. Because of the consideration of both the school and the family, it was not possible to know to what extent this creation of a new scenario represented a form of reenactment of past intergenerational trauma. Omar's story, however, shows how the representations of the host country can be activated in powerful ways within family means of action.

Including Structural Competence and Legal Consciousness in Self-Awareness when Working with Refugee Families

Difficult or ambivalent clinical experiences are often an invitation to reexamine our representations and basic assumptions. Case formulations are complex processes in which diverse threads of academic, professional and experiential knowledge are woven together in a unique way [21]. Systemic theories orient the gaze toward family and institutional dynamics, while cultural formulation approaches propose to identify the gaps and the interactions between the representations mobilized by the family and those which are at stake for the treatment team. Through this series of small case studies which all have ambiguous outcomes, I wished to draw some attention to the clinical and institutional blind spots about our legal consciousness and about the consequences of this for traumatized refugee families.

The first three stories (Meriem, Juana and Hamid) illustrate different forms of traumatic reenactment which had important legal consequences for these refugee families. For Meriem, her risk-taking endangered herself. In the cases of Juana and Hamid, traumatic reenactment was replayed among family members with a direct jeopardy of physical integrity. In all these cases, family members had an ambivalent relationship toward the protection which was offered to – or imposed on – them by host country institutions. Also, in all cases, issues of meaning are associated with what the family considers a legitimate way to provide protection.

The stories of Abdi and Omar focus more on the ways in which host country representations can evoke trauma repetition scenarios. In the case of Abdi, his psychiatric diagnosis was seen as reinforcing the prejudices about the violence of black Muslim young men. For Omar, however, the host country representations became a powerful way to mobilize services around his family. This second group of stories illustrates how host country representations can interfere with clinical intervention, can cause harm in some cases but can also be reappropriated and subverted by refugees to provoke familial transformations.

This case series is by no means comprehensive. Reenactment patterns may also emerge through silence, deprivation and neglect. The violence of the absence, or of the void, may be difficult to disentangle from other forms of transmission, for example, those associated with the psychic unavailability of parents. Although institutions often, as shown in the case studies, reflect host country hegemonic discourses, they may also sometimes become a place of resistance and critique of those discourses (see, for example, the Migrant-Friendly Hospital movement). These stories open different lines of reflection.

The first line of reflection concerns the relationship between hegemonic law and trauma repetition. This could be at stake when the host country concept of legal protection interacts with racial, ethnic or religious prejudices and leads to a reification of ethnocentric norms, which may result in interventions which erode refugee families' legitimacy. One could wonder if these processes could also be conceptualized as a form of trauma reenactment on the host country's part, in which internalized expectations about refugees who are constructed as potential threats are projected onto the families, who are represented as aggressors. The institutions and clinicians may then subsequently position themselves into savior positions in which iconic victims are identified along gender and age lines.

The second area which requires attention is the relationship between reenactment of past trauma (and intergenerational trauma) in refugee families, with its associated risk-taking and chains of acting out, and the use of legality by host country institutions to constrain or punish the youth or families. In those situations, there is often, on one hand, a missed explicit recognition of the trauma experience which does not manifest itself through the classic PTSD symptoms (nightmares and flashbacks). On the other hand, the professionals may react to the internal pain provoked in them by the trauma transmission, which may be interpreted by them as an aggression, confirming implicitly their stereotypical understanding of the family dynamics as transgressive or violent.

In a review of research with immigrant and refugee families, Glick [22] emphasizes the emergence of integrative models to address the interactions of attitudes and values with structural conditions in receiving and sending societies. This attention to structural determinants should consider the interaction between legality, legal consciousness and clinical interventions addressing protection issues for refugee families in order to better circumscribe the dynamics which are at stake. It would also be interesting to introduce discussions around legal pluralism, the legitimacy of societal and familial rules and ethical dilemmas for clinicians and trainees working with refugee families in order to raise awareness about the importance of these issues for this population.

At the clinical level, these reflections invite the opening of a dialogue with refugee families around what defines the family, what constitutes violence and how past traumas may reemerge in daily experiences. These topics are sensitive, and a conversation about them requires the establishment of cultural safety. The acknowledgment by clinicians of the diverse forms of structural discrimination that families may encounter in the host country and of the ways in which those may constitute a reminder of their experiences of organized violence before exile is often a cornerstone. For clinicians, mourning the idealized benevolence of their institutions and society is often both difficult and painful. Symbolically, the acknowledgement of the hidden or "clean" violence of our societies represents, beyond the "us and them" split, the fact that a shared humanity includes both a darker side and a common investment in loved ones.

References

1. V. M. Esses, L. K. Hamilton and D. Gaucher, The global refugee crisis: Empirical evidence and policy implications for improving public attitudes and facilitating refugee resettlement. *Social Issues and Policy Review*, 11(1) (2017), 78–123.

2. M. Beiser and F. Hou, Mental health effects of premigration trauma and postmigration discrimination on refugee youth in Canada. *The Journal of Nervous and Mental Disease*, 204(6) (2016), 464–70.

3. S. S. Silbey, After legal consciousness. *Annual Review of Law and Social Science*, 1 (2005), 323–68.

4. S. E. Merry, *Getting Justice and Getting Even: Legal Consciousness among Working-Class Americans* (Chicago, IL: University of Chicago Press, 1990).

5. L. J. Kirmayer, R. Kronick and C. Rousseau, Advocacy as a key to structural competence in psychiatry. *JAMA Psychiatry*, 75(2) (2017), 119–20.

6. B. de Sousa Santos and C. A. Rodríguez-Garavito, *Law and Globalization from Below: Towards a Cosmopolitan Legality* (Cambridge University Press, 2005).

7. F. von Benda-Beckman, K. von Benda-Beckman and A. Griffiths, *The Power of Law in a Transnational World: Anthropological Enquiries* (New York: Berghahn Books, 2012).

8. C. Rousseau, U. Jamil, T. Ferradji and A. Mekki-Berrada, North African Muslim immigrant families in Canada: Giving meaning and coping with the war on terror. *Journal of Immigrant & Refugee Studies*, 11(2) (2013), 136–56.

9. C. Rousseau and U. Jamil, Muslim families understanding and reacting to 'The War on Terror'. *American Journal of Orthopsychiatry*, 80(4) (2010), 601–9.

10. M. Darvishpour, Immigrant women challenge the role of men: How the changing power relationship within Iranian families in Sweden intensifies family conflicts after immigration. *Journal of Comparative Family Studies*, 33(2) (2002), 271–96.

11. L. Tingvold, A.-L. Middelthon, J. Allen and E. Hauff, Parents and children only? Acculturation and the influence of extended family members among Vietnamese refugees. *International Journal of Intercultural Relations*, 36(2) (2012), 260–70.

12. G. Hassan, B. Thombs, C. Rousseau, L. J. Kirmayer, J. Feightner, E. Ueffing et al., Intimate partner violence: Evidence review for newly arriving immigrants and refugees. *Canadian Medical Association Journal*, 183 (2011), Appendix 13. www.cmaj.ca/lookup/suppl/doi:10.1503/cmaj.090313/-/DC1

13. G. Hassan, B. D. Thombs, C. Rousseau, L. J. Kirmayer, J. Feightner, E. Ueffing et al., Child maltreatment: Evidence review for newly arriving immigrants and refugees. *Canadian Medical Association Journal*, 183 (2011), Appendix 12. www.cmaj.ca/lookup/suppl/doi:10.1503/cmaj.090313/-/DC1

14. N. K. Aggarwal, Men*tal Health in the War on Terror: Culture, Science, and Statecraft* (New York: Columbia University Press, 2015).

15. J. Zine, Unveiled sentiments: Gendered Islamophobia and experiences of veiling among Muslim girls in a Canadian Islamic school. *Equity and Excellence in Education*, 39(3) (2006), 239–52.

16. A. Kleinman and J. Kleinman, The appeal of experience, the dismay of images: Cultural appropriations of suffering in our times. In V. D. Arthur Kleinman and M. Lock, eds., *Social Suffering* (Berkeley, CA: University of California Press, 1997), pp. 1–24.

17. K. Kishi, *Anti-Muslim Assaults Reach 9/11-Era Levels, FBI Data Show* (Washington, DC: Pew Research Center, 2016), p. 21.

18. S. P. Huntington, The clash of civilizations? In L. Crothers and C. Lockhart, eds., *Culture and Politics* (New York: Palgrave Macmillan, 2000), pp. 99–118.

19. M. de Certeau, Corps torturés, paroles capturées. In L. Giard, ed., '*Michel de Certeau' sous la direction de cahiers pour un temps* (Paris: Centre Georges Pompidou, 1987), pp. 61–70.

20. R. S. Pynoos, A. M. Steinberg, C. M. Layne, E. C. Briggs, S. A. Ostrowski and J. A. Fairbank, DSM-V PTSD diagnostic criteria for children and adolescents: A developmental perspective and recommendations. *Journal of Traumatic Stress*, 22(5) (2009), 391–8.

21. K. Manassis, *Case Formulation with Children and Adolescents* (New York: Guilford Press, 2014).

22. J. E. Glick, Connecting complex processes: A decade of research on immigrant families. *Journal of Marriage and Family*, 72(3) (2010), 498–515.

Amplifying Our Engagement with Refugee Families Beyond the Therapeutic Space

Cécile Rousseau and Lucia De Haene

Approaching Complexity through a Diversity of Voices

Through a collection of clinical and academic voices, this book has aimed to regroup and further shape knowledge on refugee families and their role in coping with traumatic migration histories and diasporic identities in its members. Across the volume, contributions in Part I account for the growing empirical interest in documenting the refugee family unit as a dynamic system of interacting personal, transgenerational, and collective meaning systems, imbuing family relationships in exile with forms of relational and cultural dynamics of trauma coping and resilience. Parts II and III shift this systemic understanding into clinical practice, with contributions that provide a window into diverging modalities of working with refugee families, with contributions including different client system compositions, sectors, and systems-theoretical inspirations, located within particular national and local settings.

In developing this volume, our aim was not to present this collection of voices as a comprehensive state of the art of evidence-based practice in clinical work with refugee family systems. Rather, we aimed to engage with a particular niche of refugee family clinical and academic work developing in the margins of the broad field of psychosocial refugee studies. Hence, the volume reflects the relatively marginal position of systemic clinical practice with refugee families. This position at the margins is marked by a multilayered clinical wisdom fueled by the growing empirical knowledge of refugee family relationships in coping with trauma and social and cultural resettlement in exile and rooted in an innovative integration of notions from within the fields of family and systems therapy, trauma care, transcultural psychiatry, and social and community approaches. Yet, this rich experiential and clinical knowledge remains seminal and is not yet systematically supported by solid empirical evidence based on valid and culturally sensitive outcome measures and on the identification of process parameters of clinical work with refugee families. In different ways, this volume reflects this pioneering mode and position of the field. Strengthening the reach of systemic clinical wisdom in the broader field of refugee care, the volume forms an invitation to further root clinical, experiential wisdom within empirical knowledge in learning from our clinical encounters with refugee families.

How could a call for developing an empirical base for clinical practice with refugee families coexist with an orientation on acknowledging and validating the complexity and divergence of this experiential wisdom? Importantly, our call for further developing empirical evidence on systemic work with refugee families does not rest on a certain interest in shifting the experiential character into more standardized, protocolled approaches to working with refugee family systems. What is shared across the contributions is a broad lens on clinical practice with family systems, yet this core orientation throughout the volume does certainly not support (or converge into) a standardized perspective on clinical intervention with refugee families. Across the volume, divergent therapeutic and psychosocial approaches coexist. This multiplicity of voices, resisting a 'one size fits all' approach in clinical intervention with refugee families, reflects an explicit editorial choice. It is not only rooted in an orientation towards representing divergence within the field of systemic refugee care, but most importantly echoes our editorial interest in inviting reflection and acknowledgement of how this multiplicity of clinical voices reflects divergent forms of anchorage imbuing the therapeutic position, shaping how we see, feel, understand, and act as clinicians. The diverse constructions of meaning across the book are relational, shaped by each participant's experience and inner voices and entering into a dynamic interaction and ongoing dialogue with others' voices.

It is this engagement with anchorage and positioning that lies at the heart of systemic practice itself [1–3], reflecting the core orientation on working from within an understanding of the relational nature of understanding and meaning, constructed between participants partaking in therapeutic dialogue. From a systemic perspective, acknowledging the clinician's anchorage in personal experience and professional knowledge implies an understanding of the therapeutic positioning beyond the notion of the neutral expert. Indeed, validating how the clinician's anchorage enters into dialogue with clients' voices invokes an understanding of the therapeutic position that resists an adherence to objectifying categories of suffering or to normative concepts of normalcy, leading the expert to intervene in the dysfunctional system from a position external to that system in order to fix it. Acknowledging our anchorage as clinicians implies a reflection on how what we experience and understand within the clinical encounter is shaped by our personal and professional positioning and how this positioning enters into interaction with family members' voices in therapeutic dialogue [4, 5].

In this volume, our editorial orientation on representing divergent clinical voices from different national and local settings is shaped by an interest in including a reflection on our own anchorages and positioning as clinicians as integral to each therapeutic encounter. As clinicians, we are all situated in one or in multiple cultures that we reclaim or that we prefer to forget. We represent a range of professions, but we may be more homogeneous in terms of social class. Age, gender and life trajectories also differentiate us and tint our perspectives. And, maybe most importantly, we all have internalized families: past, present, or future families who look over our shoulders and influence the ways in which we listen, understand, and sometimes do not understand. This plurality of voices can be heard or perceived as a subtext across the volume, inviting us to reflect on how, between the lines, our multiple identities frame and transform a knowledge which cannot be seen as neutral or objective. Crossing all these divergent gazes across the volume aims to provides a prismatic vision of family work with refugees that may inform and inspire the readers. Hopefully, this diversity will not create a cacophony but rather an encounter with divergent or contrasting perspectives that mobilize reflection on the reader's personal stance and anchors.

In essence, this orientation on acknowledging and articulating anchorage and its intrapersonal and interpersonal resonance involves a mentalizing exercise that mirrors the mentalizing process with refugee family clients in therapeutic practice itself. Indeed, engaging with these different clinical gazes across the volume and its related reflection on the relational construction of meaning may indeed provide a mirror reflection of what is implied in working with refugee family systems.

First, as amply indicated across the volume, working with refugee families requires the development of a holding relational context that enables the containment of family members' multiplicity of anchorages, to explore the multiple personal, transgenerational, transnational, social, and cultural voices present in family and therapeutic interaction, and to negotiate the fluidity of anchorage in their life histories of exile. In engaging with these multiple voices shifting over time and place, the clinical encounter aims at developing a holding context that locates family members' experiences within meaningful narratives, providing a mentalizing language for lived experience, and at creating an open welcome for layers of experiences that are yet untold. This responsive interaction between family members aims at shaping a conversational space that contains family members' inner voices that are yet unspoken and difficult to express and that supports attunement between family members' voices. Here, the relational shaping of meaning within the therapeutic encounter becomes an important locus of therapeutic change: in validating inner voices and supporting a relational holding and meaning of these voices lies the promise of reshaping meaningful stories in the face of injustice and suffering. Reconstructing restorative narratives on living in exile may equally be part of those clinical processes where therapeutic or intersectoral intervention aims at supporting refugee families' coping with ongoing resettlement stressors. Through enhancing family-school interaction, promoting the mobilization of social support, or negotiating access to housing or employment, therapeutic intervention is oriented at supporting refugee families in navigating exile-related stressors and simultaneously reconstructs narratives of living in exile through reshaping social positions of agency and solidarity and allowing refugees' personal, familial, transgenerational, or cultural voices to enter social spaces. In this process, the holding and containment of the therapeutic dialogue may be extended and amplified within the broader social fabric.

Second, the diversity of voices across the volume also evokes the core tension between narrative versus political testimony that often characterizes clinical work with refugee families. Indeed, a systemic clinical approach is imbued with the importance of narrative [6], with an emphasis on how narrative shapes experience and the world we live in. Yet, precisely this emphasis on meaning-making and narration may at times present important clinical dilemmas in clinical work with survivors of collective violence living in exile. A clinical approach rooted in the premise of the relational construction of meaning may at times sit uneasily with refugees' moral imperative to provide testimony of the historical truths and social conditions that shaped their lives in home and host societies. Indeed, while an orientation on narration and meaning-making carries an understanding of how life histories are relational constructions that may shift across time and social spaces, the impetus of political testimony may be bound by an orientation on recounting historical facts and social conditions. Such accounts may require social spaces of witnessing and listening communities rather than the intimate space between the walls of the consultation room and may at times invite clinicians to develop testimony themselves in public engagements or to support refugee families in mobilizing social spaces of testimony. Where clinicians balance between a narrative, relational meaning-making approach and supporting the healing role of refugees' historical testimony on human rights abuses, persecution, and collective violence in their transgenerational life histories, a delicate clinical theme refers to the fragile trade-offs between collective and personal narratives. Indeed, communal accounts of historical conditions of violence may deny some of the more singular experiences of family members [7]. Across the volume, different contributions have engaged with this tension between narrative meaning-making and social and political testimony and have reflected on shifting the clinical space towards the threshold of intimate and political spaces.

Third, although an interest in the relational construction of understanding and meaning may implicitly suggest the equality and nonhierarchical position of multiple voices, the coexistence of a myriad of voices precisely calls for a reflection on subtle power differences in the resonances of each of these voices. Across the volume, the divergence of voices does not erase the implicit hierarchies between those voices, as the different chapters both reflect familiar western theoretical frameworks and more unsettling voices from within postcolonial writings. Engaging with these implicit hierarchies is mirroring clinical work with refugee families, as our dialogue with refugee family members is always imbued with a negotiation of power positions, not only between family members (in addressing intergenerational or cultural change issues) but equally elements of power disparities imbuing our clinical position and the institutions we represent. Important in this reflection is how the collection of professional voices in this volume does not leave a space for parents, grandparents, children, and overall the families' voices. This has been a debate between us when planning the book: mixing voices was our goal, but what impact would the establishment of different levels of voices, testimonies, and expert knowledge have? Would it be respectful or patronizing? Could it be an empowerment process, or was it an instrumentalization on our part of the subject voices? Reflecting on those questions with refugee families and with children, whose voices are so often forgotten, would have taken a lot of time. It will be, we hope, a necessary second step to invite resettled refugee families to enlarge and challenge the conversation we are having about them. While editing this book, we have sometimes tried to weave together the stories which were told from one chapter to another. At other times, on the contrary, we have resisted our tendency to homogenize the content, leaving space for dissent and contradictions. We believe that gaps and paradoxes can be fruitful to destabilize our theoretical premises and to question our clinical practice. They reflect our ignorance and the fact that the capacity to survive our uncertainties may help us to resist the push toward standardization of practices, which in the present stage of knowledge would probably be a form of violence for many of the families we accompany.

Training in Family Systems Practice across Disciplines

Although working with families is often part of the daily work of most health and social services professionals, it is not always recognized as such. Among some of the reasons for this nonrecognition could be the fact that family work is considered difficult and that many practitioners who do not feel adequately equipped to do family therapy will minimize the importance of the family interventions that they engage in. In this book, we have illustrated how professionals from a wide range of disciplines can contribute to understanding, supporting, and advocating for refugee families. At the same time, in order to do so in the best interests of refugee families and to avoid some of the harmful effects of interventions in a context lacking cultural safety, trainees and professionals need to be sensitized to and trained in this form of intervention.

Introducing refugee family and community work as key elements of intervention in the health and social sciences curricula of trainees in countries who receive many refugees is a necessary first step. Very often, the refugee experience is reduced to premigratory trauma, presented through the frame of posttraumatic stress disorder as the main category of suffering. In terms of content, the training should address the contextual conditions associated with resettlement in order to reflect the systemic challenges that the refugee family will face in specific national contexts. This includes, among other things, family reunification laws and procedures, asylum determination processes, access to health care, education, and social benefits for asylum claimants, and, of course, discrimination against and ostracism of refugees and certain religious, racial, or ethnic groups. Further, the impact of exile, traumatization, separation, and the resettlement trajectory on family roles and dynamics should take center stage in basic training. Without expecting all trainees to have extensive expertise on these issues, their introduction should elicit the reflex to think always in terms of family, without, however, forgetting the singularity of individuals' voices and trajectories.

In terms of skills, system theory and ecosystemic approaches are certainly key to supporting intervention, but beyond useful theories, working with diverse families together with experienced clinicians encourages learning through modeling and acquiring hands-on skills for all the trainees who have not had family therapy training [8]. Learning to work with interpreters and cultural brokers is another basic skill which should be part of trainees' curricula and rotations. This is important because of the institutionalized tendency to use family members as interpreters for economic reasons, a practice which is proven to be harmful, in particular when children or youth are asked to interpret for their parents [9].

However, training should not only address content and skills (which may differ from discipline to discipline); it should convey a certain posture of reflexivity and respect, which is essential to fostering cultural safety. Experiential learning may support a decentering reflection which invites the trainees to become conscious of their premises, prejudices, biases, and privileges [10]. Overall, even minimal training should succeed in transmitting the idea that family intervention is a shared responsibility among professionals and that, although complex, family work is possible to do with respect and sensitivity and is very rewarding.

Among experienced clinicians, continuing education can enhance and complete the skills and knowledge needed to engage refugee families. Interdisciplinary and interinstitutional case discussions have been shown to be good collective tools to master the involved complexity [11]. These regular case discussions propose inverting the usual learning approach, which transmits theoretical and clinical knowledge before applying it to the clinician's daily work. Rather, the group begins to work around a case presented by one of the participants, which is progressively unfolded by the whole group through an inquiry which reveals participants' professional and cultural premises, which are then subsequently situated in different theoretical fields. The case discussion process thus reveals the plurality of institutional mandates and disciplinary frames and their interaction with the personal worlds of clinicians. The resulting understanding usually integrates these different visions to define what is possible in terms of a systemic intervention for the family. Unfortunately, such case discussion time is increasingly difficult to protect of administrative imperatives, but different, less formalized, formats for clinical reflection involving teams may support a continuous co-construction of knowledge, which involves a safe space to reflect on our failures, sense of impotence, and counter-transference.

Moving from the Academic and Therapeutic Space into Social Action and Advocacy

A number of chapters in this book have illustrated how receiving societies are often sources of hurt and distress for the refugee families: Asylum determination procedures are always stress-provoking and may be humiliating and retraumatizing or favor the persistence of psychopathology [12], family members may be detained for various lengths of time and separated because of immigration reasons, a severe stress which almost always reactivates past traumas [13], or family reunification may require years because of procedural and financial obstacles. In addition, refugee families in most countries do not have access to daycare or to college or university education for the older siblings. In some countries, children are encouraged to learn the host country language while parents are de facto discouraged from doing so; in others, families or youth are resettled in camps with very little agency. Furthermore, refugee families may continue to encounter limitations affecting their access to health care [14]. All of these obstacles and limitations send a powerful message to refugee families, who resent these forms of exclusion from the common wealth, increasing their sense of distrust. Although as clinicians our role is to heal, support, and comfort, we also have a role in preventing suffering and supporting wellbeing and development through all developmental stages, and especially so for children. Thus, clinicians working with refugee families may play a key role in mobilizing stakeholders, community representatives, and policymakers to shift policies and institutional procedures restricting the access of refugee families to justice or the social benefits of the majority.

In times of increasing xenophobia and anti-immigrant and anti-refugee feelings, these collective actions to preserve or increase the social safety net for refugee families have at least two important functions. First, they may help to limit harmful policies. This has, for example, been the case recently in the United States when the American Association of Pediatrics strongly opposed family separation of asylum claimants in detention, joining in with diverse parts of society in a successful advocacy movement to condemn and reverse a migration policy [15]. It has also been the case in Canada when many health professional associations successfully pressurized the government to abolish the cuts to refugee health care which were affecting asylum claimant adults and children [16]. Second, they convey a strong message of solidarity, which may become a strong support for families and enable them to have a more nuanced perception of the host society. These collective mobilizations require time and energy and are sometimes seen as political and thus not the mandate of clinicians. However, health professionals have the capacity to mobilize public opinion and are key members of advocacy coalitions. While abstaining from partisan political involvement (which we may choose to engage in as citizens), we need to learn how to develop advocacy work to promote policy changes rather than accepting the status quo when we know that some harm may be avoided. This is, however, not a solitary adventure, and the coalition should be strategic and build on robust alliances with diverse milieus and on a comprehensive analysis of the targeted reform. Denunciations through political protest, although honest and legitimate, may paradoxically harm the vulnerable communities that we wish to preserve unless they are carefully planned in order not to increase polarization and provoke different forms of social retaliation. For example, in a context of economic uncertainty and of mounting xenophobia, public demonstrations in favor of equity in health care access for refugees may fire up critics focusing on the fact that refugees are a socioeconomic burden to the host societies and justify more repressive migratory policies.

In this context, the advocacy coalition may decide to work instead with allies within health institutions and the health ministry in a low-key manner. At the opposite extreme, after wide media coverage of painful stories of children separated from their parents at the border, advocates may choose to surf the public empathy wave to promote better family reunification policies.

Finally, in a globalized world, protest and transformation may also take advantage of international networks. This has been the case at a certain point in time in Australia, where international pressure supported internal mobilization to improve inhumane detention conditions for asylum seekers [17]. We clinicians and researchers working with refugee families thus need to support each other in this long and demanding process of constructing and preserving just and welcoming societies.

Strengthening Engagement with Refugee Family Systems in Research

The contributors to this book have in different ways illustrated the central importance of families as the first circle supporting or challenging reconstruction after enduring the challenges of war, persecution, and exile. We have also shown that clinical, social, educational, and intersectoral intervention practices need to take into account family transformations in exile and sometimes support internal processes of (partial or modulated) transmission of trauma, trauma- and culture-related meaning-making, and shifting dynamics to preserve both the family unit and its members in their developmental trajectories of adaptation in resettlement. Yet, in contrast to this salience, research has often neglected to consider family variables except for at times documenting household composition and parent-child or couple relationships. Furthermore, very few refugee family interventions have been evaluated, leaving a void that, unfortunately, good clinical practices cannot bridge and that is a major obstacle to the formulation of guidelines and training in emphasizing evidence-based practices. Beyond recognizing the value of the available evidence based on experiential and clinical knowledge, it is more than time to begin to address this gap in knowledge through rigorous scientific studies.

A first step would be to encourage existing and future studies with refugees to introduce family variables in their designs. At the sociodemographic level, there is often a tendency to reduce the family unit to the persons who reside in the host country or to the nuclear family. Rather, considering the premigratory household provides a far more exact idea of the losses and relational challenges that family members may face. Similarly, documenting the extended family present in exile may provide an excellent measure of support and sometimes of the burdens and obligations that the family may have. Among other family variables, some are relatively easy to collect and, although simple, provide a first appraisal of family functioning. For example, family conflict and cohesion are often very good predictors of mental health and can be operationalized through transculturally valid instruments. Other constructs like attachment, while highly pertinent, are far more difficult to measure, will only be considered in studies centered on familial and relational issues, and need to include an exploration of particular parameters of proximity and responsivity in the context of cultural practices of parenting, extended family networks, and living through ongoing separation [18]. In sum, the main idea is to think in terms of family when documenting the experience of individuals throughout the life cycle, from toddlers to the elderly, and to challenge the idea that this is necessarily a cumbersome process.

A second step is to refine our models of the multilevel transformations experienced by refugee families in order to be able to study these processes concurrently rather than in parallel. This raises important dilemmas related to the relative burden that research may represent for a family which is already overstretched. Thus, a methodological move toward designs aiming at capturing more complexity should go hand in hand with an ethical reflection on the researcher's stance in front of families or subjects who may be in a survival mode [18]. To what extent is a posture of neutrality ethical? To what degree should the research team move out of an observer position and provide empathic support and liaison with resources? What are the risks of a paternalistic stance which does not fully recognize the agency of the refugee family members? Research itself thus needs to be rethought as a relational adventure with affective (supportive and hurtful) components that cannot be minimized [18, 20, 21].

The third step has to do with the urgent need to develop evaluative studies of family interventions. A number of difficulties emerge in these types of studies. On the first level, these challenges are related to technical and material obstacles: Every family being a unit, quantitative studies, which are often more credible to decision-makers, very rapidly become huge and very costly, or, alternatively, they stay small-scale and are considered pilots. Second, determining appropriate family and/or individual outcomes is another major challenge. Furthermore, as in the case of other psychotherapies, trying to identify the active ingredients responsible for therapeutic change or recovery may be difficult, given the complexity of the intervention. This limit, however, may interfere with the replication and transferability of innovative interventions. In spite of all these obstacles, compounded by the added challenges of working with a hard-to-reach population, evaluation is an absolute must if we want to transfer and perpetuate the meaningful clinical work which is going on. At first sight, the systemic focus on the relational construction of understanding and meaning may seem to set limitations on the set-up of intervention studies, as this processual nature of meaning-making and its roots in multiple forms of personal, social, and cultural anchorage may seem what should be controlled for in shifting towards evidence-based practice. Yet, we argue that another possible stance in the design of intervention studies regarding working with refugee families would consist precisely of documenting rather than controlling these anchorages. Here, intervention process and outcome studies can engage in analyzing how therapeutic change and restoration are shaped by working with a diversity of voices within the therapeutic space, including the clinician's anchorage, in both the resonances of personal experience and multiple sources of knowledge, playing a role in therapeutic interaction and trajectories. In this modality, intervention studies may succeed in accounting for the complexity of systemic practice and provide a window into the dynamic richness and intricate personal, familial, cultural, and social multivocality of working with refugee families.

Working with and for Refugee Families: We Need to Join Forces

As we are finishing this book, anti-refugee rhetoric is growing and obstacles to asylum are multiplying. In the present refugee predicament, working to protect refugee families may first entail creating international networks to advocate for the right to asylum and to preserve family reunification policies. Improving services and psychosocial support will always remain an important task, in particular in a context where refugees' access and entitlement to services and social benefits is increasingly questioned. Our present and future clinical and research knowledge can become a precious tool to argue for and justify measures which will enhance refugees' and their families' wellbeing and agency. We hope to pursue with you not only this conversation but a firm common commitment in favor of our shared humanity.

References

1. E. Mony, *Si tu m'aimes, ne m'aime pas* (Paris: Points, 1989).

2. M. Elkaïm, À propos du concept de résonance. *Cahiers critiques de thérapie familiale et de pratiques de réseaux*, 45(2) (2010), 171–2.

3. P. Rober, The therapist's inner conversation in family therapy practice: Some ideas about the self of the therapist, therapeutic impasse, and the process of reflection. *Family Process*, 38(2) (1999), 209–28.

4. P. Rober, The therapist's self in dialogical family therapy: Some ideas about not-knowing and the therapist's inner conversation. *Family Process*, 44(4) (2005), 477–95.

5. P. Rober, *In Therapy Together: Family Therapy as a Dialogue* (London: Palgrave Macmillan, 2017).

6. T. Malinen, S. J. Cooper and F. N. Thomas, *Masters of Narrative and Collaborative Therapies: The Voices of Andersen, Anderson, and White* (New York: Routledge, 2013).

7. L. Atlani and C. Rousseau, The politics of culture in humanitarian aid to women refugees who have experienced sexual violence. *Transcultural Psychiatry*, 37(3) (2000), 435–49.

8. C. Rousseau and J. Guzder, Teaching cultural formulation. *Journal of the American Academy of Child and Adolescent Psychiatry*, 54(8) (2015), 611–12.

9. Y. Leanza, I. Boivin, M.-R. Moro, C. Rousseau, C. Brisset, E. Rosenberg et al., Integration of interpreters in mental health interventions with children and adolescents: The need for a framework. *Transcultural Psychiatry*, 52(3) (2014), 353–75.

10. L. J. Kirmayer, C. Rousseau and J. Guzder, The place of culture in mental health services (introduction). In L. J. Kirmayer, J. Guzder and C. Rousseau, eds., *Cultural Consultation: Encountering the Other in Mental Health Care* (New York: Springer, 2014), pp. 1–20.

11. C. Rousseau, J. Jonhson-Lafleur, G. Papazian-Zohrabian and T. Measham, Interdisciplinary case discussions as a training modality to teach cultural formulation in child mental health. *Transcultural Psychiatry*, (2018). https://doi.org/10.1177/1363461518794033

12. G. Bodegård, Life-threatening loss of function in refugee children: Another expression of pervasive refusal syndrome? *Clinical Child Psychology and Psychiatry*, 10(3) (2005), 337–50.

13. J. Cleveland and C. Rousseau, Mental health impact of detention and temporary status for refugee claimants under Bill C-31. *Canadian Medical Association Journal*, 184(15) (2012), 1663–4.

14. C. Rousseau, Y. Oulhote, M. Ruiz-Casares, J. Cleveland and C. Greenaway, Encouraging understanding or increasing prejudices: A cross-sectional survey of institutional influence on health personnel attitudes about refugee claimant' access to health care. *PLoS One*, 12(2) (2017), e0170910.

15. American Academy of Pediatrics, (2018). *Protecting Immigrant Children*. www.aap.org/en-us/advocacy-and-policy/federal-advocacy/Pages/ImmigrationReform.aspx

16. J. Cleveland and J. Hanley, *We Won the Battle but Lost the War: Lack of Access to Health Care for Asylum Seekers Following Reinstatement of the Interim Federal Health Program* (Ottawa: Canadian Association for Refugee and Forced Migration Studies, 2018).

17. Z. Steel, D. Silove, R. Brooks, S. Momartin, B. Alzuhairi and I. Susljik, Impact of immigration detention and temporary protection on the mental health of

refugees. *The British Journal of Psychiatry*, 188(1) (2006), 58–64.

18. L. De Haene, H. Grietens and K. Verschueren, Adult attachment in the context of refugee traumatisation: The impact of organized violence and forced separation on parental states of mind regarding attachment. *Attachment & Human Development*, 12(3) (2010), 249–64.

19. C. Rousseau and L. J. Kirmayer, From complicity to advocacy: The necessity of

refugee research. *The American Journal of Bioethics*, 10(2) (2010), 65–7.

20. L. De Haene, H. Grietens and K. Verschueren, Holding harm: Narrative methods in mental health research on refugee trauma. *Qualitative Health Research*, 20(12) (2010), 1664–76.

21. A. Mekki-Berrada, C. Rousseau and J. Bertot, Research on refugees: Means of transmitting suffering and forging social bonds. *International Journal of Mental Health*, 30(2) (2001), 41–57.

Index